Being Doctor

MBBS FOUNDATION

Your First Book of Medicine

Lokesh Tiwari

Jyoti Chaturvedi

Welcome to the World of Medicine

The first year of MBBS quietly shapes the kind of doctor a student will become. Most students enter medical college unprepared for the cognitive overload, emotional strain, communication challenges, and clinical skills needed far earlier than they expect. MBBS Foundation: Your First Book of Medicine is written for that moment when guidance matters most. Aligned with the NMC Foundation Course and AETCOM competencies, this evidence-based handbook integrates life-saving skills such as CPR and First Aid, essential soft skills, and real-world clinical wisdom that are rarely taught but deeply needed from the beginning. It does not merely help students survive and thrive in MBBS; it prepares them to stand steady when knowledge alone is not enough. While firmly grounded in the competency-based curriculum, it goes beyond checklists to address the hidden curriculum of medicine: how to think, how to act, how to care, and how to remain stable under pressure. For students, this book offers the compass every new doctor needs, but few are given. For parents, it provides a quiet yet powerful assurance—that alongside academic excellence, their child is being guided toward responsibility, compassion, professional integrity and self-care.

Medicine is not only about what a student learns; it is about who they become.

Made with ♥ on the Notion Press Platform
www.notionpress.com

Disclaimer

Some illustrations in this book were generated with the assistance of artificial intelligence tools. All AI-generated visuals in this publication were created specifically for this publication and do not represent real individuals, hospitals, or events unless explicitly stated. These visuals are used solely for educational and illustrative purposes. The drowning chain of survival image is reproduced with permission from the International Life Saving Federation. © International Life Saving Federation. The WHO medical resuscitation algorithm, the WHO trauma resuscitation algorithm, the hand wash poster, and the handrub posters are used with the permission of the WHO.

To My Father: In Honour of a Teacher

A few years ago, one of my first-year MBBS students called me late on an Eid evening, his voice trembling between shock and relief. Just days earlier, I had taught his batch CPR and how to relieve choking — the stance, the sequence, the Heimlich manoeuvre repeated until muscle and memory became one.

That night, as his family sat together, his father suddenly choked on a piece of bone. Panic broke the room open - gasping, cyanosis, fear. And yet, in that storm, something steady awakened inside him. He remembered everything. He rushed behind his father, positioned his hands, and delivered the Heimlich thrusts exactly as taught.

One. Two. Three.
And on the fourth, breath returned.
A life returned…

Something profound happened for the whole family!

"Sir… I saved my father. Because you taught us. I still can't believe it… I saved my father."

As I listened, pride rose in me.

When he lived the miracle, something shifted within me. His wow moment became mine. A moment of healing, of purpose, of continuity. A reminder that the life we cannot save in one chapter can return through the hands of those we teach in the next.

I dedicate this book to my father, Shri Bhagwati Lal Sharma.
The man who shaped my first values,
Who taught me how to care,
Who made me a teacher long before I knew I would become one.

Everything I teach,
Every lesson shared,
Every student inspired,
Carries a part of him —
The teacher of my becoming.

Foreword

Medical education marks the beginning of a lifelong journey, one that demands not only scientific rigour but also empathy, ethical clarity, and a deep sense of service to society. As young students enter the MBBS course, they are often confronted with the vastness of medicine, without sufficient guidance on integrating knowledge, skills, values, and professional identity.

MBBS Foundation: Your First Book of Medicine is a timely and meaningful contribution to undergraduate medical education in India. Aligned with the National Medical Commission's Foundation Course and AETCOM framework, this book offers students a structured and reflective introduction to medicine. It blends core scientific principles with communication skills, ethics, professionalism, life-saving competencies such as CPR and First Aid, and the often-unspoken realities of medical training.

What is particularly commendable is the book's emphasis on the human side of medicine. In an era where technology and specialisation are advancing rapidly, the values of compassion, integrity, teamwork, and leadership must be consciously nurtured. This book recognises that competency-based education is not merely about achieving outcomes, but about shaping doctors who are trustworthy, resilient, and responsive to the needs of patients and communities.

Dr Lokesh Tiwari brings to this work his rich experience as a clinician, educator, and leader in pediatric critical care and resuscitation science. His engagement with medical students, training programs, and national and international professional bodies is reflected in the book's practical insights and global perspective. I am confident that this book will be of great value not only to MBBS students, but also to educators and institutions seeking to strengthen the foundational years of medical training. It is a sincere effort to remind us that while medicine is grounded in science, it is ultimately practiced with humanity.

I wish the authors every success and hope this book inspires a generation of doctors to learn with curiosity, serve with compassion, and lead with integrity.

Prof Meenu Singh

Executive Director,

All India Institute of Medical Sciences Rishikesh

Message from a Mentor

Medical education has traditionally emphasised the acquisition of knowledge and clinical skills. The journey from school to medical college represents a critical psychological and professional transition. Students arrive with intelligence and aspiration, but often without a clear framework to interpret the complexity of health, illness, and care in the real world. Too frequently, this understanding is left to chance.

MBBS Foundation: Your First Book of Medicine addresses this gap with clarity and intention.

What distinguishes this work is its recognition that the foundations of medical training extend beyond early clinical exposure and must address both the professional and personal realities of becoming a doctor. Alongside introducing students to life-saving skills and core clinical competencies, the book engages with the inner demands of the medical journey—time and energy management, stress and emotional regulation, seeking help, building support systems, and remaining connected to the human roots of medicine through family, friendships, and diverse traditions of care. In doing so, it prepares students not only to treat illness but to sustain themselves through the long and demanding years of medical training. At the same time, it orients them to the broader healthcare ecosystem, including health financing, public programs, ethics, communication, patient safety, and population health.

The formative years of medical training are where values are set, attitudes are shaped, and professional identity begins to crystallise. Guidance at this stage can influence not only individuals but also the future culture of healthcare itself. This book provides a structured, humane orientation to medicine—one that balances scientific rigour with social responsibility, and competence with compassion.

I believe this book will help young doctors see beyond diseases to determinants, beyond procedures to people, and beyond hospitals to health systems. It will encourage them to ask not only *"What is the diagnosis?"* but also *"What is fair, feasible, and right?"*

This work is timely, thoughtful, and deeply necessary.

Prof C M Singh

Director,

Ram Manohar Lohia Institute of Medical Sciences, Lucknow

Prologue

Dear student,

You may not fully realise it now, but by choosing a career in medicine, you have entered a sacred space—not only a career, but a calling. Healing others is a privilege. Being trusted when life hangs in the balance is a grace few professions offer.

The beauty: you will not only learn how to treat, but you will slowly learn how to see the flicker of fear in a mother's eyes, the hopeful breath in a silent child and your own dedication to navigate through all challenges.

What you can expect

If you commit fully, medicine will open doors beyond imagination: academia that shapes the next generation, innovation that becomes lifesaving technology, public health that serves communities, and global arenas where an Indian doctor becomes a changemaker. Socially, you become a voice of reason and compassion. Financially, it is a stable profession; although not the highest-paid everywhere, it is a dignified and widely respected field. Above all, medicine offers a legacy: lives touched, trust restored, and generations healed.

The challenges ahead: scientific & clinical

Let's be honest: this is one of the most demanding journeys. The doctor-to-population ratio in India remains short of the WHO's 1:1000 benchmark, resulting in overburdened healthcare systems. The MBBS program lasts 5½ years, with many students pursuing an additional 3-10 years of training. Non-communicable diseases now cause over 60% of deaths, requiring long-term, team-based care rather than quick fixes. Technology advances faster than curricula, so you will absorb large amounts of knowledge, make time-critical decisions, and sometimes do both with little sleep.

The challenges ahead: soul, ethics, and self

The tougher truths are quieter. Many doctors report moral distress and burnout; resident doctors in Indian studies show significant symptoms of depression and even suicidal thoughts. Violence against healthcare workers has been documented quite often in recent years, often driven by mistrust and poor communication. You will be trained to restart a failing heart, but not always how to cope with your own heartache. This book takes care of your soft skills, too.

Your North Star: AETCOM

From day one, connect yourself to AETCOM- Attitude, Ethics, and Communication. Attitude and professionalism are based on humility, reliability, and respect for every team member. Ethics encompass autonomy, beneficence, non-maleficence, justice, informed consent, confidentiality, and fair use of resources. Communication involves clear, kind, and culturally sensitive conversations; shared decision-making; and documentation that tells the truth.

These are not "soft extras." They are vital clinical skills. They prevent conflict, reduce errors, and build trust, saving lives and time in a crisis.

Life-saving basics every student must carry

You will study advanced science, in reality, simple disciplines save more lives: Bystander CPR can double or triple survival in sudden cardiac arrest. Learn it, practice it, teach it. Check response and breathing; call for help. Start chest compressions at 100–120 compressions per minute, with a depth of 5–6 cm, full recoil, and minimal pauses. Use an AED at the earliest opportunity; defibrillation within 3-5 minutes can increase survival to 50-70%. Carry this skill like you carry your stethoscope. CPR and First Aid help ensure patients survive to receive advanced care. Apply direct pressure for bleeding and add a tourniquet for life-threatening limb haemorrhage. If someone is choking, encourage coughing, give abdominal thrusts and back blows suitable for their age and size, and start CPR if unresponsive. In burns, fractures, and medical emergencies, simple actions can prevent deterioration while definitive care reaches the patient.

"Be a doctor not only of the body, but of broken trust, unheard pain, and unseen wounds."
We wish you a meaningful journey. When in doubt, return to this book.

With love and deep trust in your becoming,

— **Dr. L. T.**

— **Dr. J. C.**

Table of Contents

List of Figures

List of Tables

Part 1: Foundations of Understanding Medicine

Threshold

A *Threshold* is a small space between what was and what is about to come.

To step across it is to leave behind the familiar and explore a new realm.

This book invites you to pause

and learn what comes as pages unfold

at this threshold

between the school and the medical college.

It is a crossing-over:

into responsibility,

into compassion and

into the lifelong identity of being a doctor.

Step mindfully, and what lies beyond will shape

not only your studies,

but your life.

Forever!

Chapter 1: Threshold

Between the First Step and the First Life You Save

Take a Deep Breath.

You are standing at the edge of a transformation - a threshold between what you were and what you are going to be. The letters M.B.B.S. may be small in their physical appearance, but the weight these letters carry is of a lifetime commitment. Beyond the textbooks and examinations, this journey will teach you to hold trembling hands, to listen to the heartbeats, and to see the feelings beyond illness. Welcome to medicine, not just as a profession, but as a way of life, to see the world from a different view.

A New Start

As you enter this world, you are not only learning about cells, tissues, organ systems, diseases, investigations, and treatments, but you are also entering an ancient commitment between science and humanity. You are joining the profession of thinkers, doers and innovators. This group embodies compassion and precision in its service to humanity, following scientific evidence to treat every life with dignity. This book is your first companion on the journey through, and will be relevant forever in the medical profession. It will not promise certainty, because medicine is a continuous evolution, but it will take you to clarity, character, and competence.

Purpose of Book

The National Medical Commission (NMC) has envisioned the Foundation Course for Indian Medical Graduates (IMGs) to prepare the doctors who blend medical knowledge with professional attitude, ethical reasoning, communication skills, and social accountability. This book reflects that intent in the design of each chapter, integrating the values of the medical profession, orientation to the structure of the curriculum, and an introduction to the healthcare ecosystem, along with training in CPR, life-saving, and first-aid skills updated to 2026. It also effectively addresses empathy, discipline, and leadership qualities essential for students in their journey through medical training.

Becoming a doctor is not a linear path; it is a spiral of learning that involves the mind, hands, and heart throughout one's career.

Structure

This book unites the two halves of your professional evolution: 'Understanding Medicine' and 'Living Medicine', each comprising seven sections.

Part I: Foundations of Understanding Medicine

This part takes you through the ethical and value system to understand what medicine is and why it matters. It unfolds with **Threshold,** a pause before the journey begins.

Inception is a formal initiation into the medical world that shapes your identity as a student doctor. You understand the structure of the MBBS curriculum and the principles of medical education. It orients you to self-directed learning, early clinical exposure and horizontal and vertical integration across subjects.

Genesis is the soul of medicine. It includes the history, philosophy and ethical principles of this profession. The genesis of a doctor's identity happens in the understanding of autonomy, beneficence, non-maleficence, and justice.

Synthesis orients you to the healing heritage of India including Ayurveda, Yoga, Unani, Siddha, and Homeopathy, and its integration with modern medicine. Understand how to balance tradition with evidence and heritage with hypothesis.

Matrix is an introduction to the architecture of healthcare delivery in India, spanning from sub-centres to tertiary hospitals, and governed by policies and systems. It reveals how inequities persist and how various stakeholders impact this system.

Covenant takes you to the moral fabric, legal responsibilities, professional codes, and ethical dilemmas that test judgment and ethics.

Ultimately, **Crossroads** brings theory to life. Real-world case studies and ethical dilemmas navigate when beneficence conflicts with non-maleficence, and the right answer is not easy.

These seven sections help you understand medicine as both a scientific fact and a moral guide.

Part II: The Foundations of Living Medicine

The first half of the book builds your mind; the second half trains your hands and heart to translate values into action and guidance into competence.

It unfolds with **Revive**, where you meet *Sanjeevani Vidya*, the science and spirit of saving lives. You will learn CPR, chain of survival, and how to save victims from choking who could die if you do not act fast and provide Basic Life Support.

The rescue section introduces you to first aid and emergency care. Not to treat but to start the most important actions to save in life-threatening conditions, ranging from heart attacks to snakebites and from syncope to anaphylaxis. You will learn to stay calm and act when others panic. This section builds confidence through clarity on what to do and how to think when seconds matter.

Impact shows the aftermath of trauma. You learn to handle bleeding, fractures, head and spinal injuries from the site of injury to the hospital emergency department. Each protocol and skill you master adds to your capability of managing situations when life hangs in the balance.

Tempest prepares you to manage situations when natural forces converge, creating an imbalance. Disasters occur when the disharmony of the five elements in nature, i.e., *Agni, Jal, Vayu, Prithvi, and Aakash*, leads to fires, floods, smoke, earthquakes, and lightning. This is the time for a doctor to test their clinical skills, courage, and composure. This section teaches disaster preparedness, triage, teamwork, and the calm within chaos that defines every emergency physician.

Illumination is enlightening about the science of safety, infection control, immunization, biomedical waste management, research methodology, and evidence-based medicine. You will also learn to search, appraise, and apply scientific knowledge and evidence in clinical practice.

Resonance brings back the human element in the journey ahead, soft skills that are hard to learn. You will learn concepts of professional communication, empathy, time management, teamwork, mentorship, and self-care. This section unfolds the *hidden curriculum*. Stay curious.

And finally, **Continuum** beyond college - toward a culture of lifelong learning and global relevance as a doctor, researcher, and scientist.

How to Use This Book

A Note For Students

This book is not your syllabus. It's your companion in your journey to becoming a doctor. Read it as a story. Don't rush to connect chapters to competencies or checklists on your first reading. Read it thoroughly to understand how medicine affects patients, the community, and doctors.

When you need to revisit a concept or prepare for assessments, turn to the Competency Mapping Table placed in the Continuum section. It links each competency with the corresponding chapters.

The map will help you navigate, but the story will help you transform.

This book is designed to be your companion throughout your journey. Each time you revisit, it reveals a little more of what you need to become a doctor.

A Note For Faculty

Before using this as a teaching tool, we invite you to read and walk through its sections with curiosity, reflection, and rediscovery. Feel the pulse of the profession; this book tries to revive through values, empathy, and evidence. The 'Competency Mapping Table' at the end will help you connect every chapter to its relevant NMC-defined outcomes. You can use it to plan your sessions with contextual examples.

Use it to identify learning resources (e.g., interactive discussions, reflections, simulations, community visits) for each competency. Encourage students to engage in reflection-based, self-directed learning and to integrate a portfolio and logbook into their learning.

This book aligns with the competency-based curriculum, yet it offers far more than a list can capture. It is built to reawaken the art in medical education, re-enforcing that while competencies define what we teach, humanity defines why we teach. As mentors, let us read not only to teach better but to feel the wonder of learning.

Learning Beyond the Page

Each section combines science, skill, and ethics. The rigour of the curriculum is combined with the rhythm of storytelling.

Case studies make you think like a clinician.

Coffee Moments are brief pauses to connect ideas with emotions.

Concept notes and mini-skills to strengthen competencies.

QR codes and digital extensions linking certification modules, demonstrations, and learning resources.

Whether you're subtly becoming a doctor, preparing for an exam, planning a project, or sitting by a patient's bed, return to this book and find relevance.

The Mentor's Promise

This book will not lecture; it will remind you to be curious and correct, and it will challenge you-
To think and reflect when others memorize.
To be attentive when others rush.
To act when others can't decide.
The world needs better doctors, practising evidence-based medicine and guided by ethics and compassion.

Medicine will test you, but it will also transform you. You will witness the vulnerability of life and the energy of the human will. Somewhere between your first book of medicine and your first patient, you'll discover something precious, something powerful and something holy. keep exploring.

Welcome to the journey.
Welcome to the fraternity of doctors.
Welcome to the **MBBS Foundation - Your First Book of Medicine.**

Inception

Inception is the conscious start of your journey,

the first footsteps towards becoming a doctor.

Here, you learn that a doctor's journey begins not with machines or prescriptions,

but with values, respect, empathy, ethics, and responsibility.

You will take your first steps:

your beginning,

your first date with medicine,

the MBBS curriculum,

the ways doctors learn,

a guided tour of your campus and a

Community Health Centre,

and lessons beyond your classroom.

Take a pause.

Look at your white coat.

Ahead lies a journey that will test your patience, shape your character, and awaken your purpose.
By the time you finish it,

You will not only know how to heal others, but you will have discovered who you are meant to become.

S No.	Inception: At a Glance
1.	**Chapter 2** Inception: A Story They Won't Teach You in Lectures Your first human encounter with medicine: presence before prescriptions; the white-coat awakening.
2.	**Chapter 3** My First Date with Medicine Why the Foundation Course exists; the IMG roles and the pledge to grow.
3.	**Chapter 4** The MBBS Curriculum CBME spiral, ECE, integration, assessments, internship, and real career pathways.
4.	**Chapter 5** How Doctors Learn SDL, PBL/CBL, flipped class, simulation, collaborative & integrative learning; reflection and recall.
5.	**Chapter 6** A Guided Tour of Your Medical Campus From lecture theatres to simulation labs, ICU, libraries, wellness & counselling bays.
6.	**Chapter 7** A Walk Through a Community Health Centre CHC/IPHS reality: OPD, labour room, minor OT, cold-chain, ASHA/ANM, records.
7.	**Chapter 8** Beyond the Classroom Culture, conduct, rules, professionalism, consequences, and bridging to Genesis–Synthesis–Matrix.

Chapter 2: Inception

A Story They Won't Teach You in Lectures

He was maybe eight. Thin. Feverish. Curled like a question mark under a worn-out blanket in the emergency observation bay. You spotted him during your clinical posting. Nobody had assigned him to you; he was not a 'case.' He was just there.

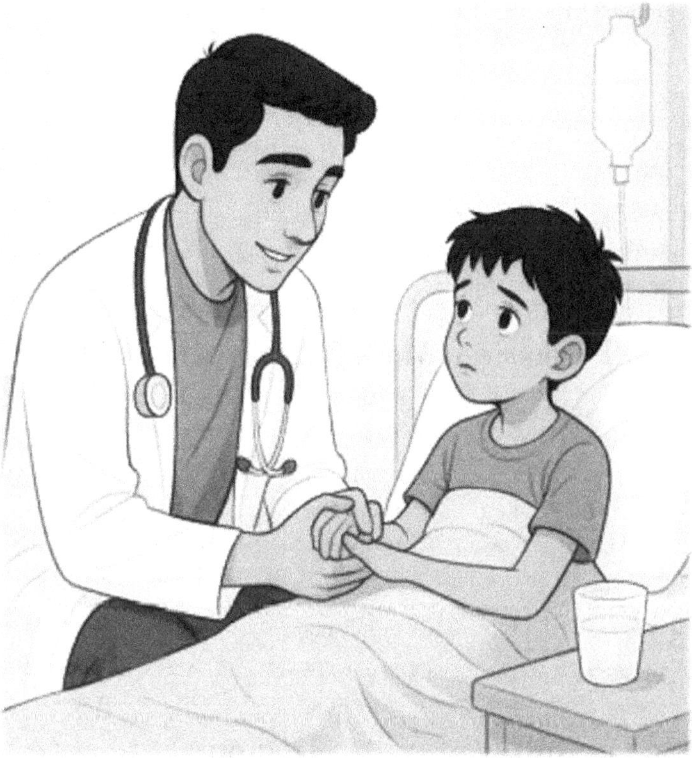

Figure 2.1: A Child in Emergency Room

You hesitated. You were new, still learning where to stand, how much to ask. But his eyes found yours.
And that was enough.

You knelt beside him. *"Kya hua champ?"* (What happened, Champ?)
No reply. Eyes full of fear. Father stood nearby, silent, anxious, unsure whether to speak or not. You checked his chart. Dengue. Low platelets. Waiting for repeat labs. You brought him a cup of ORS and a smile that said, *I see you.*

Later that evening, after helping insert an IV and adjust his bed, you walked past again. He gripped your finger and whispered, *"Aap kal bhi aayenge na? Papa bolte hain doctor acche hone pe jaldi chhutti de dete hain…"* (You will come again tomorrow? Father says that doctors discharge home early as I improve)

You smiled, blinked faster than usual, and nodded.

The next day, you came back. Not because you had to. But because you were already becoming a doctor, not by books, but by presence.

You didn't administer a life-saving drug.
You didn't perform a heroic procedure.
But you offered what every patient secretly hopes for, *Someone who cares, Someone who listens.* And that, too… is medicine!

Your introduction to the Most Human of Professions

Alongside the formal syllabus, you will encounter the values, attitudes, and habits you learn silently from seniors, mentors, and even the system itself. (1) These lessons often shape you as much as textbooks and lectures. The global journey of Indian doctors further reminds us that our profession belongs not only to hospitals here but also to communities worldwide (2).

Medical Profession: More than Science

Becoming a doctor is not only about knowledge. It is about witnessing humanity in its various forms, in birth, in pain, in fear, in recovery, and sometimes, in the goodbye. You will be there when someone hears the word "cancer" for the first time. You will be the one they look at during labour, during distress and at the time of fear of death, hoping you know what to do. You will witness gratitude, anger, helplessness, and faith, all in the same 10 minutes.

Yes, medicine is tough. But it's also deeply human.

And in the toughest places, you'll find your soul, not only your skills.

Global Footprints of Indian Doctors

India is producing doctors and also nurturing global healers living up to the विश्व आरोग्यं हि धर्मो नः Viśvārogyaṃ hi dharmo nah (Global health is our spiritual duty).

Over 80,000 Indian doctors practice in the USA, UK, Canada, and Australia, often holding top clinical, academic, or research positions.

Indian doctors comprise one of the largest groups of international medical graduates in the UK's National Health Service (NHS). (3,4)

Many Indian-origin doctors have led COVID-19 response units, cancer research labs, and robotic surgery programs worldwide. Indian doctors are known for clinical acumen, emotional resilience, and dedication. You're walking into a legacy that already shines. (3)

In Rhythm with the Nation's Pulse

Doctors are among the most respected professions, ahead of bureaucrats, engineers, and celebrities in surveys. Every doctor in a government setting serves thousands, sometimes millions, over the course of a lifetime.

A single neonatal resuscitation you perform gives more than 70 life-years, and a single CPR you perform may change the destiny of the whole family. A single counselling session may prevent suicide, abuse, or disease.

They may forget your name, but they'll never forget how you made them feel in those crucial moments. You may not remember all the people you treat. But for them, the moments spent in the hospital will get imprinted in their memories forever, and they will never forget the way you treated them during this period.

Okay to Dream Big

Being a doctor opens doors to financial stability, global mobility, careers in research, health policy, AI in medicine, telehealth, entrepreneurship, and leadership. There are incredible opportunities to publish, travel, mentor, and inspire, but the real richness comes from something else.

What the Future Demands from You

You will wear multiple stethoscopes in the form of

- A rural PHC doctor,
- A disease outbreak warrior,
- A telehealth specialist.
- A public health advocate and
- A changemaker.

To do justice with different roles, be a healer, not just a service provider and reflect on how you can contribute to improving the system in your area of influence. The doctor in India must

- Understand systems, not only symptoms,
- Communicate with patients as well as policymakers and
- Understand community health with clinical medicine.

Think Globally, Act Locally: You may evolve into a change maker within your system, train abroad to learn different models and technologies, and then return to serve or stay back. You can work with NGOs, policy teams, or on AI platforms, or create your own model of change. You should also understand global health policies, international partnerships (WHO, UNICEF) and medical migration and exchange.

Every patient you treat reflects the success or failure of the system. Don't ignore the broken system, but fix it and don't excuse injustice; you should question it. As a student doctor, you can

- Bring an innovative change,
- Develop a data-driven project with your mentor or
- Volunteer in a health camp or school CPR training.

☕ Coffee Moment

You pause with your first cup of coffee on campus, taking a slow breath. This is your journey to become a doctor. Ahead lie sleepless nights, days full of doubts, and years of tireless effort. Throughout this journey, you will experience moments of awe while learning and a sense of quiet victory that will transform you. This is your white coat moment, the first page of a story that will test and shape you. Welcome, dear doctor-in-the-making. The journey has begun.

References

1. Brownell AK, Côté L. Senior residents' views on the meaning of professionalism and how they learn about it. Acad Med. 2001;76(7):734-7.
2. Mullan F. Doctors for the world: Indian physician migration. Health Aff. 2006;25(2):380-93.
3. OECD. Recent Trends in International Migration of Doctors, Nurses and Medical Students. Paris: OECD Publishing; 2019.
4. Sheikh A, Naqvi HA. Indian doctors abroad: boon or bane for healthcare? BMJ. 2017;356:j634.

Chapter 3: My First Date with Medicine

You are not entering a classroom; you are stepping into the culture of science, skills, and service.

A New Beginning

Do you remember your first visit to a hospital as a kid? The smell, the crowd, the anxiety in your mind and the calm voice that said, 'You'll be okay.'

That voice? That was a doctor.

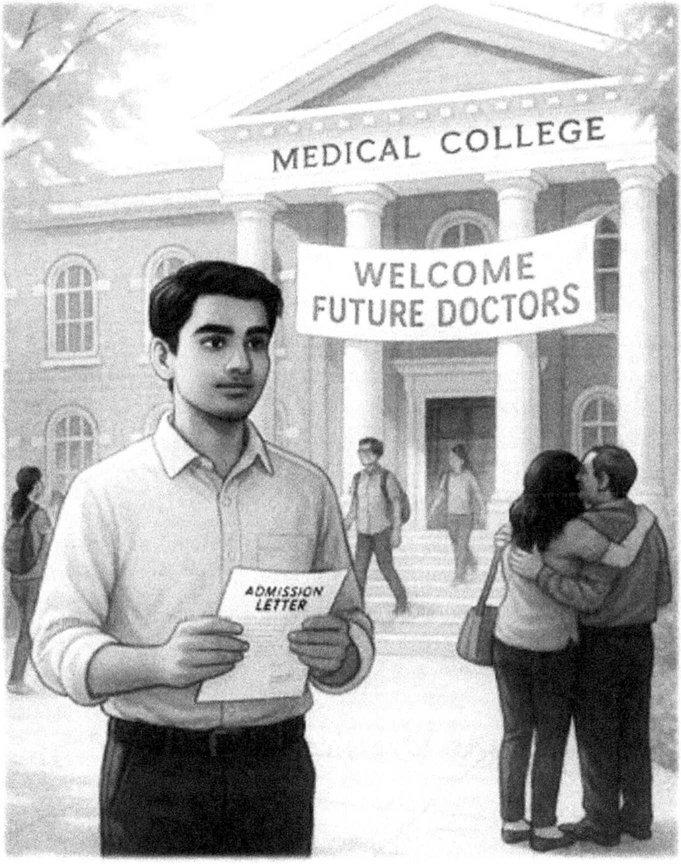

Figure 3.1 My First Day in Medical College

You crossed a significant threshold when you became eligible to study in the medical college. You are not only a student; you have joined the legacy of a respected and continually evolving profession. This is not a simple academic journey, but a transformation into a doctor.

Why a Foundation Course?

The National Medical Commission (NMC) introduced the Foundation Course to bridge the gap between school education and MBBS. Medicine is not just a profession; it is a way of life. It requires an open attitude, ethical clarity, emotional intelligence, and communication skills. (1)

This transformation is profound and demands not only knowledge and skill, but also compassion, integrity, and humility. This Foundation Course is your first step into a medical mindset. A good doctor begins with a good human being.

Indian Medical Graduate

The NMC defines an Indian Medical Graduate (IMG) as someone who is clinically competent, ethically grounded, socially sensitive, a lifelong learner, a communicator and a leader.

Table 3.1: Roles of an Indian Medical Graduate

Role	Core Purpose	Societal Impact
1. Clinician	Provide preventive, promotive, curative, palliative, and holistic care	Reduces disease burden and saves lives with evidence-based, patient-centered care
2. Leader and a team member	Coordinate with nurses, technicians, administrators, and community workers	Ensures efficient teamwork, equitable resource use, and safe healthcare delivery
3. Communicator	Convey empathy, information, and reassurance	Builds trust with patients, families, and society
4. Lifelong Learner	Keep updating medical knowledge and skills	Sustains innovation, patient safety, and high-quality care
5. Professional (Ethical & Accountable)	Uphold integrity, empathy, and respect for human dignity	Strengthens public trust in the medical profession and fosters social justice

What to Expect: An Overview of the Foundation Course

Here's a broad outline the NMC has designed for Indian Medical Graduates to explore during the Foundation Course. (2)

Orientation Module (30 hours)

- History and philosophy of medicine
- Role of doctors in society
- Introduction to the MBBS curriculum and expectations

- Principles of family practice
- Time management and study skills
- Introduction to medical ethics

Skills Module (35 hours)

- Basic Life Support (BLS)
- First aid, immunization practices
- Hand hygiene and biomedical waste disposal
- Documentation and medical records

Community Orientation (10 hours)

- Visit to a Primary Health Centre (PHC)
- Understanding healthcare delivery in rural/urban India

Professional Development & Ethics (AETCOM) (40 hours)

- Empathy, altruism, and professional behaviour
- Basics of bioethics: autonomy, beneficence, justice, non-maleficence

Computer Skills (40 hours)

- Using digital tools for learning and research
- Word processing, data handling, and online medical resources

Stress and Language (25 hours)

- Stress management and emotional resilience
- Effective communication in English and regional languages
- During the foundation course, you are expected to achieve specific competencies to a certain level. (3,4)

Levels of competency

- Know – Awareness of concepts (can explain them)
- Know How – Can apply the concept to solve or relate
- Show – Can demonstrate the skill or behaviour
- Show How – Performs under observation in a real or simulated setting

List of Competencies

The NMC provides a comprehensive list of competencies for IMGs. For natural learning, you are advised to first go through the book without thinking about competencies. The continuum section revisits the list of competencies, mapped to different sections and chapters in this book, to refer for a specific competency.

Table 3.2: List of competencies

Code	Competency	Domain-
FC 1	**Orientation**	Level
FC 1.1	Demonstrate understanding of the role of doctors in the society and their impact.	A- KH
FC 1.2	Demonstrate understanding of the Roles of an Indian Medical Graduate and relate it to the societal impact.	A- KH
FC 1.3	Discuss and appreciate the expectations of the students from the Nation, society, Institution, peers, colleagues and patients and vice versa.	A- KH
FC 1.4	Understands rules and regulations of the institution.	A- SH
FC 1.5	Orient themselves to the college campus, facilities, faculty, administrative structure, support systems and processes of the institution.	A- KH
FC 1.6	Discuss the various career pathways and opportunities for personal growth.	A- KH
FC 1.7	Demonstrate understanding of the overview of MBBS curriculum, its structure and outcomes and its relation to the career pathways.	K- KH
FC 1.8	Demonstrate understanding the role of physician at various levels of Health care delivery.	K- KH
FC 1.9	Discuss the principles of family practice.	K- KH
FC 1.10	Demonstrate awareness of the History of Medicine and alternate systems of Medicine.	K- K
FC 2	**Skills**	
FC 2.1	Perform Basic Life support in Skills lab.	Skill- SH
FC 2.2	Perform First Aid in a simulated environment.	Skill- SH
FC 2.3	Follow bio-safety and universal precautions.	Skill- SH
FC 2.4	Demonstrate handling and safe disposal of Biohazardous materials in a simulated environment.	Skill- SH
FC 2.5	Demonstrate proper hand washing and use of PPE.	Skill- SH
FC 2.6	Demonstrate proper response to needle stick injuries.	Skill- SH
FC 2.7	Demonstrate Biomedical Waste segregation (BMW), observe and explain the process of management of BMW in accordance with National Regulations.	Skill- SH
FC 2.8	Discuss the Immunization requirements of HCWs.	K- KH
FC 2.9	Demonstrate awareness of documentation in patient care and the proper method of documentation.	Skill- SH
FC 3	**Community Orientation**	

FC 3.1	Demonstrate understanding of the National Health Goals and Policies.	K- KH
FC 3.2	Discuss the national health scenario, demographic, socio-cultural and epidemiological issues.	K- KH
FC 3.3	Demonstrate understanding of the health care systems in India with reference to primary, secondary and tertiary level care.	K- KH
FC 3.4	Discuss the basic principles of community health and its impact on health and disease.	Skill- SH
FC 3.5	Demonstrate understanding of structure and functioning of the community health center.	K- KH
FC 3.6	Demonstrate ability to obtain patient experiences through patient and family interactions and relate these experiences to impact of environment and diseases.	Skill- SH
FC 4	**Professional Development**	
FC 4.1	Demonstrate the concept of professionalism and ethics among health care professionals and consequences of unprofessional and unethical behaviour.	Skill-KH
FC 4.2	Demonstrate understanding that compassion, altruism, integrity, duty, responsibility and trust are the core values that defines the nature of the physician's work.	K- KH
FC 4.3	Discuss the value, honesty and respect in interaction with peers, seniors, faculty, healthcare workers and patients.	Skill KH
FC 4.4	Discuss the significance of teamwork in a health care.	Skill-KH
FC 4.5	Discuss disability competencies.	K-KH
FC 4.6	Demonstrate respect for cultural diversities and interact with those with different cultural values.	K/A-KH
FC 4.7	Discuss the significance and methods of stress management and risk-taking behaviour.	K KH
FC 4.8	Understand role of Yoga & meditation in self health.	Skill- S
FC 4.9	Discuss the significance and appropriate ways of Time management.	K-KH
FC 4.10	Demonstrate importance of interpersonal relationship while working in a health care team.	Skill-KH
FC 4.11	Understand the role of mentoring.	Skill-KH
FC 4.12	Demonstrates understanding of the process of group learning and group dynamics.	Skill-KH
FC 4.13	Comprehend the learning pedagogy and learning skills.	Skill-KH
FC 4.14	Understands methods of self-directed learning.	Skill-KH
FC 4.15	Understand collaborative learning.	Skill-KH
FC 5	**Communication- Demonstrates ability to-**	

FC 5.1	Communicate with patient and families, be aware of barriers to communication and appropriate response.	C- SH
FC 5.2	Use of local language in patient and peer interactions.	C- SH
FC 5.3	Communicate and learn in English.	C- SH
FC 5.4	Use basic computer skills.	Skill- SH
FC 5.5	Accessing online resources.	Skill- SH

Reflect and Write

What does becoming a doctor mean to you ? Write your answers

- Why do I want to become a doctor? ------------------------------
- What does being a doctor mean to me? --------------------------
- What are the qualities I admire most in a physician? -----------

Coffee Moment

During your orientation module, your facilitators and teachers will introduce you to the institution, campus, and facilities. Get oriented to walls, paths, plants, and people, and rise together in love with them. You can write down your memories from your first day here or paste a picture. These words or pictures you will keep close to your heart. Forever!

My First Day…

References

1. Cruess RL, Cruess SR. Professionalism must be taught. BMJ. 1997;315:1674–1677.
2. Medical Council of India. Competency-Based Undergraduate Curriculum for the Indian Medical Graduate. Vol. 1. New Delhi: MCI; 2018.
3. Frank JR, Snell L, Sherbino J. CanMEDS 2015 Physician Competency Framework. Ottawa: Royal College of Physicians and Surgeons of Canada; 2015.
4. Harden RM. Outcome-based education: the future is today. Med Teach. 2007;29(7):625–629.
5. Association of American Medical Colleges (AAMC). Careers in Medicine: Pathways and Planning. Washington, DC; 2021.

Chapter 4: The MBBS Curriculum- Science, Skills, and Service

Introduction

The MBBS curriculum is not a collection of subjects to be memorised; it is a carefully structured journey that transforms a student into a competent, compassionate doctor. You will move from understanding the fundamentals of the human body to applying knowledge at the bedside, in communities, and during moments of crisis. The curriculum blends scientific reasoning with clinical skills, ethical practice, and service to society. Understanding this structure helps students navigate medical school with clarity, confidence, and purpose.

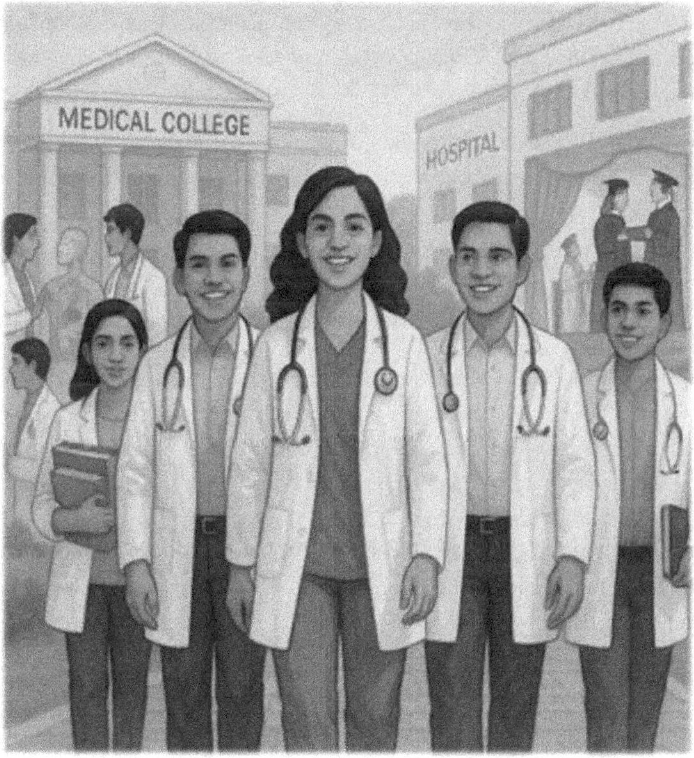

Figure 4.1 Medicine is not Simply a Course. It is a Commitment to Life.

Unlocking the Universe of Possibilities

Medicine is a career that profoundly impacts human life, affecting physical, emotional, social, and even spiritual aspects. As a future doctor, you are not just training to treat diseases; you are entering into a universe of possibilities:

Global Mobility and Recognition: MBBS from India is recognized in many countries. With licensing exams such as the USMLE (USA), PLAB (UK), AMC (Australia), and DHA (UAE), doctors can work and grow in various countries.

Financial Stability and Growth: Doctors can earn handsomely in different specializations. Earnings are not only generated through clinical practice, but also via medical entrepreneurship, telemedicine, research, health technology, and writing.

Social Respect and Legacy: No profession enjoys the lifelong social respect that doctors do. They inspire others. They are admired and remembered by many.

Diverse Career Pathways: In surgery, space medicine, critical care, and creative medical education, as well as in AI-driven diagnostics and policy-making, doctors can reinvent their roles as often as they like.

Real Impact on Human Lives: Doctors are in the profession of saving lives, holding hands during grief, bringing hope during despair, and witnessing the shades of human behaviour.

Innovation and Research Potential: Today's medical student will be tomorrow's inventor of therapies, devices, protocols, and systems.

Contribution to Nation-Building: Working as a doctor is a patriotic act, whether you are working in a village, in an institute of national importance, in war zones or in research labs. Doctors serve the people, uphold scientific knowledge, and contribute to the health of a country.

Let this excite you. Let this humble you. Let this fuel you through the long hours and heavy books. Your white coat is not a uniform; it is a promise, a privilege, and a passport to making a difference in the world. With the awe of possibilities that await a medical graduate, the MBBS curriculum anchors you to the structured path that makes it all possible. Designed by the NMC, the Indian MBBS curriculum is now Competency-Based Medical Education (CBME). It's not only about knowledge, but it's about building doctors who are clinically competent, ethically grounded, communicative, and lifelong learners. (1)

Overview of MBBS Curriculum

Duration: 4.5 years of academic learning plus 1 year of compulsory rotating internship, making a 5.5 years.

The Spiral of Learning: Medical knowledge is built in layers

Foundation Course – orientation, soft skills, language, and basic life support and the beginning of attitude, ethics and communication (AETCOM) module.

First Professional Year – understanding the normal human body and functions through Anatomy, Physiology and Biochemistry.

Second Professional Year – understanding mechanisms of disease and drug action in Pathology, Microbiology, Pharmacology and Forensic Medicine.

Third Professional Years: clinical management and population health in Part 1 subjects, including Community Medicine, ENT, Ophthalmology and in Part 2, i.e. Medicine, Surgery, Pediatrics, Obstetrics and Gynaecology (OBG), Psychiatry, Orthopaedics, Dermatology, and allied subjects.

Internship: Putting it all into practice. Each phase integrates clinical exposure, skills lab simulation, community immersion, electives and research projects.

The MBBS journey is competency-based, outcome-driven, and socially accountable (1,2). The upcoming *National Exit Test (NEXT)* will serve both as a final assessment and a licensure examination, aligning Indian training with global standards (3).

Key Features of CBME Curriculum

Competency-Based: Outcome-focused learning to acquire demonstrable competencies.

Early Clinical Exposure (ECE): Even first-year students interact with patients and understand the relevance of subjects.

Horizontal and Vertical Integration: Subjects like anatomy (first year) and radiology (final year), or pathology and medicine, are taught in an interconnected manner so that understanding is holistic and not in silos.

Electives and Research: Students pursue topics of interest, including audit, innovation, and social service.

Skill Labs and Assessment: Practical skills are taught in a safe environment and assessed using OSCEs and logbooks

Internship: From Learner to Doctor

The one-year internship combines theoretical knowledge with practical experience. Interns rotate through major departments, take calls, manage wards, assist in surgeries, and learn crucial skills that textbooks never taught: how to provide support - in pain, in urgency, and in hope.

Examination and Assessments

To ensure that medical graduates meet the expected competencies, the MBBS curriculum includes a well-defined examination pattern and assessment strategy for each academic year. Slight variations are possible, as per the syllabus approved by the university, institution, or college.

Internal Assessment

- Conducted through unit tests, seminars, practicals, logbooks, and attendance.
- A minimum grade of 50% in the internal assessment is required to be eligible to appear in university or professional exams.

University Examinations

Conducted at the end of each professional phase for assessment of theoretical components, including multiple-choice questions (MCQs), short-answer questions, and long-answer questions, as well as practical or clinical skills in the form of case presentations, OSCEs, OSPEs and viva.

Pass Criteria: A minimum 50% score in both the theory and practical exams.

- **First Professional Exam (End of 1st Year):** Anatomy, Physiology, Biochemistry
- **Second Professional Exam (End of 2nd Year)**: Subjects: Pathology, Microbiology, Pharmacology, Forensic Medicine.
- **Third Professional – Part 1 Exam (After 1 year)**: Subjects: Community Medicine, ENT, Ophthalmology.
- **Third Professional – Part 2 Exam (Final MBBS)**: Subjects include Medicine, Surgery, Paediatrics, Obstetrics and Gynaecology, Orthopedics, Psychiatry, and Dermatology. Also referred to as final exams, these assessments are the most comprehensive and integrated.

Skill-Based Assessment

- Includes OSCE, spotters, procedural stations, case presentations, and AETCOM-based tasks.

Logbooks and Portfolios

Evidence of acquired skills and competencies is required for certification before university examinations.

Electives and AETCOM Module

Integrate formative and summative assessments across different years, emphasizing reflection writing, case discussions, peer interactions, and team-based learning. (1)

Internship Evaluation

Daily logbooks, direct observation, and periodic assessment by mentors.

The competency-based medical education and comprehensive assessment system promotes ongoing learning, hands-on skills development, reflective thinking, and accountability. It is designed to prepare students not only to pass exams but also to practice safe, compassionate, and evidence-based medicine.

Curriculum Reflects National Health Priorities

The Indian MBBS curriculum is closely linked to National Health Programs, public health infrastructure, drugs, and social accountability. Students are sensitized to rural health, social determinants, health economics, ethical dilemmas, and emerging diseases. We will take this in detail in the coming sections. (1)

Career Pathways After MBBS

The journey after completing an MBBS can lead you in many directions: clinical practice, academia, entrepreneurship, or humanitarian work, which are the main avenues for personal and professional growth.

Postgraduate Specializations (MD, MS and DNB): Pursue a residency in internal medicine, surgery, paediatrics, obstetrics and gynaecology, psychiatry, radiology, orthopedics, and more.

DM, MCh and Fellowships: After specialization or as integrated courses, you can pursue super-specialization in fields like cardiology, neurology, gastroenterology, neurosurgery, pediatric surgery, oncology, and more.

Para-Clinical: Community medicine, pharmacology, microbiology and pathology, offering different roles in diagnostics, research, teaching, and public health.

Research and Innovation: Work as a clinical researcher, trial coordinator, or data scientist. Pursue a PhD or fellowships (ICMR, CSIR, NIH, WHO).

Administrative and Policy Roles: Become a healthcare administrator, public health officer, or work in ministries and agencies (WHO, UNICEF, NITI Aayog).

Teaching and Academia: Become a faculty member in a medical college and inspire future generations.

Global Medical Careers: Clear licensing exams such as the USMLE (USA), PLAB (UK), AMC (Australia), MCCQE (Canada), or HAAD/DHA (Middle East).

Digital Health & Medical Technology: Innovate in fields like AI in diagnostics, telemedicine, app development, digital therapeutics, and wearable health tech.

Entrepreneurship: Start your own clinic, diagnostics centre, health startup, medical consultancy, or e-learning venture.

Law, Ethics, and Journalism: Combine your degree with law, medical ethics, public policy, or health journalism.

Government and Competitive Exams: UPSC CMS, Armed Forces Medical

Services, Railways, ESI, and state PSCs open public service roles.

MBBS is not a finish line; it's a springboard for its own rewards, struggles, and meaning. With time, you will find your calling. Welcome to medicine. Welcome to a lifelong purpose. When you don the white coat, you wear the trust of a society.

Reflect and Write

What excites you most about the curriculum? --------------------------

Which clinical department are you most curious about? -------------

What challenges do you foresee in becoming a competent, caring doctor? -----------

☕ Coffee Moment

As you look at the vast MBBS curriculum, it may feel like standing at the foot of a mountain whose peak is hidden by clouds. Remember, this curriculum is not meant to overwhelm you—it is meant to *shape you.* Every subject, every lecture, every practical is a step in becoming a doctor who understands, heals, and serves. Take it one day at a time. Growth in medicine is quiet, gradual, and deeply transformative. Remember how it felt when you stood in a hall wearing a white coat for the first time.

That awe

That fear

That fire

Never lose it!

One day, someone will trust you with their life, be worthy of it.

References

1. Medical Council of India. Competency-Based Undergraduate Curriculum for the Indian Medical Graduate. Vol. 2. New Delhi: MCI; 2018.
2. Frenk J, Chen L, Bhutta ZA, Cohen J, Crisp N, Evans T, et al. Health professionals for a new century: transforming education to strengthen health systems. *Lancet.* 2010;376(9756):1923-58.
3. Kuppili S, Madala E, Kant R, Tiwari LK, Edara L. Concept Proposal for Nationalised Formative and Summative Assessments to Enhance the Preparedness of Medical Students for the National Exit Test (NExT) and Solution for Low Resource Countries: Insights from NBME Examinations in the USA: Enhancing preparedness of medical students towards NExT. Global Journal of Medical Students. 2022;2(3):28-30.
4. Harden RM, Crosby J, Davis MH, Friedman M. AMEE Guide No. 14: Outcome-based education: Part 5. *Med Teach.* 1999;21(6):546-52.

Chapter 5: How Doctors Learn

Introduction

You learned *what* to study in school, but in medical college, you must master *how* to study due to the enormous volume of information, high stakes, and the continual learning process. You'll encounter different types of situations, from biochemistry equations to breaking bad news to families. Each area requires a unique learning strategy, which we will discuss in this section.

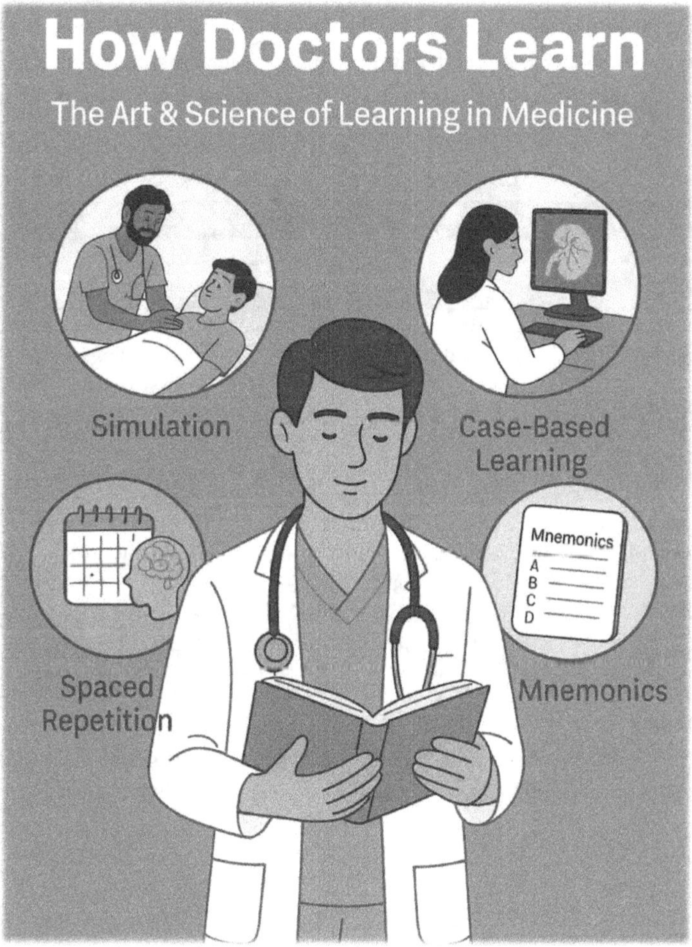

Figure 5.1: How Doctors Learn

While practising different learning methods for different requirements, ask yourself regularly:

- Am I learning actively or passively?

- What's working? What is not working?
- Am I just memorizing or understanding?
- Am I emotionally engaged with what I'm learning?

Try different techniques, apps, diagrams, models, mnemonics, and methods that work for you. (1)

Learning Pedagogy

When you enter medical school, you might feel overwhelmed by the variety of teaching methods: lectures, small group discussions, bedside clinics, simulation labs, and even self-directed learning. This variety isn't accidental; it comes from the science of pedagogy, the art and method of teaching. Pedagogy shapes not only what you learn, but also how you learn. For instance:

Table 5.1: Different types of learning methods

Method	How It Works	Example
Reading & Reflection	Read textbooks, articles, or guidelines beyond lectures.	ICMR hypertension updates.
Case-Based Learning	Explore real or simulated patient cases to identify gaps in understanding.	Anemia case - linking lab findings with physiology.
Problem-Based Learning	Start with a clinical problem → research → discuss → conclude.	Diabetic ketoacidosis scenario studied in small groups.
E-Learning & Open Online Courses	Use online platforms (e.g., SWAYAM, OpenWHO) for skill/concept building.	Completing Online IAP CPR module.
Peer-to-Peer Learning	Teach and quiz each other; Teamwork and retention.	Group explaining ECG interpretation.
Learning Portfolios	Maintain records of skills learned and feedback.	BLS logbook or case reflection portfolio.
Reflective Practice	Write reflections after patient interactions.	"What did I feel when delivering bad news?"
Micro-Research & Mini-Audits	Identify small research questions; collect and analyze data.	Audit of hand hygiene compliance in your ward.
Simulation & Skill Labs	Practice procedures in controlled environments; repeat till mastery.	Airway management on manikins.
Teaching	Teach peers and junior colleagues.	Take a bedside class on recognition of a sick child.

- Lectures help you gain a broader perspective.
- Problem-based learning trains you to think like a detective.

- Simulation helps build muscle memory for emergencies, such as CPR.
- Reflective writing deepens empathy and professional values.

Understanding pedagogy enables you to appreciate *why* your teachers choose specific methods, and more importantly, how to adapt your learning style to each one. Doctors never stop learning, and grasping pedagogy now equips you to be a better self-directed learner and, in future, a better teacher for your patients and juniors. (1)

Self-Directed Learning

To grow as a doctor, you must learn how to learn. Self-Directed Learning (SDL) means taking charge of your own learning journey, with curiosity as your compass. SDL is taking responsibility for identifying your learning needs, setting goals, finding resources, and evaluating your progress while teachers act as guides, not lecturers. (2)

Methods of Self-Directed Learning

Some learning methodologies discussed below need practice, while some methods you will grasp in your learning journey.

Problem-Based Learning (PBL)

What it is: Working in small groups to solve clinical cases, fostering inquiry and collaborative learning. (2,3)

Best For: Applying knowledge across subjects, clinical reasoning, and teamwork.

Scenario: In a PBL session, a group of students is presented with a case study of a young boy with jaundice. They brainstorm differential diagnoses, revisit liver physiology, explore investigations, and present findings. You don't only learn the case; you know how to think like a doctor.

Case-Based Learning (CBL)

What it is: Using real or simulated patient cases to anchor theory to practice.

Best For: Integrating basic science with clinical thinking

Scenario: Meher learns about nephrotic syndrome not from a textbook but from a case: A 6-year-old with swelling, frothy urine, and low albumin. As she studies the case, the clinical signs and symptoms, pathology, pharmacology, investigation plan and treatment algorithm all come alive. One typical patient to remember for a common condition.

Flipped Classroom

What it is: Watching lectures or materials before class, and using classroom time for discussion, application, or problem-solving. You can effectively use e-learning platforms before attending the offline classroom. (4,5)

Best For: Complex topics that benefit from discussion (e.g., bioethics, pharmacodynamics).

Scenario: Dr Mehta assigns a video on the mechanisms of antibiotic resistance. Instead of re-teaching it in class, he divides students into teams to analyze a case of a multidrug-resistant infection and suggest appropriate therapies. *Learn at your own pace. Apply at your peak.*

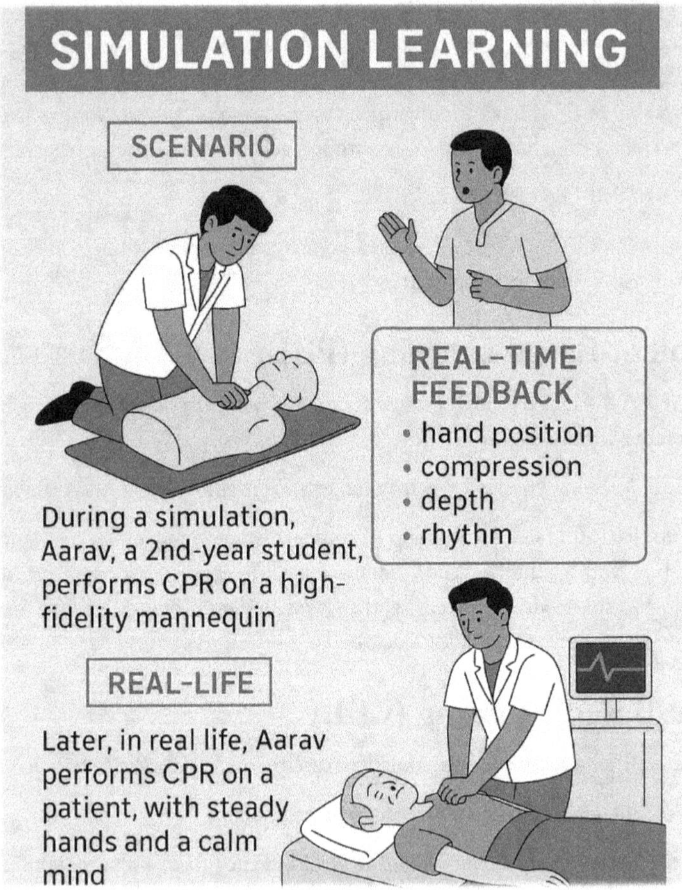

Figure 5.2: Simulation Learning

Simulation-Based Learning

What it is: Practicing clinical skills or emergency scenarios on mannequins, task trainers, or digital platforms.

Scenario: Performing CPR Practice in the skill lab, followed by actual application on a real patient.

Best For: CPR, suturing, intubation, obstetric deliveries and emergency decision-making.

Collaborative Learning - Growing Together

Collaborative learning is an educational approach in which students work together, sharing ideas, questioning, teaching, and supporting one another to achieve a common learning goal. It builds communication, teamwork, empathy, and critical thinking qualities that every future doctor needs. Every diagnosis discussed, every case analysed, every late-night group study is collaborative learning in action.

Table 5.2: Different methods of collaborative learning

Method	How It Works	Outcome
Small group discussions	Analyze a case or ethical dilemma together.	Learn multiple viewpoints.
Peer-assisted learning	Senior students mentor juniors in practical skills.	Builds confidence and leadership.
Team-based learning	Work in structured teams to solve clinical problems.	Promotes teamwork and accountability.
Journal clubs and group presentations	Review research papers collectively.	Encourages evidence-based thinking.
Interprofessional sessions	Learn with nursing, physiotherapy, or public health students.	Strengthens respect for healthcare roles.
Integrative Learning	Links concepts across subjects (e.g., anatomy, physiology, and pathology) or connects basic sciences with clinical cases.	Promotes holistic understanding, reduces compartmental learning, and enhances clinical reasoning.

Why It Matters in Medicine

Healthcare is a team effort involving doctors, nurses, technicians, administrators, and patients' families. Learning collaboratively prepares you for teamwork in procedures, surgeries, codes and projects.

- It develops leadership and communication skills, essential for interprofessional teamwork.
- Sharing perspectives improves concept retention, clinical reasoning, and emotional intelligence.

How to Make It Work

- Listen actively, not competitively.

- Respect different viewpoints.
- Share responsibilities equally.
- Reflect together on what worked and what didn't.

Group Learning

From your first small-group discussion in anatomy to managing a code blue in the ICU, learning and working in groups is part of becoming a doctor. Group learning helps you:

- Share different perspectives.
- Divide complex topics into manageable parts.
- Motivate each other to keep pace.
- Develop the teamwork skills necessary for clinical practice.

However, learning in groups also creates its own unique psychology, known as group dynamics. This is about how people interact:

- A group with clear roles and respectful communication thrives.
- A group where one person dominates or others withdraw struggles.
- Well-managed conflict sparks deeper learning; if ignored, it derails progress.

As future doctors, mastering group dynamics prepares you to collaborate effectively in healthcare teams where lives depend on clear and effective communication. The key? Listen actively, respect diverse views, maintain focus on learning and performance, and reflect together afterwards. You will learn more about this in the *Revive* section, under team dynamics, where you will discover how good team dynamics can help someone survive a code blue.

Reflective Practice

What it is: Analyzing your experiences to learn from them and improve future performance.

Best For: Ethics, communication and professionalism.

Scenario: After witnessing an argument between a doctor and a patient's family, Arjun writes a reflection: What could the doctor have done differently? How did the environment affect emotions? How will *he* respond differently in the future?

Reflection turns experience into wisdom.

Spaced Repetition and Active Recall

What it is: Reviewing material at increasing intervals (spaced repetition) and testing yourself frequently without looking at notes (active recall).

Best For: Memorizing anatomy, drugs, clinical signs, diagnostic criteria, etc.

Scenario: Remember the names of the branches of the arch of aorta. Later, you were asked the following MCQ in your exam. Which of the following arises directly from the aortic arch? You now know the answer without help.

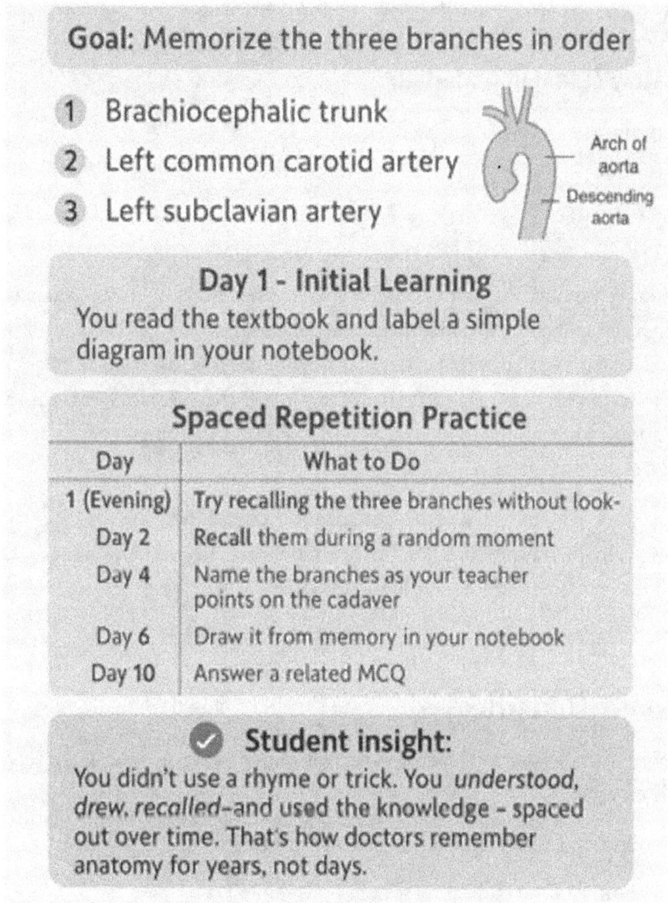

Figure 5.3: Spaced Repetition Practice

Use of Mnemonics

Things are not as easy as the branches of the arch of the aorta. Your memory and recall capabilities will be thoroughly tested here. But don't worry; handling more challenging cases is even more fun.

Scenario: Riya, a first-year student, struggles to remember all the wrist (Carpal) bones in sequence.

Proximal Row (Lateral to Medial)

- Scaphoid
- Lunate
- Triquetrum
- Pisiform

Distal Row (Lateral to Medial)

- Trapezium
- Trapezoid
- Capitate
- Hamate

She tries to remember the names of all cranial nerves, but forgets the sequence every time. She uses spaced repetition and recall, but only partially succeeds, and becomes frustrated. In the evening, when she went out with her friends to an ice cream parlour, she tried to recall, but she was blank. One of their seniors, overhearing the conversation, came smiling and said, **S**neh **L**ata **T**ried **P**ainting; **T**hen **T**hey **C**ooked **H**alwa.'

For a second, she felt awkward, but in another second, she had her sequence **S**caphoid, **L**unate, **T**riquetrum, **P**isiform, **T**rapezium, **T**rapezoid, **C**apitate, **H**amate. You will learn many more in your labs. Stay cool!

Fact fades. Recall rewires.

Books to Bedside

You'll shift from classroom learning to real patient care in your later years. New methods emerge:

Bedside clinics: Learn examination skills from real cases.

Ward rounds: Absorb clinical reasoning by watching seniors.

Internship journaling: Note down key learnings daily: symptoms, signs, errors, breakthroughs.

Case presentations: Hone communication and diagnostic clarity.

Patients don't speak in MCQs. Clinical learning is messy and magical.

Medicine Needs Multi-Modal Minds

There's no one-size-fits-all in medical learning. Some days, you will memorize enzymes, and on other days, you will hold a trembling hand. You need both the data and the depth of wisdom. Choose your tools wisely. Try new methods. Respect your own pace and style. And remember, you're not just learning for exams. You're learning for the lives you will one day touch. (6)

Discover Your Learning Style

Knowing yourself is the beginning of all wisdom. -Aristotle

A Self-Reflection Worksheet: Take 10 minutes. Be honest. No grades here, but guidance. Tick what you relate to

What do you enjoy while learning?

- I like drawing mind maps and diagrams
- I enjoy listening to podcasts or discussions
- I remember things better when I teach them
- I prefer reading in silence with a highlighter
- I like hands-on practice more than theory
- I love flashcards and quick quizzes
- I reflect better when I write about what I learned

What frustrates you most about studying?

- Too much theory
- Can't remember facts
- Not sure where to begin
- Get bored easily
- No connection to real-life medicine
- Information overload

What are your learning goals this month?

(Understand ECG basics, revise the anatomy of the heart, write one reflection)

1.____

2.____

3. ____

What do you want to try new this month?

Choose a method you've never tried: simulation, reflection, flashcards, etc.

"The goal is progress, not perfection."

☕ Coffee Moment

Medicine is not learned in one style or one classroom. You will learn from textbooks and lectures, yes—but also from patients' stories, seniors' mistakes, late-night doubts, and quiet moments of reflection. Sometimes learning feels slow, even invisible. Trust that it is happening. Every question you ask, every concept you revisit, every experience you reflect on is shaping the doctor you are becoming—often long before you realise it.

References

1. National Medical Commission. AETCOM Module: Attitude, Ethics and Communication. New Delhi: NMC; 2019.
2. Murad MH et al. Self-directed learning in health professions education: A systematic review. Med Educ. 2010;44(11):1057–68.
3. Dolmans DH, Michaelsen LK, Van Merriënboer JJ, van der Vleuten CP. Problem-based learning: future challenges. Med Educ. 2015;49(7):749–756.
4. Brown PC, Roediger HL, McDaniel MA. Make It Stick: The Science of Successful Learning. Harvard University Press; 2014.
5. Ellaway R, Masters K. AMEE Guide 32: e-Learning in medical education. Med Teach. 2008;30(5):455–473.
6. Yardley S, Teunissen PW, Dornan T. Experiential learning: AMEE Guide No. 63. Med Teach. 2012;34(2):e102–e115.

Chapter 6: A Guided Tour of Your Medical Campus

To walk through a medical college is to walk through dreams made of discipline and devotion.

Introduction

Close your eyes for a moment. Take a deep breath. Now imagine you're standing at the main gate of a sprawling campus, a place where hope is stitched together in operating rooms, where young minds debate over diagnoses, and where night lights never go out, because someone, somewhere, always needs help.

Welcome to your new home, medical college, and affiliated tertiary care hospital. This chapter offers a guided virtual tour to help you become familiar with the walls, corridors, and grounds where you'll laugh, struggle, learn, play, heal, and transform. Let's begin.

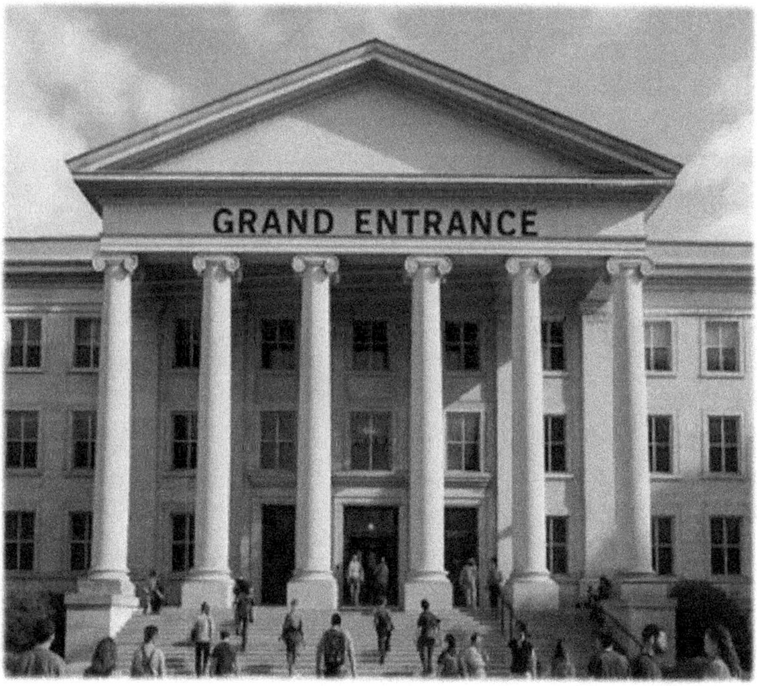

Figure 6.1: Academic Block

Academic Block

Stop 1. Entrance: Where Purpose Begins

The gates open to a broad avenue lined with trees, where you walk in with other white-coat dreamers, nervous and excited. You see security staff giving a polite nod, and a student-run help desk during orientation week. This is your first encounter with the real world of medicine.

Stop 2. The Dean's Office: Centre of Academics

You now walk toward the Dean's Office — often an elegant but quiet corner of the Academic Block. This is the medical education headquarters. The Dean is responsible for academic activities. Sometimes, you'll visit here to submit forms, discuss electives, or maybe to receive an award you never imagined. The office maintains discipline and dignity, and reminds you that professionalism is the essence of medicine.

Stop 3. Lecture Theatres - Where Minds Take Shape

Academic Block is a blend of modern architecture and timeless purpose. Classrooms are equipped with digital boards, 3D anatomy models, and interactive AV tools, and behind every screen lies a patient you may one day save.

Lecture Halls: These are the auditoriums of your awakening, where professors with decades of wisdom make you fall in love with medicine subjects.

Mini-Auditorium CME, Workshops and Conferences: Many lecture halls double as conference venues. You'll attend Continuing Medical Education (CMEs), interdisciplinary clinics, grand rounds, and medical quizzes here. Sometimes, international doctors visit, and their words spark dreams of fellowships and frontiers yet to come.

Demonstration Rooms: These are smaller, more intimate spaces for focused learning. You'll revisit these rooms during clinical postings.

Central Library: A quiet fortress of knowledge. You'll come here for more than books - peace, group study, and coffee-fuelled midnight revisions.

☕ **Coffee Moment:** In a corner of library cafeteria, a 2nd-year student smiles as she sees you holding your anatomy book. She offers coffee and the community begins.

Stop 4. The Dissection Hall - First Encounter

You walk into the Anatomy Dissection Hall**,** your first sacred lab. This space changes you. Here, under the respectful guidance of teachers, you meet your first silent mentor, the cadaver - a gift of science and sacrifice.

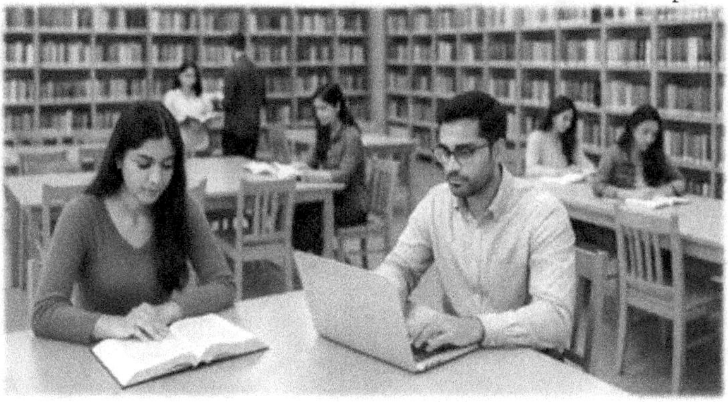

Figure 6.2: Library

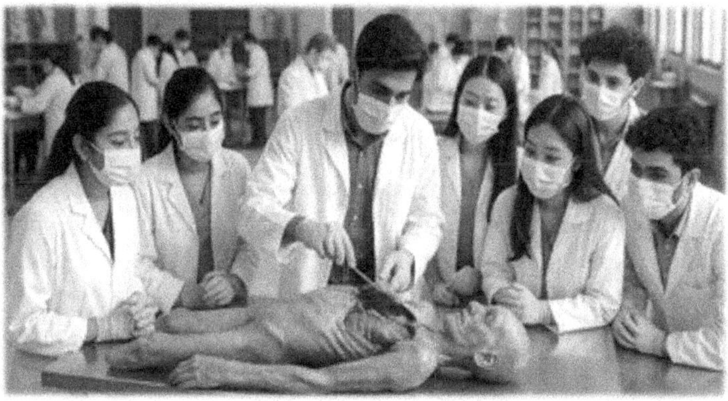

Figure 6.3: Dissection Hall

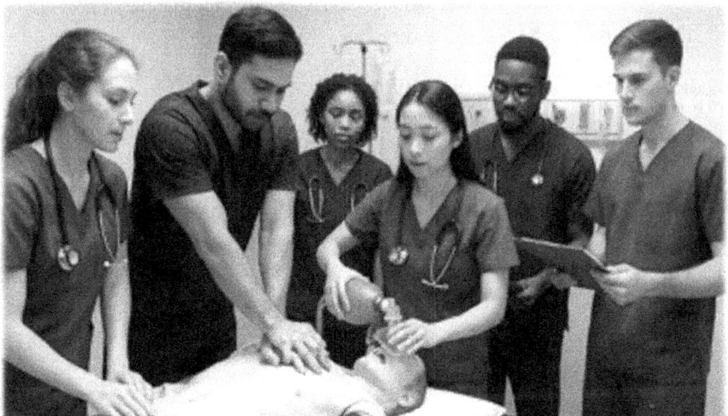

Figure 6.4: Simulation Lab

Stop 5. Skills and Simulation Lab - Learn by Doing

Here you'll practice CPR, intubation, injections, suturing, and emergency procedures until your hands have mastered what your mind has learned. It is equipped with mannequins, virtual reality setups, and task trainers. You will fail here. And you will try again. Until one day, you don't. (1)

Stop 6. Museums and Demonstrations

Pathology Museum: A hall of diseased organs, preserved forever for your learning - heart-wrenching, awe-inspiring.

Community Medicine Labs: Here you'll learn how medicine meets the masses. You'll conduct field visits, understand preventive care, and explore the heart of public health, where vaccination drives, nutrition programs, and epidemiological surveys begin.

Stop 7. Health & Wellness Centre

Students studying in the medical field also require proper care during times of illness or stress. This on-campus facility offers medical and mental health support with complete confidentiality, addressing a range of issues from the flu to managing stress or homesickness, as essential as libraries and laboratories. Burnout and stress are genuine risks in medical training, and accessing counselling, peer support, and recreational activities early is as important as achieving academic excellence. (2,3)

The Counselling Bay offers comfort without judgment. Here, trained counsellors - often clinical psychologists or psychiatry residents - gently guide patients, caregivers, or even students through emotional distress.

As a medical student, you may one day refer a patient here. Or, on a tough day, you may walk in yourself.

Hospital Block: Where Books Come Alive

As you step into the Tertiary Care Hospital, the air shifts. It smells of disinfectant, urgency, and silent prayers. This is where your knowledge finds meaning.

Stop 1. Casualty or Emergency Department

A symphony of speed and triage at the hospital's entrance on the ground floor. Red, yellow, and green zones for prioritized care, based on the patient's clinical condition. It is not a first-come, first-served area, but rather a place where the sickest receive immediate attention and stable patients can wait. You will learn what every second means.

Stop 2. Vaccination Centre - The First Line of Prevention

Near the community medicine clinic or the pediatric OPD, the Vaccination Centre is often bustling with mothers and infants. You'll see resident doctors advising vaccines, interns and nurses administering shots, and updating records. Public health quietly triumphs in this small room.

Stop 3. Outpatient Departments (OPDs)

Patients queue here daily, bringing fevers, fractures, and fears. You will shadow doctors, observe case-taking, and learn how to listen.

Stop 4. Inpatient Wards

Here, you'll learn bedside manner, respect for patients, and clinical examination.

Stop 5. ICUs, HDUs and OT Complex

You must be precise in your assessment and clinical decision-making, evaluating, identifying, and intervening at every step. In critical care, the beeping monitors and ventilators are a constant presence. In the OT Complex, you'll first observe, through glass panels, surgeons with scalpels and anaesthetists monitoring every breath. Someday, you'll scrub in to assist and then to lead the chorus.

Stop 6. Laboratories and Diagnostic Wings

Samples from the entire hospital are prepared and analysed in the central laboratory. From CBCs, LFTs, KFTs, cultures, and sepsis panels to advanced testing facilities, these services are coordinated through various departments.

Radiology: X-rays, CT scans, and MRIs to guide diagnosis and interventions.

Stop 7. Mortuary and Museum of Realizations

Some lessons are learned in silence, sometimes after death. In the mortuary and forensic museum, you witness this. It's a stop to make you gentler. Some conditions are diagnosed after death through autopsy. Sometimes it serves as an evidence lab for medico-legal cases.

System Behind Ecosystem

Faculty, Administration, and Support Systems: A medical college is more than lecture halls and wards; it is an ecosystem. Understanding its structure will help you know where to go, whom to ask, and how to keep growing.

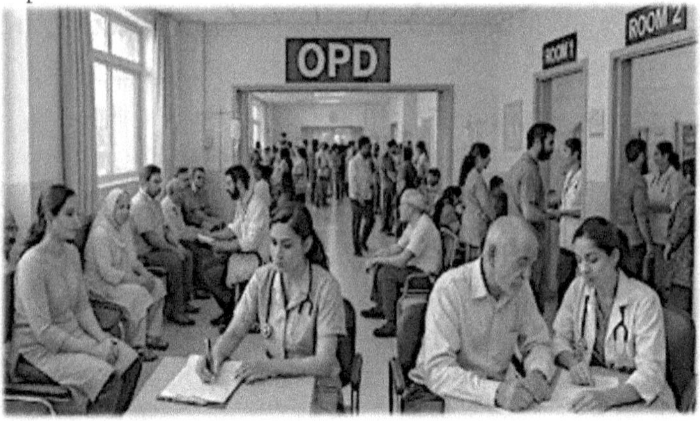

Figure 6.5: Out Patient Department

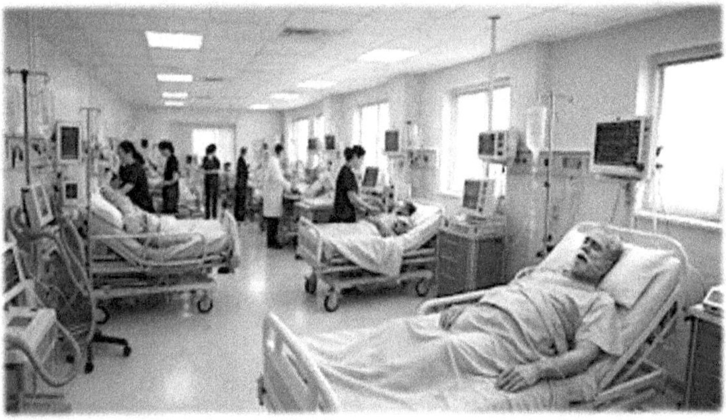

Figure 6.6: In Patient Department

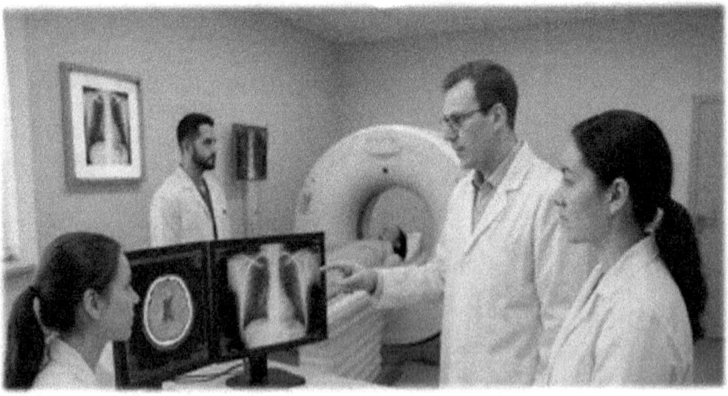

Figure 6.7: Radiology Department

Faculty Structure

Director/Principal: Head of the institution, oversees academics, hospital services, administration, and overall functioning.

Dean: Head of all academic affairs, faculty and students.

Medical Superintendent: Oversees all hospital and patient care-related services. Executive head of medical, nursing and hospital support system.

Heads of Departments (HODs): Lead each speciality (e.g., Medicine, Surgery, Pediatrics). They manage teaching, research, and patient care in their department.

Professors, Associate Professors, and Assistant Professors: Teachers, researchers, and clinicians who guide you in classrooms, labs, and wards.

Senior Residents, Tutors, Demonstrators: Middle-grade cadre in hospitals, labs and teaching departments, working after their postgraduate training (MD/MS/DNB) in a particular speciality under the direct supervision of faculty and guiding Junior Residents (post-graduate trainees)

Junior Residents: Post-graduate trainees, often your first mentors in dissection halls, clinics, and labs.

Administrative Structure

Deputy Director (Admin)/Registrar/Administrative Officer: Manages college/hospital administration, student records, exams, and official communication.

Finance and Accounts Section: Handles fees, stipends, salary, and reimbursements.

Examination Cell: Coordinates internal and university exams.

Library & Digital Learning Cell: A support system with study space and books, journals and online resources.

Hostel Office & Wardens: For accommodation and student welfare.

Student Counselling Services: Offer services related to mental health, stress management, and academic support.

Anti-Ragging & Mentorship Cell: Provides a safe and supportive environment for discussing any issues related to ragging. Seek help immediately if you need.

Skill & Simulation Labs: For hands-on practice in CPR, first aid, and procedures before facing real patients.

Hospital Support: Medical records, blood bank, pharmacy, nursing services, each vital to patient care.

Processes to Know Early

- Registration and ID card issuance.

- Access to the library and digital platforms.
- Reporting pathways for grievances or complaints.
- How to apply for leave, certificates, or research permissions.
- Use of hospital facilities: patient entry, diagnostic services, and interdepartmental referrals.

Library & Digital Learning Cell: For books, journals, online resources, and study spaces.

Mess, Matches, and Memories

Stop 1: The Hostels and Cafeteria- Second Home

Your hostel is your home away from home, where you will learn about forming friendships, managing stress, and developing time management skills. Mess & Cafeteria is a place to debrief after a tough day, where samosas and chai become a form of therapy. This is a world of shared Maggi, late-night breakdowns, guitar music, and endless case discussions.

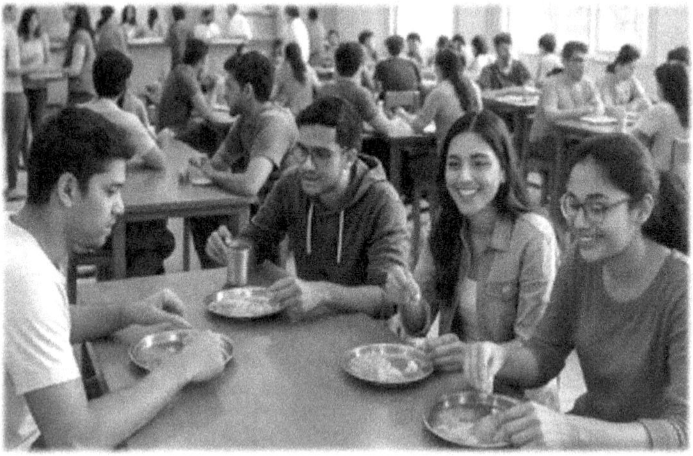

Figure 6.8: Hostel Cafeteria

Stop 2: The Sports Ground- Breathe Beyond Books

Beyond the classrooms and labs lies the green and open field. Whether you're a sprinter, a cricketer, or a daily walker, it's your space for sports, laughter, and to clear your head. Annual sports meets, friendly faculty-student matches, and early morning jogs are where stress finds an outlet and friendships grow stronger.

Stop 3: Utility & Vendor Shops

Daily needs within reach. From stationery to toiletries, mobile recharges to midnight snacks - these campus kiosks and general stores make your essential items available. Most are open till late to match the student lifestyle.

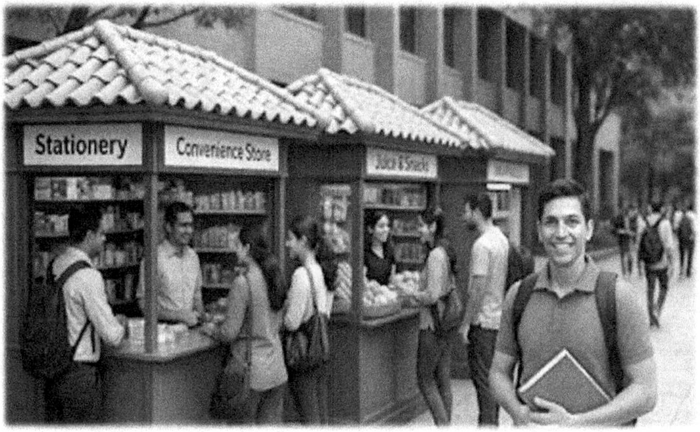

Figure 6.9: Utility and Vendor Shops

Stop 4: Centre for Yoga, Meditation and Fitness

A gentle pause in the fast-paced life. Morning and evening sessions are held here to help students build physical flexibility and emotional resilience. Many find peace here before exams or after a hectic day. Some faculty also drop by! You may go to the gym to train your body like your mind. Equipped with cardio machines, weights, and mats, this space keeps students healthy and energetic. Many make it a ritual - gym sessions after class, or a quick run before breakfast, some will go as visitors.

Stop 5: Student Activity Hub

Work hard, unwind harder. This hub includes indoor games, movie nights, music corners, and notice boards for upcoming events. It's where clubs meet, cultural programs are planned, and creativity finds space beyond the confines of textbooks. Before your annual festival, your student unions may meet and plan cultural, literary, and sports activities here.

Stop 6: The Auditorium - Where Minds Gather

A short walk from the lecture theatres, the Auditorium stands tall. Thousands of curious students and professionals sit here for CMEs, debates and discussions. This is where your white coat ceremony might happen, where you'll attend CMEs, hear visiting professors, perform skits, and cheer for batchmates during cultural events.

Sometimes, one inspiring speaker can change your career goals in this very hall.

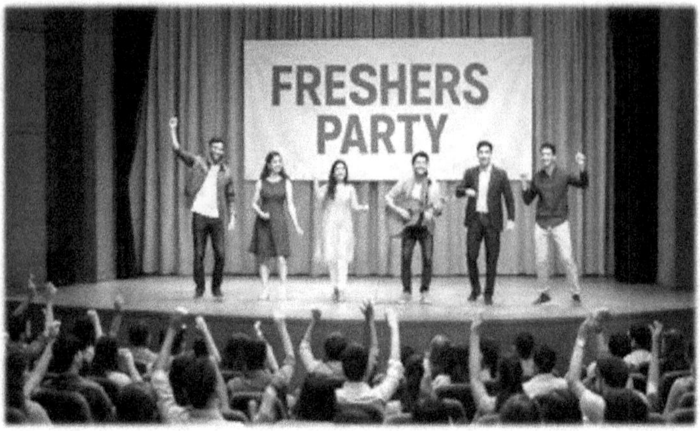

Figure 6.10: The Auditorium

Stop 7: Reflection Bench

Every good tour ends with a place to sit and think. You may find a bench near the herbal garden. Look at the hospital building in front of you. Somewhere in that building, someone is being saved, someone else is being consoled, and you have started walking through the most incredible journey of your life.

☕ Coffee Moment

This campus may seem like buildings and corridors, but within its walls, you'll find purpose, pain, growth, grace, and the unshakable courage to serve. From the dissection table to the basketball court, from the Dean's cabin to the counselling bay, every space on this campus contributes to your growth. Medicine isn't just about understanding diseases - it's about becoming a compassionate healer, and this campus is where that transformation happens.

References

1. Issenberg SB, McGaghie WC, Petrusa ER, Lee Gordon D, Scalese RJ. Features and uses of high-fidelity medical simulations that lead to effective learning. Med Teach. 2005;27(1):10–28.
2. Dyrbye LN, Shanafelt TD. A narrative review on burnout experienced by medical students and residents. Med Educ. 2016;50(1):132–149.
3. WHO. Mental health and well-being of health workers. Geneva: WHO; 2022.

Chapter 7: A Walk Through a Community Health Centre

Introduction

You have seen the medical college, the ICUs, and the lecture halls. Now, let us visit the Community Health Centre (CHC), which is often located in semi-urban towns or large villages and serves a population of 80,000 to 120,000 people. At CHCs, the healthcare system interacts with the community at its basic level. As you approach the front gate, you see a low-rise building with unevenly faded signage reading "Community Health Centre." A scooter is parked under a neem tree, and a few anxious patients and attendants wait on the bench outside. A watchman gives a friendly nod, and students and interns enter, their white coats rolled up in their hands.

Welcome to the world of rural health delivery, where CHCs serve as a bridge for most of India's population living in villages. (1,2)

Stop 1: The OPD Wing - Daily Dose of Dedication

The Outpatient Department (OPD) is the major service area of every CHC, where a medical officer manages many patients with limited time and ego. Patients with fever, cough, wounds, and pains and pregnant females, all pass through these rooms for their checkup and prescription. It's clinical skill, rather than the list of investigations, that makes a diagnosis here.

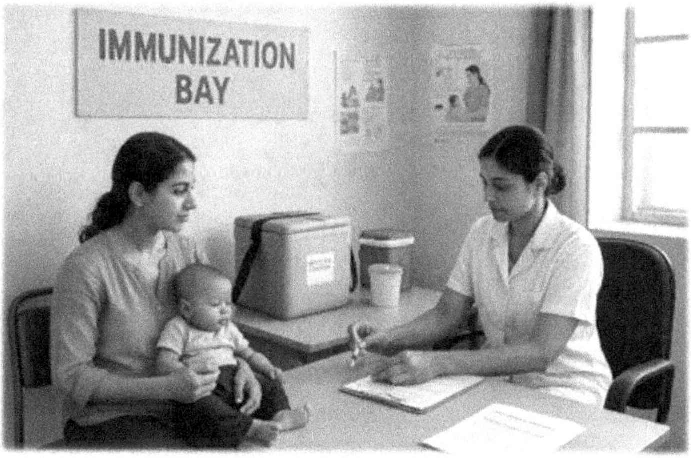

Figure 7.1: Immunization Corner

Consultation Room: A big wooden table, a stethoscope, a blood pressure machine, and maybe an ECG unit.

Immunization Room: You will see mothers holding infants swaddled in shawls,

ANMs explaining the next due vaccine, a vaccine carrier and the ever-reliable deep freezer maintaining cold chain.

Case Registers: Yes, paper records are maintained well here.

Counselling Corner and DOTS Clinic: Health education is a daily ritual of CHC. From family planning to TB counselling, a health worker or counsellor sits under a "Health for All" chart, explaining things that textbooks often skip. (4) Students often sit in, watching the art of simple language, saving lives.

Stop 2: The Labour Room

Here life begins, sometimes hardly prepared. The labour room is the place where babies are born and mothers are taken care of during the painful process of delivery. It has delivery tables, sterile trays, and an efficient nurse assisting a woman in labour. Some days, it brings joy; on others, heartbreak. You will never forget the sound of a newborn's cry here. Remember to start resuscitation if there's no cry immediately after birth. You'll soon learn resuscitation steps, a vital skill for healthcare workers.

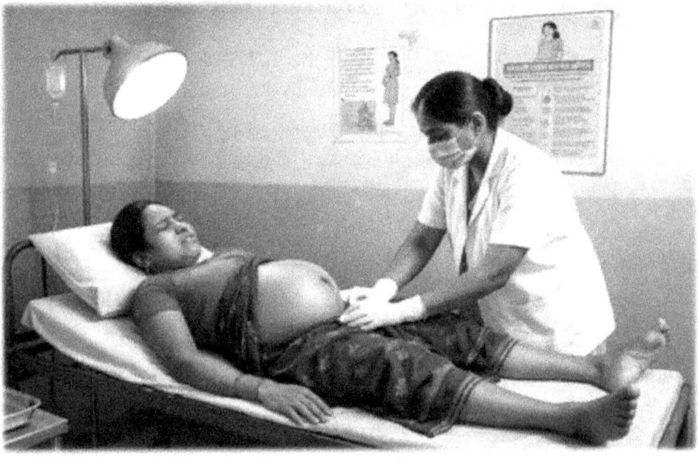

Figure 7.2: Labour Room

Stop 3: Minor OT and Dressing Room

The Minor Operation Theatre isn't what you imagine after seeing the OT Complex in your medical college. It is an isolated, restricted area used for abscess drainage, wound suturing, Incision & Drainage of boils, and sometimes for first-trimester MTPs. The sterility might feel rustic, but the compassion is spotless. In the dressing room, you will see patients with wounds, ulcers, diabetic feet, or snake bites.

Stop 4: IPD Wards - Holding Hope on Simple Beds

CHCs typically have 30 beds - male, female, maternity, and observation wards. The beds may have worn-out mattresses, but the people have deep stories. You will see:

- Patients recovering from dehydration, infections, and acute asthma
- Children with fever or seizures
- Mothers in care after babies are born
- A medical officer and a nurse do rounds together, without fanfare, but with dedication.

Stop 5: Laboratory and X-Ray Room

There's no CT or MRI facility here. There is an X-ray room, and a lab technician runs basic tests, such as haemoglobin, blood sugar, malaria smears, and urine tests, in the pathology room. At a well-equipped CHC, you may find a portable X-ray machine. This is a diagnostic reality. (3)

Stop 6: Records Room and Administrative Block

You will understand the maintenance of health data here.

- Birth and death registers.
- Malaria surveillance sheets.
- NCD screening records.
- Rogi Kalyan Samiti (RKS) files.

Stop 7: Anganwadi and ASHA Coordination Room

Here, you meet the unsung heroes: ANMs, ASHAs, and Anganwadi Workers. They are barefoot epidemiologists who walk miles to bring healthcare to every home. You'll listen to them speak about malnourished children, missed antenatal checkups, sanitation in schools, and adolescent girls needing iron pills.

This is grassroots medicine at its best.

☕ Coffee Moment

While sipping tea under the neem tree, you realize there are no shining ICUs or cutting-edge surgeries here. But what you witness in a CHC is the power of first-contact care, the dignity of service in simplicity and the urgent need for empathetic, grounded young doctors.

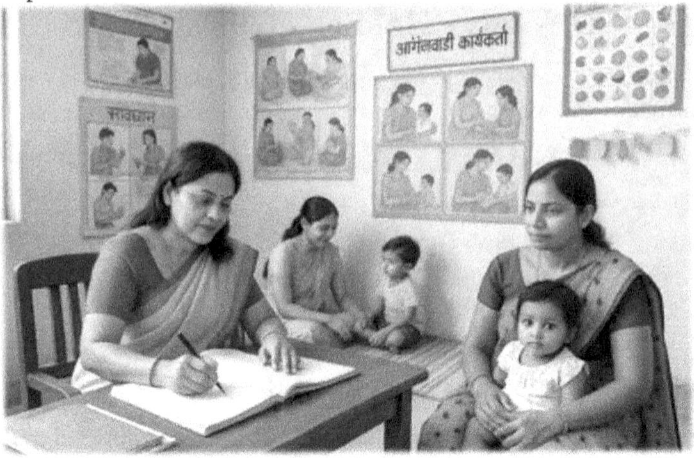

Figure 7.3: Anganwadi and ASHA Coordination Room

References

1. Ministry of Health and Family Welfare. Indian Public Health Standards (IPHS) Guidelines for CHCs. New Delhi: MoHFW; 2012.
2. National Health Systems Resource Centre. Ayushman Bharat – Comprehensive Primary Health Care through Health and Wellness Centres. MoHFW; 2018.
3. Berman P, Ahuja R, Bhandari L. The Impoverishing Effect of Healthcare Payments in India: New Methodology and Findings. Econ Polit Wkly. 2010;45(16):65–71.
4. Gupta M, Rao KD, Chandru S, et al. India's health system at a crossroads: progress and future directions. Lancet. 2022;399(10331):1947–1961.

Chapter 8: Beyond the Classroom

Introduction

The Foundation Course is your soft landing into medicine. In 'Inception', you explored the values, oath, and curriculum followed by your first campus tour and a walk through a Community Health Centre. You've seen how medicine is not only about scientific facts, but about developing clinical competence guided by ethics and social sensitivity. (1) Walking through a hospital corridor for the first time is a lifetime experience for a medical student. Patients' eyes follow you with hope, sometimes more than you deserve. The stethoscope is not only an instrument; it is a responsibility. You will explore in the coming sections that medicine is not limited to hospitals and clinics, but it lives and breathes in the larger system outside. Different systems that teach medicine in various forms are:

- The Campus & the Hospital.
- The Library: where knowledge resides in books and digital forms.
- The Simulation Lab: where mistakes are safe.
- The Wards: where mistakes are costly, and humility is mandatory.
- The Community: where medicine touches lives beyond prescriptions.

Cultural Diversities in Medicine

India's strength lies in its diversity. Patients come to the hospital with symptoms and diseases, but also with a background of beliefs, traditions, and values. Respecting these cultural differences is important for a doctor to develop trust and deliver effective patient care. Cultural competence complements clinical competence through developing

- **Trust**: Patients follow advice if they feel their beliefs are respected.
- **Accuracy**: Understanding cultural context prevents misinterpretation of symptoms or behaviour.
- **Equity**: Understanding and respecting diversity reduces discrimination and enhances care for underserved populations.
- **Professionalism**: A holistic understanding fosters empathy, justice, and respect in patient care, which are core values of medicine.

Cultural Scenarios in Healthcare

- Some patients may prefer a physician of the same gender for consultation and physical examination.
- Religious restrictions can affect treatment plans, such as a vegetarian diet and products for Hindus or Jains, and fasting patterns during Ramadan.

- Many patients combine Ayurveda, home remedies, or faith-based practices with medicine.

Recognizing these cultural beliefs and patterns is lifelong learning.

Professional interaction

- Ask clearly before planning care for the patients if there is anything important about their culture or beliefs. Do not assume.
- Use clear, simple language and avoid medical jargon. Use translators for linguistic barriers.
- Acknowledge cultural practices and allow what is not harmful. Clearly explain when something conflicts with safety. Recognize that cultural knowledge is lifelong learning.

Rules and Regulations of the Institution

Every community thrives on shared principles. A medical college is no different; its rules are not restrictions, but guidelines to help you learn safely, grow responsibly, and serve society with dignity.

Why They Matter

- **Professionalism starts now:** Discipline in attendance, assignments, and examinations is your first training in responsibility.
- **Safety and ethics:** Rules on labs, hostels, patient care, and research ensure the safety of students and the dignity of patients.
- **Fairness:** Regulations on evaluation, leave, and grievances ensure equal treatment for all.
- **Trust:** Institutional norms builds trust between students, faculty, and society.

Common Institutional Rules

Attendance: Usually 75% or higher is required as an eligibility criterion for exams. Regularity reflects professionalism.

Dress Code: White coat, ID card, and neat appearance are symbols of belonging and respect in hospital areas.

Examinations: Internal assessments, practicals, and final exams as per university regulations. Any malpractice has strict consequences.

Conduct: Display respect for faculty members, staff, patients, and colleagues. There is a zero tolerance for ragging, harassment, discrimination, smoking or drug abuse.

Hostel & Campus Discipline: Adhere to entry and exit timings, safety checks, and noise limits to maintain a safe and healthy environment.

Patient Rights: Confidentiality, respect, and consent must always be maintained.

Research & Ethics: Projects require proper approval from both the research committee and the ethics committee before data collection or patient involvement can commence.

When Lines Are Crossed

Following rules is not about avoiding punishment, but it is about building habits of accountability and integrity, qualities that society expects in every doctor.

Consequences of Unprofessional Behaviour: Medicine is built on trust. Patients trust doctors with their lives, institutions trust doctors and students with responsibility, and society trusts the profession with dignity. When rules are broken or behaviour turns unprofessional, this trust is broken, and consequences follow.

What is Unprofessional or Unethical?

- **Academic misconduct:** Cheating in exams, plagiarism in assignments.
- **Patient-related lapses:** Breaching confidentiality, ignoring consent, or disrespecting.
- **Campus misconduct:** Ragging, harassment, substance abuse and unprofessional behaviour.
- **Professional lapses:** Chronic absenteeism, rudeness to staff, and the misuse of social media with patient data.

Consequences

- **Institutional Action:** Warnings, suspension, fines, or expulsion in severe cases.
- **Legal Action:** Possible action under laws like the Anti-Ragging Act or the Rights of Persons with Disabilities Act.
- **Professional Impact:** Loss of credibility and negative references may restrict career opportunities.
- **Personal Consequence:** The erosion of respect among peers, faculty, and patients is a significant personal loss. Respect is hard to earn.

Why This Matters Early

Doctors maintain the highest standards of excellence because even small lapses can harm patients. By following rules and practising ethical conduct, you build your identity as a responsible and trustworthy professional.

Bridging Forward

Your journey so far has introduced you to a few key concepts in medicine. You understand some words, such as ethics, professionalism, learning methods, student life, and your role in society. You have stepped through the gates, worn your first white coat, and tasted the adrenaline rush of initial days in medicine. **Inception** is about that rush, the thrill of entering a world where every corridor hums with possibility. From here, your journey begins to unfold into layers you may not have even imagined. So, as *Inception* closes, remember: Ahead lies a journey through meaning, connection, systems, community, and the choices that shape them. (4) Each section is a new layer, and each layer brings you closer to becoming a doctor and a healer the world can trust.

Coffee Moment

During clinical posting, a student carelessly shares a patient's photo on social media. The patient's family complains, the faculty investigates, and the student is suspended. Over coffee that evening, classmates whisper, 'It was just one photo.' But soon, they realize that in medicine, a single careless act can cost more than grades; it can cost trust, careers, and dignity.

References

1. Bhore J. Report of the Health Survey and Development Committee, 1946. Government of India: New Delhi; 1946.
2. World Health Organization. Declaration of Alma-Ata: International Conference on Primary Health Care, Alma-Ata, USSR, 6–12 September 1978. Geneva: WHO; 1978.
3. Ministry of Health and Family Welfare. National Health Policy 2017. New Delhi: Government of India; 2017.
4. Gupta M, Rao KD, Chandru S, Jain M, Sundararaman T. India's health system at a crossroads: progress and future directions. Lancet. 2022;399(10331):1947–61.

Genesis

The spirit of beginning

"Every science has an origin.
But medicine has a soul."

Genesis is the dawn of your transformation, the moment when curiosity begins to take shape as purpose.

You awaken to the why behind medicine:

why healing matters and why humanity is essential in the context of science.

The story of medicine does not begin in the textbooks or dissections, but in the wonders of life, breath, and consciousness.

In this section, you will delve into the essence of the profession and its underlying philosophy of healing.

As you turn this page, pause for a breath –

you are stepping into the oldest tradition known to humankind.

Let this beginning remind you that before medicine became a science, it was an act of humanity.

S No	Genesis at a Glance
1	**Chapter 9** From Scrolls to Stethoscopes A journey through the history of medicine, from ancient healing traditions to modern science.
2	**Chapter 10** What Does It Mean to Be a Doctor? Explores professional identity through attitude, ethics, and communication. Being a doctor is as much about values as it is about skills.
3	**Chapter 11** The Role of Doctor in Society Highlights the doctor as healer, leader, advocate, and change-maker.
4	**Chapter 12** Respect for Life - The Cadaver as Our First Teacher Introduces the cadaver as the silent teacher of anatomy, instilling respect, humility, and professionalism at the beginning of medical training.
5	**Chapter 13** Ethics and Professionalism in Medicine Presents the core principles of medical ethics and the habits of professionalism that safeguard trust between doctor and patient.
6	**Chapter 14** Principles of Bioethics and Justice Understand the principles of autonomy, beneficence, non-maleficence, and justice, to guide the decision-making in complex scenarios.
7	**Chapter 15** The Evolution of Healthcare in India - A Journey Through Time India's healthcare journey from Ayurveda to Ayushman Bharat, helping you understand the system.

Chapter 9: From Scrolls to Stethoscopes

Introduction

You are the heir to a legacy of healing. Long before the white coat, there was the healer's touch. Before antiseptics and ventilators, there were herbs, hymns, and hope. From the Ayurvedic sutras of Charaka to Vesalius's anatomical sketches. From Sushruta Samhita to Hippocrates' oath. ***Charaka Samhita,*** written around the 1st–2nd century CE, laid the groundwork for internal medicine. ***Sushruta Samhita,*** written around the 6th century BCE, provided detailed descriptions of surgical techniques, centuries before modern surgery developed. (1,2)

Medicine has always been more than science. It is a philosophy of care, a faith in life, and a mirror of humanity. Today, as you begin your MBBS journey, your own path starts. You will learn about bones and blood, but also about trust, humility, wonder, and witnessing suffering with strength. If medicine were a river, history is its source, and you are its next stream. You are not just studying: You are becoming it.

A Timeless Lineage

The good physician treats the disease; the great physician treats the patient who has the disease. – William Osler (3)

To understand what it means to become a doctor, one must understand the origins of medicine. Medicine has evolved in its current form through the struggles of civilizations, felt in the prayers for the sick children and medical discoveries spanning centuries. It's the timeless journey of human desire to reduce suffering, preserve dignity, and give life another chance. Since ancient times, medicine has emerged through careful observations, shared wisdom, and empathy. Many parts of the world still follow the conventional healing systems that predate the modern clinical system. These traditions complement the holistic approaches that modern science is rediscovering and validating. What you're stepping into is not just a degree, it is a lineage.

From History to Humanity

Medicine is the convergence of science that explains '*how*' and humanity that reminds us '*why*'. Current medicine has evolved from the Atharvaveda shlokas to Ayurvedic sutras, from Charaka and Sushruta Samhitas to the Hippocratic Oath, and from tribal midwives and dais to high-tech ICUs. The modern history of medicine has witnessed milestones, including Pasteur and Koch's germ theory, Fleming's discovery of antibiotics, and the rise of evidence-based medicine. (4) This journey is an ever-unfolding story of innovation, discovery, and service.

Why History Matters

Understanding the past gives a roadmap that makes us wiser for the future. It illustrates how societies have faced illness and how knowledge has been gained and shared to combat diseases. The evolution of medicine has happened through

- Valuing the patient's story,
- Questioning the rigid systems,
- Respect for traditional knowledge and
- Adapting with insight, not arrogance.

India's Contribution to Global Health

India has preserved the wisdom of healing.

Ayurveda is a holistic Indian health system that emphasises a balanced diet and harmony with nature for disease prevention, as well as the use of herbal medicines and yoga for treatment.

Yoga is a timeless contribution of India to the world. It believes in the connection between the external world and the inner world. It combines breath, body, and consciousness to balance physical and mental well-being.

Sushruta is referred to as the father of surgery in India.

Charaka Samhita is an ancient medical text.

Unani, Siddha, and Homoeopathy have grown in India.

India's modern contributions are also remarkable:

- Eradication of polio.
- Development of low-cost vaccines.
- Production of generic medicines.
- Mass health campaigns.
- Global respect for doctors of Indian origin for professional excellence.
- Doctors as innovators, investigators, and academicians.

Imagine the Future

On one hand, we are advancing in genome sequencing, robotic surgery, and digital diagnostics; however, there are also rising ethical challenges, overdependence on technology, and health inequities. The future isn't only about tools but also about values. It is doctors, not devices, who can keep the compass accurate. Medicine is all set to progress in the coming decade to

- AI-assisted diagnosis.

- Tele-ICUs are linked globally.
- Personalized gene therapy.
- Community-based health coaching.
- Spiritual healing integrated into ICUs.
- AI-assisted doc-bot kiosks in hilly and remote terrains.

The Doctor's Journey: A Lifelong Transformation

As medicine evolves, every doctor's personal journey unfolds in stages, from the wide-eyed student to the seasoned healer.

Phase I: The Student
Awed, overwhelmed, and excited, the first year is all about the dissection hall, biochemistry lab, physiology concepts, endless acronyms, and the thrill of wearing a white coat for the first time. You begin to learn the language of medicine.

Phase II: The Clinical Exposure
The white coat is complemented by the stethoscope. You step into the wards and, for the first time, listen to real heartbeats. You see the wonder of the sick becoming healthy with the first prescription you assisted with. You see life, death, and everything in between. Textbook diseases now wear faces.

Phase III: The Young Doctor
As an intern and resident, you carry the responsibility of managing patients. You face fatigue, taste success and emerge through struggle. You become the doctor to whom patients come, and you learn something new each day.

Phase IV: The Specialist or Generalist
Your path narrows or widens based on your choice, surgery, medicine, research, or public health. Whatever route you choose, your core remains the same: to serve, to learn, and to lead.

Staying Human in High-Tech Healing

As technology advances, your human touch becomes increasingly essential.
Empathy cannot be automated.
Kindness cannot be coded.
Integrity cannot be outsourced.

Global Lens: The Universal Doctor

Across continents, the journey to becoming a doctor shares common themes, i.e. rigorous training, service to the underserved, and a commitment to lifelong learning. What differs are resources, policies, and public interaction. Global reforms in medical education now emphasize not only clinical excellence but also systems thinking, teamwork, and social accountability to address health inequities. (5) In India, the challenge is often volume: too many patients, too few doctors. In the West, it may be bureaucracy or burnout. But everywhere, a good doctor is defined by the same qualities.

- Listening deeply
- Speaking honestly
- Caring selflessly
- Acting wisely

The stethoscope works best when your ears are open, and your heart is receptive.

Reflect and Write

"Even in the ancient scrolls of medicine, the patient, not the prescription, remained at the centre. What will be at the centre of your practice?" ---------
What innovation do you wish to see in the next 10 years? ---------------------
How can you carry forward India's healing legacy in spirit and science? -----
What role will human touch play in the medicine of tomorrow? -------------

Coffee Moment

The art of healing has endured for centuries, thanks to the combination of science and spirit. What's one ancient healing practice that still inspires you?

References

1. Wujastyk D. The Roots of Ayurveda: Selections from Sanskrit Medical Writings. 3rd ed. New Delhi: Penguin Classics; 2003.
2. Bhishagratna KL. The Sushruta Samhita: An English Translation. Varanasi: Chowkhamba Sanskrit Series; 1963.
3. Osler W. The Principles and Practice of Medicine. New York: D. Appleton; 1892.
4. Porter R. The Cambridge Illustrated History of Medicine. Cambridge: Cambridge University Press; 2001.
5. Frenk J, Chen L, Bhutta ZA, et al. Health professionals for a new century: transforming education to strengthen health systems in an interdependent world. Lancet. 2010;376(9756):1923-58.

Chapter 10: What Does It Mean to Be a Doctor?

Introduction

Medical students are excited to don a white coat and be recognized as members of the medical profession. This is a significant transformation in their life; however, few people are aware of the obligations that accompany their new identity. Embarking on the journey to become a doctor is both an honour and a responsibility. This chapter helps you understand what it means to be a doctor, what it means to be a patient, and how the two interact. You will understand how attitude, ethics and communication shape your professional identity.

Indian Medical Graduate

The National Medical Commission (NMC) defines an Indian Medical Graduate (IMG) as someone who is clinically competent, ethically grounded, socially sensitive, a lifelong learner, a communicator and a leader. (1) There are many other qualities and expanded roles of a doctor, which develop with a professional attitude, ethical practice, and effective communication that integrate into their professional identity. The role of the doctor and its societal impact has been discussed in Chapter 3 and summarised in the following table.

Table 10.1: Roles of an IMG

Role	Core Purpose
1. Clinician	Provide preventive, promotive, curative, palliative, and holistic care
2. Leader and Team Member	Coordinate with nurses, technicians, administrators, and community workers
3. Communicator	Convey empathy, information, and reassurance
4. Lifelong Learner	Keep updating medical knowledge and skills
5. Professional	Uphold integrity, empathy, and human dignity

Professional Identity of a Doctor

Doctors are identified by their professional qualities, which include competence, honesty, and compassion. They spend their careers alleviating human suffering. A professional approach requires insight into patients' illnesses and suffering, without becoming emotionally overwhelmed and physically exhausted, in order to maintain own well-being throughout this journey.

- **Empathy versus equanimity**: Physicians must maintain compassion while maintaining sufficient emotional distance to make rational decisions.

- **Commitment to lifelong learning**: Medicine evolves rapidly, and doctors need to continually update their knowledge and skills.
- **Social responsibility**: Prioritising patient welfare, acting with integrity, and advocating for justice in healthcare is a social responsibility we carry.
- **Balancing privileges and sacrifices**: The profession brings respect and trust, but demands long hours, emotional labour, and personal sacrifice.
- **Healing versus curing**: When doctors cannot cure, they can still heal by alleviating suffering, listening, and offering comfort. Understand your limitations, but do not let them restrict patient care.

IMG and Society: Mutual Expectations

Society has its own expectations from the IMG, and you, as an IMG, have certain expectations from society. It should strike a balance, but more importantly, your own expectations of yourself will define your growth. You are expected to be sincere, not perfect; you are expected to learn, not already know, but have a lifelong learning & teaching mindset, and you are expected to respect life, not fear it.

Table 10.2: IMG and society- mutual expectations

Expectations of IMG from society	Expectations of society from IMG
Safety & dignity in hospitals; zero violence. Early, rational care-seeking and adherence. Functional systems: referral, ambulance, labs, and blood. Legal clarity: fair processes, no media trials. Public-health cooperation: vaccines, CPR, and sanitation. Respect & fair value for professional work.	Safe & competent clinical care. Ethical, equitable, transparent practice. Empathetic communication. Clear safety-net advice and QI. Teamwork & leadership for smooth referrals. Public-health and cost-consciousness in daily care. Professionalism in documentation. Ready for disasters; engaged with the community.

What It Means to Be a Patient

A patient is any individual who is awaiting or receiving medical care or treatment under the care of a healthcare provider. The word "patient" carries historical connotations of suffering and passivity, but modern medicine seeks to make patients active partners in their care, expecting clear communication, respect, and shared decision-making. (2,3)

Patient's perspective: Every doctor begins their journey studying the human body. But every patient who enters a clinic comes with something even more complex- 'hope'. To understand what it means to be a doctor, you must also understand what it means to be a patient.

Table 10.3: Expectations of patients

From Doctors	From the Institution	From Society	From the Nation
Compassion, patience, and respect	A clean, safe, and dignified environment	Awareness, empathy, and support	Access to affordable, quality healthcare
Clear communication and honesty	Timely care and transparent processes	Respect for privacy and inclusion	Health priority in national policies
Competence balanced with kindness	Accountability and ethical standards	Acceptance of the sick, not stigma	Continuity of care through a health system

To be a patient is to surrender one's body, fears, and trust into another's hands. It is to wait, often in pain, believing that someone will help, listen, and care. It is one of the most vulnerable human experiences and demands humility. In understanding what patients expect, we also begin to ask a deeper question. Is health their privilege or their right? This important question is discussed in the Covenant Section.

Doctor–Patient Relationship

Understanding patients' expectations transforms medical practice into a partnership. When patients feel heard and respected, adherence to advice improves and anxiety reduces. For empathy, doctors must understand what it feels like to have an illness.

Trust: Mutual trust is built through active listening and responding to patients' concerns. It forms the foundation of the doctor-patient relationship. Building mutual trust is a shared responsibility. Doctors have obligations to ensure autonomy, beneficence, nonmaleficence, and justice. Maintaining confidentiality, honesty, transparency, and professional boundaries in communication is crucial for establishing and maintaining trust. Patients have a right to competent care, equality, respect, confidentiality, informed consent, and freedom to refuse treatment. The patient's responsibilities include providing accurate information, following agreed-upon treatment plans, respecting healthcare workers, and adhering to public health measures. Trust in the doctor-patient relationship improves treatment adherence, increases patient satisfaction, and reduces medico-legal conflicts. (4)

Attitude, Ethics, and Communication

The journey of acquiring professional traits starts with understanding the values of empathy, ethics, and effective communication. The Attitude, Ethics, and Communication (AETCOM) module emphasises that being a doctor is not merely about treating diseases, but about understanding human experiences. (1)

1. Attitude

Attitude refers to a set of emotions, beliefs, and behaviours towards a particular object, person, or event. In the context of medicine, it encompasses:

- **Professionalism**: Upholding the dignity of the profession through integrity, accountability, and respect. Integrity is doing the right thing even when no one is watching. Professionalism is how you act when everybody is watching. Professionalism encompasses punctuality, reliability, accountability, dressing appropriately, maintaining personal hygiene, and respecting others, including colleagues, patients, and attendants. Integrity is the soul of professionalism.
- **Compassion**: Compassion is a feeling of sympathy and concern for others who are suffering, accompanied by a desire to alleviate their pain. In simple terms, it is empathy combined with action.
- **Commitment**: Dedication to continuous learning and improvement in knowledge and skills to deliver better care in medical practice.

2. Ethics

Medical ethics guides doctors in applying moral principles in their practice:

- **Autonomy**: Respecting a patient's right to make informed decisions about their medical care when they have the mental capacity to make decisions.
- **Beneficence**: Acting in the best interest of the patient.
- **Non-maleficence**: "do no harm". It means avoiding unnecessary risks to patients during treatment.
- **Justice**: It means ensuring fairness in medical decisions and resource allocation regardless of the background, ability, or status of the patient.

These principles form the foundation of modern biomedical ethics. (4,5) Ethical practice demands following the rules and balancing these principles in complex, real-world situations. If a patient refuses a life-saving procedure due to personal beliefs, the doctor should provide all necessary information to support an informed decision that respects the patient's autonomy and balances the best interests of both the patient and the medical team.

3. Communication

Effective communication is the cornerstone of medical practice. It involves

- **Active Listening**: Fully concentrating, understanding, and responding in communication with the patient.
- **Clear Expression**: Conveying information in a manner that patients and their

families easily understand.

- **Empathy:** The ability to recognize and respond to the emotional states of others. It is not simply feeling sorry for a patient but understanding their experience and demonstrating that understanding in your care. Listen actively, avoid judgment, acknowledge suffering and show presence, even in silence.

Research shows that structured communication training for doctors not only improves patient outcomes but also reduces medical errors and stress among physicians. (5) Case scenarios familiarize you with real-life situations. You will encounter complex scenarios in upcoming chapters and during clinical exposure.

Case Scenario

Mr Jain, 53, presents with chest discomfort. Evaluation suggests unstable angina. The cardiologist recommends a coronary angiogram. Mr Jain hesitates as his friend died during an angioplasty. He asks to consult his family doctor to explore other options. The cardiologist reacts defensively, asking him to sign immediately for the procedure scheduled for the next day; otherwise, he will be discharged from the hospital. Mr Jain feels frightened and considers skipping care.

Core Concepts

- **Informed consent:** Informed consent is a voluntary, patient-centred process. The clinician should explain the diagnosis, the nature of the procedure, its purpose, potential risks and benefits, reasonable alternatives, and answer questions to facilitate an informed decision.
- **Medico-Legal Concerns:** The patient's consent is required to start any treatment with reasonable alternatives (e.g., CT coronary angiography, stress imaging in this case) except in an emergency. Compelling or withholding material information invalidates consent. Document the discussion.
- **Socio-cultural issues:** Family influence and prior adverse experiences shape the patient's perception of risk. Acknowledging fear and involving a trusted family doctor can restore confidence and adherence.

Approach

The cardiologist resets the conversation:

- Acknowledge the patient's fear and express empathy.
- Explain unstable angina, role of angiography, potential need for percutaneous coronary intervention (PCI) and coronary artery bypass graft (CABG), and associated risks (bleeding, stroke, death - rare but possible).
- Discuss limitations and alternative treatments. (6)
- Offer to speak with the family doctor; provide a written summary.

Outcome

With counselling, Mr Jain agrees to proceed with angiography the next day after speaking with his family doctor; consent is appropriately documented.

Learning Points

- Building trust, consent & shared decision-making are important aspects.
- Consent is a dialogue, not just paperwork.
- Paternalism erodes trust; empathy enables safe decisions.
- Present benefits, risks, and reasonable alternatives; document them.

Reflect and Write

- What qualities are essential for a doctor? Reflect on personal experiences and observations to identify key attributes.
- How would you handle a situation if a patient refuses treatment? Consider the ethical principles and importance of patient autonomy.

☕Coffee Moment

While sipping your coffee, you realize that you consistently arrive on time in clinical postings, actively participate in discussions, and show genuine concern for patients' well-being. This reflects a positive professional attitude.

References

1. National Medical Commission. Attitude, Ethics and Communication (AETCOM) Module for Undergraduate Medical Education Program. New Delhi: NMC; 2019.
2. Neuberger J. Do we need a new word for patients? Let's do away with "patients". BMJ. 1999 Jun 26;318(7200):1756-7.
3. Rao JK, Anderson LA, Inui TS. Communication interventions make a difference in conversations between physicians and patients: a systematic review of the evidence. Med Care. 2007;45(4):340-9.
4. Beauchamp, T. L., & Childress, J. F. (1979). Principles of Biomedical Ethics. Oxford: Oxford University Press.
5. Beauchamp TL, Childress JF. Principles of Biomedical Ethics. 8th ed. Oxford: Oxford University Press; 2019.
6. Ibanez B, James S, Agewall S, et al. 2017 ESC Guidelines for the management of acute myocardial infarction in patients presenting with ST-segment elevation. Eur Heart J. 2018;39(2):119-77.

Chapter 11: Beyond Hospital Role of the Doctor in Society

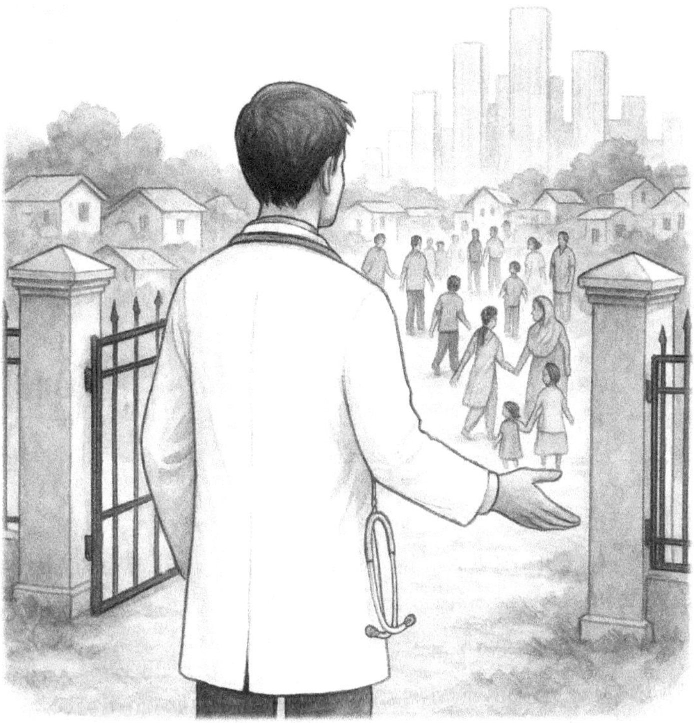

Figure 11.1: To Serve, You Must First Belong

A doctor is often imagined as a person in a white coat with a stethoscope, diagnosing diseases and prescribing medicines. In reality, a doctor wears many hats: caregiver, teacher, counsellor, community leader, researcher, and policymaker. You will realize that your role is not confined to hospitals or clinics; it extends into the community, including homes, schools, villages, and even public platforms. Doctors work at the convergence of science and humanity. Society places immense trust in doctors for their care and treatment with dignity.

Social Immersion: Doctors Beyond the Urban Citadel

The NMC highlights the concept of 'isolationism'. It is a subtle yet dangerous divide that can lead doctors to become emotionally detached from society. Often educated in urban institutions, trained and posted in high-tech settings, young doctors can inadvertently begin to operate from the 'urban citadel.' (1)

This citadel begins to separate 'us', the medical community, from 'them', the public.

This social isolation finds its roots in clinical language, profession-specific culture, long working hours, system fatigue, and burnout. Indeed, medicine demands the opposite, i.e. proximity, connection, and presence. To connect with people and profession, a doctor must break this divide. Patients are not statistics. Their villages, dialects, and struggles are part of your clinical wisdom. Let your white coat open doors, not erect the walls.

Expanded Roles of a Doctor

A healthcare system reflects the values of its nation. Doctors serve not only as clinicians but also as sources of accurate information, community welfare, and frontline leadership. (2) A doctor's role can be felt in different situations:

- Writing a clear and error-free prescription.
- Counselling a worried parent about a child's fever.
- Sitting through a difficult night monitoring a sick patient.
- Comforting a family after their loss.

These quiet acts create positive ripples. The NMC emphasizes that a doctor's role is multifaceted and extends beyond clinics and hospitals.

Social Justice

Your white coat gives you the power to speak for those who are unheard. You will witness health disparities. Some patients may reach you late due to the distance from the hospital. Some may not understand prescriptions because they are illiterate. Some people might fear hospitals due to past experiences with discrimination. By understanding such situations and finding effective solutions, doctors play a crucial role in promoting social equity. Beyond individual patient care, doctors can shape preventive health programs, influence policies, and advocate for structural changes that reduce health inequities. (3)

Health Advocacy

- Make decisions in the patient's best interest.
- Advocate for vulnerable populations and health equity.
- Promote health literacy.

Educator and Communicator

- Educate families on the prevention of diseases.
- Simplify medical language for laypeople.
- Clarify myths, promote healthy habits, and address public forums.

Role Model and Leader

- Demonstrate integrity and humility.
- Mentor team members and lead by example.

Change Agent and Policy Influencer

- Participate in the planning of health policies.
- Recommend improvements in patient safety and access to healthcare.

First Responder

- Lead efforts during epidemics, accidents, and disasters.
- Provide triage, resuscitation, and psychosocial support.

The Human Face of Science

- Balance technology with ethics.
- Bring emotional intelligence into patient care.

Surveys indicate that doctors rank among the top three most trusted professions worldwide. This trust is not automatic; it is earned through every interaction, every word, and every decision you make. (4) Being punctual, speaking kindly, respecting privacy, and acknowledging your limitations are small habits that protect this trust. Once broken, it is difficult to rebuild.

From the Clinic to the Community

Health doesn't begin in hospitals; it begins in homes, schools, kitchens, and workplaces. As a doctor, your voice has influence:

- You can educate mothers on nutrition.
- You can conduct awareness camps on hygiene.
- You can help debunk medical myths and stigma.
- You can counsel youth on mental health.
- You can conduct CPR awareness and training for the community.

You don't have to be a public health expert to make a public impact; your sincerity and science are enough. In your journey, never forget the human being in the white coat who once dreamed of healing others. The one who finds joy in small recoveries and strength in difficult nights.

☕ Coffee Moment

In a remote town, Dr Arjun, on his internship rotation, assisted with the functioning of a CHC. For two weeks, he coordinated COVID testing, arranged oxygen cylinders, and managed mild cases, earning the villagers' love and the admiration of peers. Dr Arjun raised the concern of a lack of oxygen in the second wave of COVID. The next day, a group of social workers and a recovered patient named Ravi came with three donated oxygen concentrators. That act reminded the team why they must never give up.

Reflect and Write

- What type of doctor do I wish to become? ------------------------------------
- How can I resist the pull of isolationism and remain connected in my community? --
- What invisible acts of care make a significant difference? ----------------------
- How can I use my role to impact lives beyond medicine? ---------------------

References

1. National Medical Commission. Competency-Based Undergraduate Curriculum for the Indian Medical Graduate. New Delhi: NMC; 2019.
2. The Lancet COVID-19 Commission. Public health and social measures to end the COVID-19 pandemic. Lancet. 2021;398(10318):1015-26.
3. World Health Organization. Doctors as advocates: the role of physicians in health equity and social determinants. Geneva: WHO; 2016.
4. Ipsos. Global Trust in Professions Survey 2022. London: Ipsos; 2022.

Chapter 12: Respect for Life - Cadaver as Our First Teacher

Introduction

The practice of medicine requires deep respect for human life, both in its beginning and at its end. Medical students encounter this respect in different contexts. It can be through the cadaver that teaches anatomy or through the patients and families who confront death. This chapter explores how respect for the human body translates into compassionate care of the dying.

At the beginning of the medical education, students are introduced to the cadaver in the Anatomy dissection hall to make them understand the architecture of the human body. This initial exposure is not just an academic exercise, but an encounter with mortality. This is a bridge between theoretical knowledge and practical application. The cadaver is a silent yet cogent instructor, imparting lessons that textbooks cannot convey. Cadavers may be unclaimed bodies or altruistic donations. Proper handling of cadavers and tissues is a display of respect for donors and families.

The Significance of Cadaveric Dissection

Cadaveric dissection has been a part of medical education since the 3rd century BC. It remains essential for anatomy training worldwide due to its unique role in spatial learning and tactile familiarity. (1) It connects students to the human body, enabling them to explore anatomical structures in three dimensions. There have been periodic debates about modern technical alternatives. Virtual reality, 3D images, and techniques like the Anatomage table enable interactive, virtual exploration, but are still unable to fully reproduce the complexities of human anatomy. It has been found that students exposed to cadaveric dissection perform better in clinical anatomy and surgical skill acquisition in comparison to those trained on virtual models alone. (2) Beyond anatomy, dissection helps in developing skills such as attention to detail, manual dexterity, and teamwork. It promotes a sense of responsibility and respect for the human body, reinforcing the ethical principles of medical practice.

Professional Behaviour in the Dissection Hall

The dissection hall (DH) is a space where students first engage with the human body in a respectful and professional manner. All doctors remember their 'DH days' forever for different reasons. Ethical guidelines and professional etiquette ensure that the learning environment remains a dignified and conducive space for education. The NMC Foundation Course (2019) guidelines emphasise respect, dignity, and professionalism in the DH. (3)

1. Respect and Reverence

- View the cadaver as a teacher and recognize the body as a generous gift from the donor, which facilitates your learning.
- Maintain dignity by covering the cadaver when not in use and avoiding unnecessary exposure to prevent tissue drying.
- Handle with care: Use instruments appropriately and avoid causing damage to the cadaver.

2. Professional Conduct

- Dress appropriately: Wear lab coats, gloves, and face protection to maintain safety, hygiene and professionalism.
- Maintain cleanliness: Ensure the dissection area is kept tidy, and dispose of waste materials properly. Follow the biomedical waste management protocol (Chapter 92)
- Limit distractions: Refrain from using mobile phones in DH. Take the opportunity of such a big group for face-to-face discussions. You will also remember DH as the most beautiful place of your life for face-to-face discussion and gossip when academics are over.

3. Confidentiality and Discretion

- Privacy: Avoid photography in the DH to maintain privacy and respect.
- Confidentiality: Treat all details about the donor's identity and medical history with utmost confidentiality.
- Professional demeanour: Refrain from making disrespectful jokes or comments.

4. Cultural Sensitivity

- Acknowledge diversity: Be aware of and respect cultural differences regarding death and body handling. Some of your colleagues may take a bath after coming from DH for cultural reasons.
- Inclusive practices: Ensure peers feel comfortable and respected in the dissection environment.

Emotional and Ethical Dimensions

The first encounter with a cadaver often evokes a mix of emotions, of curiosity, awe, discomfort, and reverence. It is natural and signifies the beginning of this transformative journey. Acknowledging the cadaver as a donor who has contributed to medical education instils a sense of gratitude and ethical responsibility. Medical colleges often honour families of body donors through memorial services or gratitude ceremonies, reinforcing to students that their first teacher deserves lifelong respect. (4)

Real-World Applications

The lessons learned from cadaveric dissection extend beyond the DH and anatomy exam. They influence clinical practice by enhancing skills, improving surgical techniques, and promoting patient-centred care. Surgeons return to DH to understand the complex anatomy of the targeted body parts. It enables medical professionals to approach patient care with empathy and precision.

Case Scenario: The First Teacher

It was the first day of anatomy dissection. A group of wide-eyed first-year MBBS students entered the big dissection hall, the sharp scent of formalin filling the air. Nervous and chaotic whispers echoed for a while. You are divided into 10 groups. Your group is assigned to table no 7, where you all gather. In the centre lay the cadaver - silent, still, yet about to be your very first teacher. Students are unsure whether to feel awe or fear. The professor paused before starting the session. "This," he said softly, "is not just a body. It is a gift, someone who, even in death, chose to teach you the art of healing. Treat your first teacher with utmost respect."

The students bowed their heads in silence. A few students giggled nervously during the session, reached for selfies, but stopped by the demonstrator. Ravi placed his hand quietly on the table and whispered, "Thank you, teacher."

Core Concepts

Dissection extends beyond anatomy; it is the beginning of professional values-

- **Respect:** A cadaver is treated with the dignity of a teacher.
- **Confidentiality:** No photos, jokes, or casual remarks that violate the donor's dignity.
- **Professionalism**: Every patient, living or departed, deserves respect and professional behaviour.

Learning Points

- Cadavers are often referred to as the "first teachers" of medical students.
- Professional behaviour in the DH sets the tone for future doctor–patient relationships.
- Respect, confidentiality, and cultural sensitivity are core values that should be carried throughout one's medical life.

Reflect and Write

Reflect on your first experience in the dissection hall. How did it shape your perception of the human body and your role as a medical professional? Discuss with peers to gain diverse perspectives.

☕ Coffee Moment

While sipping his tea, Ravi shared with his friends: "I realized today that the cadavers have no name, no religion, or other identity, but they are the donors who have given even their bodies for our learning. Let us honour them with dignity and respect."

References

1. McLachlan JC, Patten D. Anatomy teaching: ghosts of the past, present and future. Med Educ. 2006;40(3):243-53.
2. Azer SA, Eizenberg N. Do we need dissection in an integrated problem-based learning medical course? Perceptions of first- and second-year students. Surg Radiol Anat. 2007;29(2):173-80.
3. National Medical Commission. Competency-Based Undergraduate Curriculum for the Indian Medical Graduate. New Delhi: NMC; 2019.
4. Cahill KC, Ettarh RR. Student attitudes to whole body donation are influenced by dissection. Anat Sci Educ. 2008;1(6):212-6.

Chapter 13: Ethics and Professionalism in Medicine

Introduction

The foundation of medicine is knowledge, character and conscience. The white coat is not just a uniform but a symbol of trust, responsibility, and integrity. Ethics and professionalism are not merely concepts to know, but are integral to good clinical practice. This chapter introduces the moral framework that every doctor must adhere to. From patient confidentiality to standing firm in the face of litigation or violence, it's about who you are when no one is watching and how you must act when everyone depends on you.

Medical Ethics

Medical ethics is a system of moral principles and values that guides healthcare professionals in decision-making across clinical practice, biomedical research, and healthcare policy. The foundation of medical ethics rests on four cardinal principles:

- **Autonomy**: Respecting the patient's right to make their own decisions.
- **Beneficence**: Acting in the best interest of the patient.
- **Non-maleficence**: "Do no harm", avoiding unnecessary risks during treatment.
- **Justice**: Fairness in treatment and distribution of resources.

These principles apply whether you're prescribing medication, conducting research, or managing a challenging conversation with a family. (1)

Professionalism in Medicine

Dignity of the profession is upheld through integrity, accountability, and respect. Professionalism is reflected in various ways, including punctuality, reliability, accountability for one's actions, appropriate attire, personal hygiene, and respect for others. It is the commitment to carrying out one's duties with excellence, empathy, and accountability. (2) Key elements include:

- **Honesty**: Admitting when you don't know; never fake a diagnosis or data.
- **Integrity**: Standing by ethical principles, even under pressure.
- **Confidentiality**: Respecting patients' privacy.
- **Altruism**: Serving selflessly, especially when others will not.
- **Respect**: For patients, colleagues, juniors, seniors, and yourself.
- **Competence**: Continuous learning and updating knowledge.

Patient Rights and Responsibilities

Patients are not passive recipients of care, but rather partners in the treatment process. They have certain rights and responsibilities as active partners.

- **Patient Rights:** Patients have the right to informed consent, privacy and confidentiality, a second opinion, dignity and respect, and the right to refuse treatment.
- **Patient Responsibilities:** At the same time, patients are responsible for providing accurate information, following agreed treatment plans, being respectful to HCWs and adhering to advice and public health measures.

Confidentiality and Consent

Informed consent means that patients understand the risks, benefits, and options, and this understanding is documented. Maintain confidentiality and obtain consent before any examination or procedure, regardless of workload. Discuss sensitive matters in private, and avoid sharing patient details without permission. In teaching settings, de-identify patient data. For minors or those unable to consent, there is a provision of legal guardianship. (3)

Disability Competencies in Medicine

Disability encompasses not only a medical condition, but also health, rights, and dignity. IMGs must learn to respect, empower, and include people with disabilities (PwDs) in healthcare and society. Follow updated NMC principles and legal directions on this sensitive issue. Disability competence matters for several reasons.

- **Prevalence:** Over 2.2% of India's population lives with disabilities as per the census 2011and recent estimates suggest even higher.
- **Equity:** PwDs face barriers to access, affordability, and respectful care.
- **Legal framework:** The Rights of Persons with Disabilities (RPwD) Act, 2016, protects the rights and dignity of PwDs. It also mandates equality and non-discrimination in the healthcare sector.
- **Professional duty:** Inclusive care is an integral part of the ethics and professionalism expected from every professional.

Core Competencies

- **Clinical Sensitivity**: Recognize specific health needs of PwDs (e.g., higher risk of pressure sores, epilepsy, infections).
- **Communication Skills**: Use simple language, visual aids, or involve interpreters for individuals with hearing and speech impairments.
- **Environmental Awareness**: Identify physical barriers in hospitals (e.g., stairs,

narrow doors, and a lack of ramps) and advocate for accessibility improvements.

- **Holistic Approach**: Look beyond illness and consider a multi-sectoral strategy that includes rehabilitation, assistive devices, occupational support, and community integration.
- **Person-Centred Care:** Treat the patient as an individual, not just disability.

Practical Examples: Respect the pace of a child with cerebral palsy in OPD. For a hearing-impaired patient, write down instructions clearly. During history-taking, ask about daily challenges, not only medical symptoms. In the emergency room, ensure wheelchair access, stretcher-friendly ramps, and proper signage.

Navigating a Changing Society

With social media, instant news, and greater public scrutiny, doctors must uphold ethical behaviour both online and offline. A doctor is a role model in society. (4) Do not share patient details on social media platforms, maintain boundaries with patients and report unethical practices you may observe.

What would you do when ethics get tested

Real life isn't always black and white; you will face complex situations. You face a dilemma when a parent refuses vaccination for their child, a terminally ill patient asks to stop all treatment or a colleague is prescribing unnecessary investigations. Such dilemmas test your training, compassion, and clarity. Such dilemmas are included in the coming sections to help you navigate with precision. When unsure, seek help from mentors, ethics committees, or trusted seniors.

Case Scenario

Mrs Fatima, a 62-year-old woman with stable angina, is advised by her cardiologist to undergo elective coronary angioplasty. She is otherwise active, caring for her grandchildren, and manages her daily activities independently. After a detailed discussion about benefits, risks, and alternatives, Mrs Fatima expresses her preference to try lifestyle changes and medicines first, rather than immediate surgery. Her family is concerned that she is 'refusing treatment,' and urges the doctor to convince her to undergo surgery.

Core Concepts

Autonomy: The right of patients to make informed decisions about their healthcare. They should be given adequate information without coercion.

Shared Responsibility: Patient care is a partnership, where doctors provide accurate diagnoses, advice, and treatment, while patients are responsible for understanding instructions, adhering to the agreed-upon plan, and communicating any concerns. (5)

Approach

Information Sharing and Autonomy: Explain in plain language the nature of her condition, the pros and cons of each option, the likely outcomes and potential risks if treatment is delayed. Accept her decision if it is informed and made without undue pressure. Document the discussion and her preference.

Establish Shared Responsibility: Agree on a follow-up schedule and a plan for medication adherence. Encourage her to contact the hospital immediately if she experiences red-flag symptoms.

Family Involvement: Involve family members in the discussion to ensure they understand that her choice is medically reasonable, provided it is closely monitored.

Outcome: Mrs Fatima initiated lifestyle changes, adhered to her medications, and attended regular check-ups. Her symptoms improved, and the trust between her and her treating doctor grew stronger as they both respected each other's roles.

Learning Points

- Autonomy empowers patients and builds trust.
- Shared responsibility ensures safety and effective decision-making.
- Clear communication with both patient and family prevents conflict.

☕ Coffee Moment

A boy with a spinal injury arrives in your OPD. Instead of rushing, you sit at eye level, smile, and ask the boy directly about school and friends before discussing treatment. His face lights up. In that moment, you have given more than medicine: you have given dignity.

References

1. Beauchamp TL, Childress JF. Principles of Biomedical Ethics. 8th ed. Oxford: Oxford University Press; 2019.
2. National Medical Commission. Competency-Based Undergraduate Curriculum for the Indian Medical Graduate. New Delhi: NMC; 2019.
3. Bismark MM, Morris JM, Thomas LA, Loh E, Phelps G, Spittal MJ. Reasons and remedies for patient complaints in Australian hospitals: a retrospective, cross-sectional study. Med J Aust. 2020;212(9):418-24.
4. Medical Council of India. Code of Ethics Regulations, 2002 (Amended up to 2020). New Delhi: MCI/NMC; 2020.
5. Gillon R. Defending the four principles approach as a good basis for good medical practice and therefore for good medical ethics. J Med Ethics. 2015;41(1):111-6.

Chapter 14: Principles of Bioethics and Justice in Health Care

Introduction

Medicine has both scientific and ethical values. Physicians often face situations where they must balance conflicting values, respect individual choices, do what is best, avoid harm, and distribute resources fairly. This chapter discusses the ethical framework guiding these decisions and a physician's social obligations.

The four pillars of bioethics

We have discussed the guiding principles of bioethics, which include autonomy, beneficence, non-maleficence, and justice, forming the cardinal pillars of ethical medical practice. (1)

- **Autonomy**: Respecting a patient's right to decide about their body and life.
- **Beneficence**: Acting in the best interest of the patient and promoting their well-being.
- **Non-maleficence**: "Do no harm" means avoiding actions that could cause unnecessary injury or suffering.
- **Justice**: Treating individuals fairly with equitable distribution of health resources.

Patient autonomy and decision-making

Autonomy means that competent patients have the right to make decisions about their care, including the right to accept or refuse the treatment recommended by their treating physicians. Key concepts include:

Informed consent and refusal: Physicians must provide adequate information about the diagnosis, proposed interventions, benefits, risks and alternatives, and obtain voluntary agreement. Patients have the right to decline treatment, and doctors must respect such decisions unless overridden by law.

Competence versus capacity: Competence is a legal determination of a person's ability to make decisions. Capacity is a clinical assessment of whether a patient can understand, appreciate and have reasoning about their choices. Decision-making may shift to a surrogate decision-maker when the patient's capacity is lost.

Surrogate decision-making: When patients are unable to make decisions, family members or legally designated surrogates are consulted. The doctor's role becomes crucial in eliciting the patient's known wishes and balancing family desires with the patient's best interests.

Decision-making in special situations

Respect for patient autonomy is a core ethical principle, but patient autonomy is not absolute. Physicians must balance patient choices with the principles of beneficence, their professional duties, public health, and legal frameworks related to special situations.

Assent and consent for minors: A guardian's consent is required for legality, and a child's assent for ethics. Those under 18 lack full legal capacity, so parents provide consent; however, involving the child through their assent respects their autonomy. Assent involves explaining, encouraging questions, and acknowledging fears. It fosters trust, alleviates anxiety, and preserves the child's dignity. (3)

Child Protection: Sometimes, parents' refusal of treatment for their child based on faith raises questions about when clinicians can override parental decisions to protect the child. Certain legal conditions have clear directions in India; however, most situations are grey in this regard.

End-of-life decisions: Patients may request the withholding or withdrawal of treatments. Students should be aware of the principles behind do-not-resuscitate orders and refusal of ventilation. These complex decisions involve numerous stakeholders and necessitate meticulous adherence to relevant policies and laws.

Confidentiality and its limits

Patients must feel safe while disclosing personal and sensitive information. Patient-related information is confidential, but not in absolute terms. There are situations when it can be breached.

Keep patient information private: Only share with health-care team members who need to know.

Seek consent before disclosure: If disclosure is necessary, patients should be informed of who will receive their information and the reason.

Know exceptions: Partial or full disclosure may be required to protect third parties in the event of communicable diseases, to comply with legal reporting obligations, or to ensure public safety. (4)

Case scenarios illustrate how autonomy works in practice, the decision-making process when patients are unable to decide, and how confidentiality is maintained or breached within legal frameworks for the greater good.

Autonomy and confidentiality are fundamental principles of medical ethics, but their application is complex. Physicians must assess decision-making capacity, respect refusals, and involve surrogates. They must also balance confidentiality with described exceptions to protect others.

Case Scenario: "Do not tell my wife"

Salman, a 28-year-old man, is diagnosed with pulmonary tuberculosis and HIV. Knowing his positive HIV status, he becomes distressed and pleads not to disclose to his wife, fearing humiliation.

Core Concepts

Confidentiality and Its Limits: Confidentiality is a cornerstone of medical ethics, but not absolute. Confidentiality may be breached when:

- There is a risk of harm to others.
- The patient lacks decision-making capacity.
- Legal obligations require disclosure (e.g., communicable diseases).

Autonomy vs. Beneficence: Salman's request to withhold information from his wife puts the ethical principles of autonomy in conflict with beneficence. Respecting autonomy is important, but the potential harm to his pregnant wife and unborn child justifies breaching confidentiality.

Decision-Making Process

Capacity: Assess Salman's understanding of his disease and its impact on his family.

Counselling: Provide him with information about HIV transmission and the potential risks to his wife and the unborn child. Address his fears and emphasise the importance of informing his wife, offering support, and providing resources.

Encourage Voluntary Disclosure: Encourage him to disclose his disease status to his wife voluntarily.

Plan for Mandatory Reporting: If Salman refuses to disclose, inform him of the legal obligations to report HIV to public health authorities.

Document the Process: Document all discussions, decisions, and actions taken in Salman's medical record, maintaining patient dignity.

Outcome

After thorough counselling, Salman agrees to inform his wife, Rukhsana, of his HIV status. He is thankful for the support and resources that have been provided. Rukhsana undergoes HIV testing and receives appropriate care. Their child is born healthy, and the family receives ongoing support to navigate the challenges.

Coffee Moment

Over coffee, students reflected that while respecting patient autonomy is important, we must also act in the best interest of their social contacts, who may be at risk.

References

1. Beauchamp TL, Childress JF. Principles of Biomedical Ethics. 8th ed. Oxford: Oxford University Press; 2019.
2. Aruna Shanbaug v. Union of India, (2011) 4 SCC 454; Common Cause v. Union of India, (2018) 5 SCC 1. Supreme Court of India.
3. Alderson P. In the genes or in the stars? Children's competence to consent. J Med Ethics. 1992;18(3):119-24.
4. Government of India. HIV/AIDS (Prevention and Control) Act, 2017. New Delhi: Gazette of India; 2017.

Chapter 15: The Evolution of Healthcare in India

Introduction

This chapter provides a comprehensive overview of India's extensive healthcare system, including its historical, constitutional, and functional aspects. The Indian healthcare system originated thousands of years ago, in ashrams through healing chants and procedures and has evolved into a modern healthcare system with cutting-edge technology. This chapter presents the timeline of Indian medicine, an ongoing story that has influenced patients and the system.

Glorious Past: Ayurveda, Yoga and Science of Life

India's medical roots are deep, arguably more ancient than those of most civilizations. Systems such as Ayurveda and Yoga emphasize healing and promoting harmony in the body, mind, and spirit.

Charaka Samhita dates back to around the 2nd century CE. It is one of the oldest and most comprehensive texts on internal medicine. (1)

The Sushruta Samhita, dating back to approximately the 6th century BCE, describes over 300 surgical procedures, including cataract surgery and skin grafting, which were remarkably advanced for their time. (1)

Healers were highly respected figures in the community, as healthcare was seen as a spiritual duty and a sacred responsibility. Millions continue to turn to these traditions for chronic illnesses, wellness, and cultural comfort.

Colonial Turn: Medicine, Military, and Missionaries

The British era had a profound impact on the course of healthcare in India. Western medicine mainly focused on colonial officials, military personnel and specific areas. The Indian Medical Service (IMS), although notable for figures like Sir Ronald Ross, Sir Benjamin Franklin, and Dr Henry Vandyke Carter, primarily served colonial officers. The primary objective of IMS was to safeguard British officers in India from common diseases such as cholera, plague, and malaria, while leaving large rural populations underserved. Rural India remained consistently underserved, and indigenous systems were marginalized. This period marked the beginning of public health efforts, but the focus was not on equity but on serving the empire. (2)

The People Rise: Nationalism and Health as a Right

By the early 20th century, Mahatma Gandhi and Dr B.C. Roy began advocating for healthcare for national empowerment. Mahatma Gandhi included cleanliness and community health in his movement for political freedom. Voluntary organisations and local movements provided primary care in underserved areas, and the concept of health as a public good, rather than a private luxury, began to gain traction.

Post-Independence: Bhore Committee & Beyond

Chaired by Sir Joseph Bhore in 1946, the committee made the blueprint for India's public health. The committee advocated for universal, free, and equitable healthcare through a three-tier system. Although it was not fully implemented, it became the foundation of India's public health framework after independence in 1947. The Bhore Committee Report presented a revolutionary vision for establishing a comprehensive healthcare system for India. (3)

Global Influence: Alma-Ata and 'Health for All'

In 1978, India became a signatory to the Alma-Ata Declaration, a landmark global commitment to Primary Health Care (PHC) as the key to achieving Health for All by 2000. This declaration emphasizes community participation in health and supports low-cost, high-impact interventions such as immunization and ORS. This inspired India's missions, such as UIP, ICDS, and later the NHM. India's alignment with global health movements marked its unique place in international public health. (4,5)

Modern Turn: Digital, Diagnostic, Decentralised

The 21st century brought new challenges, energy and demands. Health policies have evolved (1983, 2002, 2017) to address emerging challenges, including non-communicable diseases, ageing, and mental health. Flagship programs such as Ayushman Bharat, the National Digital Health Mission, and the COVID-19 vaccination drive have significantly transformed access to and awareness of healthcare. India's clinical expertise, pharmaceutical capabilities, affordability and diplomacy have established it as an emerging global health leader. (6)

What This Means for Student Doctor

You are entering a system that is still healing from its past wounds and working to bridge its divides, yet it holds great potential. Understanding this progress makes you a grounded physician, builds respect for diverse healing traditions, and helps you relate to your role for individuals, communities, and systems.

☕Coffee Moment

Imagine meeting a tribal healer in Bastar, a government doctor in Bikaner, and a founder of a telemedicine startup in Patna in the same week. They are not opposites. They are chapters of the same story. And now, you are part of it.

Timeline: A Journey Through Time

From Colonial Roots to a Global Medical Powerhouse.

1764: Military medical departments in Bengal and Bombay Presidencies, precursor to the Indian Medical Service (IMS).

1835: Calcutta Medical College, the first medical college in Asia, opens.

1835: Madras Medical College (Chennai)

1845: Grant Medical College (Mumbai)

1874: Temple Medical School (Now PMCH) Patna

1885: St. Stephen's Hospital, Delhi

1897: Dr Ronald Ross discovers the mosquito-malaria link in India.

1900: CMC Vellore started as a single-bed dispensary

1911: Indian Research Fund Association (IRFA) Redesignated as Indian Council of Medical Research (ICMR) in 1949

1912: KGMC (now KGMU) Lucknow

1916: Lady Hardinge Medical College, Delhi. The first one dedicated for women.

1926: Seth G.S. Medical College & KEM Hospital, Mumbai, a public-private model.

1941: Tata Memorial Hospital, Mumbai

1946: The Bhore Committee provided the first national health policy document, advocating free and universal health care, PHCs, and district-level hospitals.

1947: SMS Medical College, Jaipur

1950: Bombay Hospital, Mumbai

1954: Sir Ganga Ram Hospital, Delhi

1956: AIIMS, New Delhi, established.

1960: Institute of Medical Sciences at Banaras Hindu University (BHU)

1962: PGIMER, Chandigarh, was founded.

1962: Jawaharlal Nehru Medical College at Aligarh Muslim University.

1964: JIPMER, Puducherry, autonomous status.

1975: National Board of Examinations (NBE). Now, NBEMS.

1980s–2000s: Rapid Expansion of state and private medical colleges and super-speciality hospitals such as Apollo (1983), Manipal Hospitals (1991), Fortis Healthcare (1996), Max Healthcare (2001).

2010s onwards: Medical Education Boom

Massive investment in medical infrastructure:

- Over 300 new medical colleges were established.
- Over 1.1 lakh MBBS seats and 75000 PG seats in different specialities.
- 22 new AIIMS institutions created.
- Expansion of corporate hospital chains contributing to postgraduate training, evidence-based care and health tourism.

2019: National Medical Commission (NMC), replacing the MCI.

2025: Comprehensive guidance for medical students and doctors. **MBBS Foundation: Your First Book of Medicine** is in your hands, and you become a partner in this journey.

From St. Stephen's legacy of service to PGIMER Chandigarh clinical excellence and AIIMS leadership in research and academics, the healthcare journey demonstrates a unique blend of service, science, and scale. There is a growing call to establish an Indian Medical Service (IMS) cadre, similar to the Indian Administrative Service (IAS), to strengthening India's public healthcare system.

References

1. Sharma PV. Charaka Samhita: Text with English Translation. Varanasi: Chaukhambha Orientalia; 1981.
2. Harrison M. Public health in British India: Anglo-Indian preventive medicine 1859–1914. Cambridge: Cambridge University Press; 1994.
3. Government of India. Report of the Health Survey and Development Committee (Bhore Committee Report). New Delhi: GOI, 1946.
4. World Health Organization & UNICEF. Declaration of Alma-Ata, 1978. Geneva: WHO; 1978.
5. World Health Organization. Declaration of Astana on Primary Health Care, 2018. Geneva: WHO; 2018.
6. NITI Aayog. Health Systems for a New India: Building Blocks — Potential Pathways to Reform. New Delhi: NITI Aayog; 2019.

Synthesis

The Harmony of Healing

Where science seeks proof, tradition seeks meaning, and medicine gives both.

This section is an invitation to explore medicine beyond boundaries to see healing not as an argument between systems, but as a conversation between wisdoms.

Ayurveda meets anatomy,

Yoga meets neuroscience, and

Empathy meets evidence.

Synthesis reminds you that there is a bridge

between ancient insight and modern science,

between prevention and cure,

between the body and the soul.

Every culture, every science, every practice that moves humanity toward reducing the suffering deserves understanding, study, and respect.

So, breathe in curiosity.

Step beyond silos.

Learn to listen to nature, to history, and to the patient before you become a part of this timeless harmony.

S No.	Synthesis: At a Glance
1.	**Chapter 16** Introduction to Alternative Systems of Medicine Understand the landscape of AYUSH and global complementary systems, their principles, and their coexistence with modern medicine.
2.	**Chapter 17** Ayurveda: Deep Roots and Modern Relevance Explore the philosophical and biological foundations of Ayurveda, its evidence base, and its integration with Yoga and preventive health.
3.	**Chapter 18** Yoga: Breath of the Body, Anchor for the Mind Discover the science, philosophy, and global evidence behind Yoga as a therapeutic and transformative practice.
4.	**Chapter 19** Other Systems: Unani, Siddha, and Homeopathy Gain awareness of traditional systems coexisting in India, their principles, uses, and scientific evaluation.
5.	**Chapter 20** Evidence-Based Appraisal for Alternative Systems of Medicine Learn how to evaluate traditional practices through the lens of modern research and critical appraisal.
6.	**Chapter 21** Real-Life Integration of Modern and Alternative Medicine Understand integrative care models and their role in patient-centred, holistic healthcare.
7.	**Chapter 22** Principles of Family Practice Appreciate how family medicine unites science and sensitivity, carrying forward the synthesis of personal care, continuity, and compassion.

Chapter 16: Introduction to Alternative Systems of Medicine

Introduction

Millions of Indians, and billions of people worldwide, rely on traditional, complementary, and alternative medicine every day. Indian medical graduates (IMGs) should understand that healing does not always start or end in an allopathic clinic; there is a wide spectrum of therapies and systems that people can access and complement modern medicine. (1) Ayurveda, Yoga & Naturopathy, Unani, Siddha, and Homeopathy (AYUSH) carry their historical, cultural, and practical relevance. Understanding these systems does not require practising them. It requires respecting patient choices, recognizing cross-referrals, and appreciating the holistic principles related to health. (2)

Modern Medicine

Allopathy, or modern medicine, focuses on pathophysiology, diagnosis, and specific treatment, utilising pharmaceuticals or surgery. It emphasizes standardization, evidence, and acute care.

Alternative Medicine

Alternative medicine refers to health practices used *instead of* conventional modern medical treatments. These can include herbal remedies, acupuncture, Ayurvedic medicine, traditional Chinese medicine, homeopathy, and more. The term 'alternative' implies that these therapies are used as standalone options outside mainstream biomedical systems.

Complementary Medicine

Complementary medicine involves using alternative practices in conjunction with conventional modern medical treatments. For example, a cancer patient undergoing surgery, chemotherapy, or radiotherapy may also follow yoga or meditation to manage stress. The goal is not to replace modern medicine but to improve the patient's overall well-being and recovery.

Evidence-Based Medicine

Evidence-Based Medicine (EBM) is the practice of making clinical decisions using the best current scientific evidence, combined with clinical expertise and patient preferences. (3) It involves:

- Systematic research and trials
- Critical appraisal of data and
- Application in real-world and patient-centred contexts

Complementary and Alternative Medicine

Complementary and Alternative Medicine (CAM) focuses on balance, prevention, and individual constitution. It frequently combines mind-body techniques, herbal treatments, and lifestyle modification. Globally, the term CAM is common, but 'Integrative Medicine' is preferred because it emphasizes collaboration rather than opposition with mainstream care. It is helpful to understand that, by applying principles of evidence-based medicine, safe and effective practices can be identified and integrated as complementary medicine to support the individual's overall well-being. A significant amount of progress is currently being made in this field, allowing you to focus on your area of interest. We will discuss about integrative medicine.

AYUSH at a Glance

Ayurveda

India's indigenous system has roots dating back over 3,000 years.
Emphasizes balance in body elements (doshas), diet, lifestyle, and herbs.
Used for chronic conditions, wellness, and prevention.

Yoga and Naturopathy

Yoga: A physical, mental, and spiritual practice for benefits in stress reduction, flexibility, breathing disorders, and mental health. It is a holistic approach towards balance and harmony at different levels..

Naturopathy: Treat the whole person, including mind, body, and spirit, and address the root cause of illness rather than merely suppressing symptoms. Diet schedules, fasting, hydrotherapy, and other non-invasive methods are used to promote self-healing.

Unani Medicine

It is a traditional system of medicine with roots in ancient Greek and Arabic teachings. It focuses on balancing the body's natural fluids (called humours) to maintain health. It is practised widely in India and parts of the Middle East.

Siddha

Siddha is one of the oldest healing systems in India, with its roots in Tamil. It utilises herbs, minerals, a balanced diet, and lifestyle practices. Siddha emphasizes long-term well-being and views disease as a consequence of an imbalance in the natural forces within the body.

Homeopathy

Based on the "like cures like" principle, using ultra-dilute substances. It is popular across India for acute and chronic ailments.

Factors Deciding a Patient's Choice

- Cultural beliefs and family traditions.
- Affordability and accessibility.
- Chronic conditions where modern medicine offers limited relief.
- Emphasis on "natural" or "holistic" care.

As a doctor, you must understand these motivations, rather than dismissing. Patients often combine therapies without fully understanding the safety and risks associated with such combinations. It is essential to inform your patients about the potential safety and risks associated with unproven practices when used in conjunction with modern medicine. Say and document, 'I don't know' if you don't know.

Integrative and Collaborative Medicine

Across India, many government and private health setups, including AIIMS, offer co-located AYUSH and allopathic services. (4) You may work alongside AYUSH practitioners or receive referrals from them. Collaborative practice requires open-mindedness, inter-system respect, and a shared goal: healing the patient. (5) Evidence-based approaches are being studied to integrate the best of both worlds, particularly in:

- Chronic pain.
- Lifestyle disorders such as diabetes and hypertension.
- Mental health.
- Palliative care.

Student Takeaway

Other systems of medicine can complement clinical practice, particularly in lifestyle counselling, preventive care, and support for chronic illnesses. India is one of the few countries with a diverse range of medical languages. Understanding this improves your ability to communicate effectively with patients, families, and community leaders. You may collaborate in integrative research, help bridge systems, or even develop new models of care.

☕ Coffee Moment

As a medical student, you will encounter many paths to healing—some rooted in modern science, others in centuries of lived experience. Understanding alternative systems of medicine does not mean abandoning scientific rigor; it means learning to listen with curiosity and humility. A good doctor knows when to question, when to integrate, and when to guide patients gently and safely. Respect for different healing traditions begins with respect for the patient who believes in them.

References

1. Ernst E. Complementary/alternative medicine for medical students: towards evidence-based teaching. Med Educ. 2000;34(3):196–200.
2. World Health Organization. WHO global report on traditional and complementary medicine 2019. Geneva: WHO; 2019.
3. Sackett DL, Rosenberg WM, Gray JA, Haynes RB, Richardson WS. Evidence-based medicine: what it is and what it isn't. *BMJ*. 1996;312(7023):71–2.
4. National Health Policy 2017. Ministry of Health and Family Welfare, Government of India.
5. Weil A, Jonas WB, Blumberg JB. *Integrative Medicine.* 5th ed. New York: Oxford University Press, 2023.

Chapter 17: Ayurveda- Deep Roots and Modern Relevance

Introduction

Centuries before blood tests, CT scans, and ICUs, medicine took a gentler yet profound form. It viewed the patient not as a body to be fixed but as a living, breathing being in balance with the universe. The foundations of Ayurveda, the "science of life," date back over 5,000 years, as encoded in ancient Indian texts such as the *Charaka Samhita*, *Sushruta Samhita*, and *Ashtanga Hridaya.* The *Atharva Veda* is the primary Veda associated with Ayurveda. Preventive care, immunity, gut health, and the mind-body connection are central to Ayurvedic thinking.

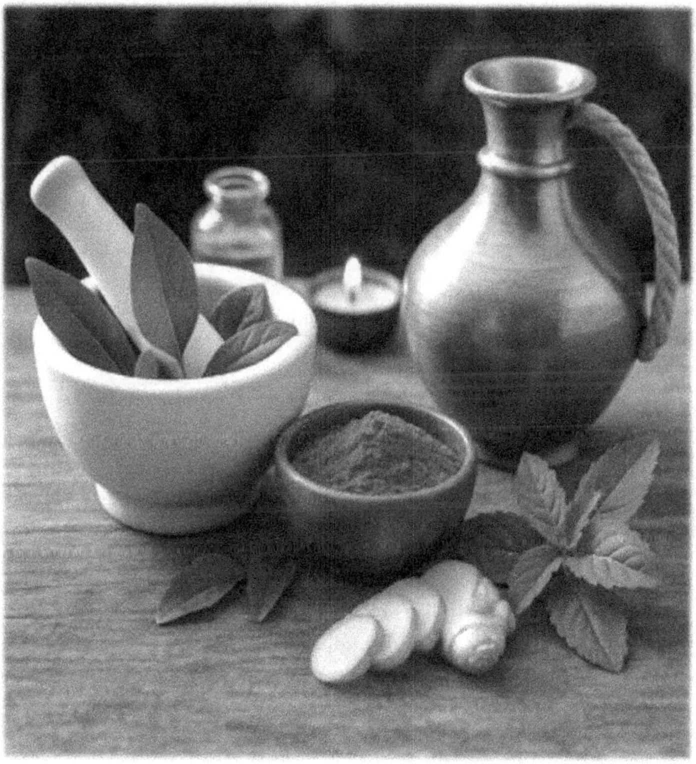

Figure 17.1: Ayurveda

Charaka had documented over 500 medicinal plants, diagnostics, and therapies tailored to the patient. (1)

Sushruta described cataract surgeries, rhinoplasty, and wound suturing techniques that resemble modern plastic surgery. (2)

Core Principles of Ayurveda

Here, the core idea is "restoring harmony" rather than "fixing a disease." Ayurveda sees health as a balance between:

- Sharir (Body)
- Manas (Mind)
- Atma (Soul)
- Kala and Desh (Environment and Season)

When any of these are out of synchrony, disease follows.

The Tridosha Theory

Every person has a unique constitution or their Prakriti (nature). This constitution is governed by three doshas. An imbalance in doshas, caused by lifestyle, diet, environment, or emotions, results in illness. The goal of treatment is to restore internal balance (1-3) and rebuild strength after illness, with a focus on enhancing immunity, promoting longevity, and enhancing vitality.

Table 17.1: Tridosh theory of Ayurved

Dosha	Elemental Nature	Functions
Vata	Air + Ether	Movement, nerve impulses, circulation
Pitta	Fire + Water	Digestion, metabolism, transformation
Kapha	Earth + Water	Stability, structure, lubrication

Ayurvedic Concepts That Mirror Modern Science

Many Ayurvedic principles align with modern biology and medicine:

- Agni (digestive fire): Gut enzymes and metabolism.
- Ama (toxins): Undigested residues, inflammatory by-products.
- Dinacharya & Ritucharya: Circadian and seasonal rhythms.
- Ojas (vital energy): Resilience or immune tone.
- Srotas (channels): Circulatory and lymphatic systems.
- Mind-body medicine: Stress and immunity links.

Tools of Healing in Ayurveda (1,3,4)

Aahara (Diet)

- Food is considered the first medicine.
- Individualized diets based on Prakriti and season.
- Spices such as turmeric, ginger, and cumin promote digestion and immunity.

Vihara (Lifestyle)

- **Dinacharya** (daily routine): waking early, tongue scraping, oil pulling, warm water rituals.
- **Ritucharya** (seasonal regimen): adjustments in diet and habits in response to climate shifts.
- **Sleep hygiene**: minimise screen exposure and practice mindfulness.

Aushadhi (Herbs and Medicines)

- Herbal decoctions, churnas (powders), and tablets made from natural sources.
- Formulations like Triphala, Ashwagandha, Brahmi, Arjuna, and Guduchi.
- Panchakarma (Detox Therapies)

Five procedures for deep cleansing of the body:

- Vamana (therapeutic emesis)
- Virechana (purgation)
- Basti (medicated enemas)
- Nasya (nasal therapy)
- Raktamokshana (bloodletting)
- Rasayana (Rejuvenation)

Integration with Yoga and Mindfulness

Ayurveda is often practised alongside Yoga, meditation, pranayama, and mantra therapy, all of which aim to align the physical body with mental and spiritual well-being. (5) This integration forms the holistic triad:

- Ayurveda (body and lifestyle)
- Yoga (movement and breath)
- Dhyana (meditation and focus)

Scientific Recognition and Global Rise

- In recent years, Ayurveda has entered mainstream wellness and medical research:
- India's Ministry of AYUSH supports clinical trials and standardization for broader international recognition. All AIIMS have an AYUSH department and are integrating patient care, education, and research.
- Harvard, Stanford, Johns Hopkins and many other global centres have been conducting research on many Ayurvedic herbs and therapies.
- Ayurvedic centres are thriving in Europe, the USA, and Australia, driven by a growing demand for personalized, preventive health solutions.

Areas of Ongoing Research

Immunity and Adaptogens: *Ashwagandha, Giloy*, and *Tulsi* have shown immunomodulatory properties. (6)

Diabetes and Metabolic Syndrome: Ayurvedic lifestyle and herbal combinations are being studied for glucose control. (1,3)

Neuroprotection: *Brahmi, Shankhpushpi*, and other *medhya rasayanas* are explored for dementia, anxiety, and cognition.

Gut-Brain Axis: *Trikatu* and *Triphala* combinations are being researched for modulation of the gut microbiota.

Student Takeaway

- Ayurveda is not anti-modern; it's pro-balance.
- Ayurveda teaches you how to prevent illness in the first place.
- Understanding Ayurveda is decoding India's medical soul.
- When chronic diseases are on the rise and modern medicine alone is not enough, Ayurveda teaches you to look at health not as an emergency but as a way of life.

☕ Coffee Moment

Ayurveda reminds us that medicine did not begin in laboratories—it began with observation, reflection, and care for the whole person. As you learn its principles, see them as a language through which generations tried to understand balance, health, and disease. You do not need to accept everything unquestioningly, nor dismiss it hastily. A wise doctor learns to appreciate ideas in their context, while remaining anchored in evidence, ethics, and patient safety.

References

1. Sharma PV. Charaka Samhita. Varanasi: Chaukhamba Orientalia; reprint 2014.
2. Sharma PV, editor. Sushruta Samhita: Text with English Translation. Varanasi: Chaukhambha Visvabharati; 2001.
3. Murthy KRS, editor. Astanga Hridayam of Vagbhata: Text, English Translation, Notes & Index. Varanasi: Chaukhambha Krishnadas Academy; 2017.
4. Lad V. Ayurveda: The science of self-healing. Delhi: Motilal Banarsidass; 2002.
5. Patwardhan B, Mutalik G, Tillu G. Integrative Approaches for Health: Biomedical Research, Ayurveda and Yoga. London: Academic Press; 2015.
6. Patwardhan B. Bridging Ayurveda with evidence-based scientific approaches in medicine. EPMA J. 2014;5(1):19.

Chapter 18: Yoga- Breath of the Body, Anchor for the Mind

Introduction

In your first year of medicine, you study the human body in detail, covering bones, nerves, hormones, and organs. One key element that connects them beyond anatomy and physiology is your breath, a fundamental aspect of yoga.

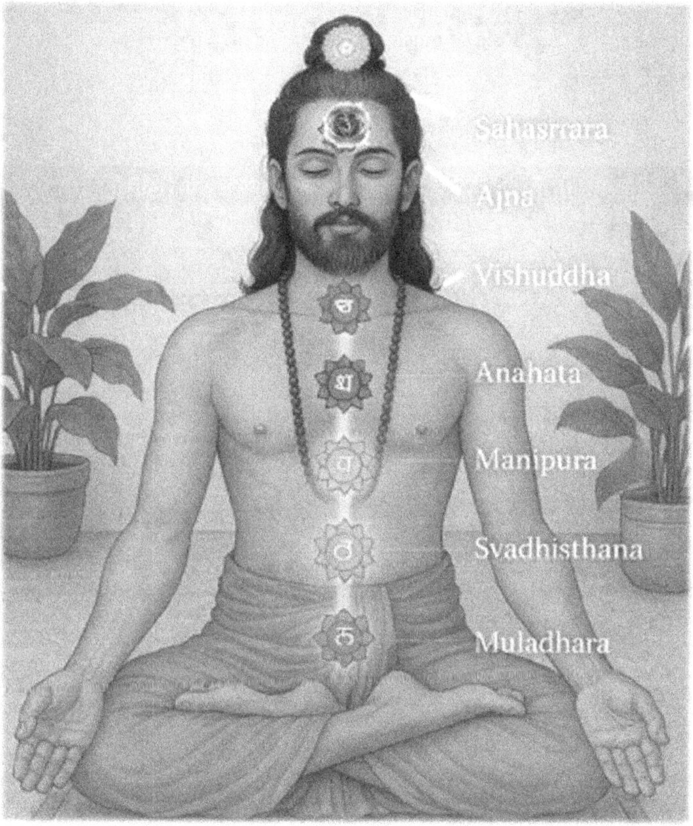

Figure 18.1: The Seven Chakras

Yoga: A Legacy Older Than Medicine

Yoga is as old as India's civilization, with references in the Rigveda and a full elaboration in the Upanishads, the Bhagavad Gita, and Patanjali's Yoga Sutras. The Bhagavad Gita explains Rajyog, Karmyog, and Jnanayog (also known as Gyanyog). Here we are focusing on the Rajyog. 'Yoga' comes from the Sanskrit root 'yuj', meaning to join or to unite, the union of body, mind, and soul. It is both a discipline and a destination. At its core, Yoga is about:

- Connecting the inner world with the outer world.
- Moving from chaos to clarity.
- Achieving harmony between physiology, pathology and psychology.

Table 18.1: Different types of Yoga

Form	Focus
Hatha Yoga	Physical postures and breath control
Raja Yoga	Mental discipline and meditation
Kundalini Yoga	Awakening energy through movement and mantra
Naad Yoga	Role of music and sound in therapy and well-being.
Therapeutic Yoga	Customized sequences for specific medical needs

Table 18.2: Seven Chakras- Energy centres of the body

Chakra Name	Location	Associated Traits
Root Chakra ***Muladhara***	Base of spine	Stability, safety, grounding
Sacral Chakra ***Svadhisthana***	Below navel	Emotions, creativity, sexuality
Solar Plexus Chakra ***Manipura***	Stomach area	Confidence, willpower, digestion
Heart Chakra ***Anahata***	Center of chest	Love, compassion, emotional healing
Throat Chakra ***Vishuddha***	Throat	Communication, truth, expression
Third Eye Chakra ***Ajna (Aagya)***	Between eyebrows	Intuition, insight, clarity
Crown Chakra ***Sahasrara***	Top of head	Spiritual connection, enlightenment

Eight Limbs of Ashtanga Yoga (Ashta-Anga Yoga)

- **Yama** (ethical restraints): non-violence, truth, non-stealing, celibacy, non-possessiveness.
- **Niyama** (observances): cleanliness, contentment, discipline, self-study, surrender to a higher power.
- **Asana** (physical postures): stability and comfort in the body.
- **Pranayama** (breath regulation): energy control through breath.
- **Pratyahara** (withdrawal of senses): turning inward.
- **Dharana** (concentration): focus on a single point or idea.
- **Dhyana** (meditation): unbroken flow of concentration.

- **Samadhi** (absorption): transcendental state of bliss and unity. (1)

The Science Behind the Silence

Is yoga a scientific practice? Yes. Over 4,000 research articles have explored the effects of Yoga. Studies on yoga in India and globally over the past two decades have demonstrated that it enhances both physical and mental health outcomes. Regular practice has been linked to reductions in cardiovascular risk factors, including blood pressure, lipid levels, body mass index, and health-related risk scores, in high-risk individuals. Evidence highlights the mental health benefits, a reduction in depressive symptoms, and improved emotional well-being. For individuals with chronic low back pain and musculoskeletal conditions, yoga has been shown to reduce pain intensity and improve function. Evidence suggests that yoga may downregulate inflammatory markers and improve immune regulation, providing a physiological basis for its benefits. Overall, these findings support yoga as a safe, affordable, and culturally adaptable supplement to standard healthcare. It works through neuroplasticity, vagal stimulation, hormonal balance, and parasympathetic activation, concepts you will learn more about in physiology and pathology. (2–6)

Global Journey of Yoga

Yoga is one of India's greatest gifts to the world. It is recognized by UNESCO as Intangible Cultural Heritage. The International Day of Yoga is celebrated globally on June 21. (7) Yoga is taught in schools, rehabilitation centres, hospitals and prisons and integrated into modern healthcare systems in countries like the USA, UK, Germany, Japan, and Australia. (2)

Student Takeaway: Begin With the Breath

Yoga is not only about flexibility, but also about stability; it is not only about movement, but also about stillness. It is not only about the body, but about your being. Even 15 minutes a day of simple practice can change how you study, sleep, and feel.

Table 18.3: Integrating yoga in life

Challenge	How Yoga Helps
Long working hours	Asanas correct posture and relieve back/neck strain
Academic stress	Pranayama calms the nervous system
Sleep disturbances	Meditation and yoga nidra improve sleep quality
Exam anxiety	Breath focus enhances focus and emotional regulation
Burnout	Mindful movement restores energy and optimism

As an MBBS student, here's what Yoga can offer you:

Whether you teach, practice, or understand it, Yoga will make you a better doctor who treats the disease and the whole person.
"Yoga is the journey of the self, through the self, to the self.": *Bhagavad Gita*
Let that journey begin with you, the future healer of others, and of yourself.

☕ Coffee Moment

A fellow student once told me: 'When I added 15 minutes of yoga before class, I was able to sit straighter and I think clearly.' That's when I realized yoga isn't for fitness alone, it's for staying in the presence. Let's bring this closer to home.

References

1. Iyengar BKS. Light on Yoga. New York: Schocken Books; 1995.
2. Cramer H, Lauche R, Haller H, Dobos G. A systematic review and meta-analysis of yoga for hypertension. Am J Hypertens. 2014;27(9):1146-51.
3. Prathikanti S, Rivera R, Cochran A, Tungol JG, Fayazmanesh N, Weinmann E. Treating major depression with yoga: a prospective, randomized, controlled pilot trial. J Affect Disord. 2017;213:208-13.
4. Saper RB, Lemaster C, Delitto A, Sherman KJ, Herman PM, Sadikova E, et al. Yoga, physical therapy, or education for chronic low back pain: a randomized noninferiority trial. Ann Intern Med. 2017;167(2):85-94.
5. Pascoe MC, Thompson DR, Ski CF. Yoga, mindfulness-based stress reduction and stress-related physiological measures: a meta-analysis. Psychoneuroendocrinology. 2017;86:152-68.
6. Bussing A, Michalsen A, Khalsa SB, Telles S, Sherman KJ. Effects of yoga on mental and physical health: a short summary of reviews. Evid Based Complement Alternat Med. 2012;2012:165410.
7. United Nations. Resolution adopted by the General Assembly on 11 December 2014: International Day of Yoga. UN; 2014.

Chapter 19: Other Systems- Unani, Siddha, and Homeopathy

Introduction

Along with Ayurveda and Yoga, which are intricately woven into the fabric of Indian civilization, India is also home to Unani, Siddha, and Homeopathy. In your career, you will encounter patients who:

- Combine allopathy with Unani or Siddha.
- Prefer homeopathic remedies for their children.
- Will ask you if they can continue Ayurvedic tonics alongside antibiotics.

Instead of dismissing these questions, your awareness and sensitivity will guide you. Understanding the diversity of Indian healthcare systems enables you to be a more connected clinician and effective communicator.

Unani Medicine: Healing Through Balance

Unani medicine, also known as Greco-Arabic medicine, has its roots in ancient Greece and was later enriched by Persian and Arab scholars, including Hippocrates, Galen, and Avicenna (Ibn Sina).

Guiding Principles

- Health is a state of equilibrium between the four bodily humours (fluids): Dam (blood), Balgham (phlegm), Safra (yellow bile), Sauda (black bile).
- Imbalance in humours due to diet, lifestyle, emotions, or environment causes disease.
- The body has an innate ability to heal, and the physician's role is to support the body's natural forces.

Tools of Healing

- **Ilaj-bit-Tadbeer** (Regimenal therapy): massage, cupping, sweat therapy, exercise, etc.
- **Ilaj-bit-Ghiza** (Diet therapy): personalized nutrition.
- **Ilaj-bit-Dawa** (Pharmacotherapy): use of herbs, minerals, and animal products.

Modern Relevance

Unani is widely practiced in Uttar Pradesh, Delhi, Hyderabad, and Kashmir, with dedicated colleges and hospitals. It is primarily used in the treatment of chronic illnesses, skin diseases, musculoskeletal disorders, and reproductive health issues. (1)

Siddha Medicine: The Ancient Southern Stream

Siddha is one of the oldest systems of medicine. It is indigenous to Tamil Nadu and attributed to sage-physicians known as Siddhas. It shares similarities with Ayurveda but has unique practices, particularly in alchemy, mineral medicine, and spiritual healing. (2)

Guiding Principles

- Health is a balance between three humours: Vata (air), Pitta (fire), and Kapha (water), similar to Ayurveda but with subtle distinctions.
- Disease is caused by imbalances in these humours, which are aggravated by diet, lifestyle, seasonal factors, and spiritual disconnection.

Tools of healing

- Use of herbo-mineral preparations and metals, such as mercury and sulphur, after purification techniques.
- Emphasis on Kayakalpa therapy, rejuvenation, and anti-ageing.
- Pulse diagnosis, varmam therapy (pressure point treatment), and siddha yoga are employed for healing and spiritual development.

Modern Relevance

Claimed to be effective in treating arthritis, chronic skin diseases, asthma, metabolic disorders, and menstrual issues, but needs scientific evidence.

Homeopathy: Like Cures Like

Homeopathy was developed by German physician Dr Samuel Hahnemann in the late 18th century. Based on the principle of "Similia Similibus Curentur" (let like be cured by like), it proposes that a substance causing symptoms in a healthy person can, in highly diluted form, treat similar symptoms in a sick person. (3)

Guiding Principles

- Individualized treatment: no two patients are treated the same, even for the same condition.
- Minimum dose: Medicines are diluted to the point where no molecules may remain, yet they are believed to carry energy or a vital force.
- Vital force concept: illness is a disturbance in the body's energy field.

Tools of Healing

- Remedies are prepared from plants, minerals, or animal substances, diluted through serial potentization (e.g., 30C, 200C).

- Given as sweet pills or tinctures.
- No side effects reported in traditional doses; however, insufficient data.

Modern Relevance

- Homeopathy is popular in India, Germany, France, and South America.
- In India, it is widely used to treat fevers, allergies, skin conditions, migraines, behavioural issues in children, and post-viral recovery; however, major scientific studies do not support its use.
- Systematic reviews by the Australian NHMRC and the UK House of Commons concluded that homeopathy should not be recommended for any condition due to a lack of efficacy beyond placebo. (4)

Table 19.1: Comparing Unani, Siddha and Homeopathy

System	Key Philosophy	Common Use Cases
Unani	Balance of 4 humours.	Skin diseases, metabolic issues.
Siddha	Balance of 3 doshas; mineral therapy.	Rheumatology, geriatrics, varmam.
Homeopathy	"Like cures like"; minimum dose.	Allergies, chronic conditions.

Controversy and Considerations

While widely used, scientific debate continues about the mode of action in all three systems. Many users report subjective improvement, leading to growing interest in placebo research, nanomedicine, and bioenergetics.

Student Takeaway

- Educate patients on the safety and potential drug interactions.
- Respect their choices while offering evidence-based advice.
- When it is appropriate to collaborate, do so with a qualified AYUSH practitioner for integrative care.

☕ Coffee Moment

As you encounter Unani, Siddha, and Homeopathy, remember that medicine evolves within cultures, histories, and beliefs. These systems reflect humanity's enduring search for healing and meaning. As a doctor trained in modern medicine, your role is not to judge hastily, but to understand thoughtfully—recognizing where evidence is strong, where it is limited, and how patient beliefs shape health choices. Compassionate care often begins with respectful understanding.

References

1. Unani System of Medicine: The Science of Health and Healing. Ministry of AYUSH, Govt of India. 2016.
2. Banerjee A, Debnath P, Debnath PK. Siddha medicine: an overview. Anc Sci Life. 2002;21(4):182–6.
3. Hahnemann S. Organon of Medicine. 6th ed. New Delhi: B Jain Publishers; 2002.
4. National Health and Medical Research Council (NHMRC). Statement on Homeopathy. Canberra: NHMRC; 2015.

Chapter 20: Evidence Appraisal for Alternative Systems

Introduction

It may seem paradoxical to test an ancient system like Yoga against the relatively young framework of evidence-based medicine. However, the truth is timeless, and any practice claiming to heal must withstand scrutiny, regardless of its origin or age. Science is not opposed to tradition; it is a tool for revealing what truly works.

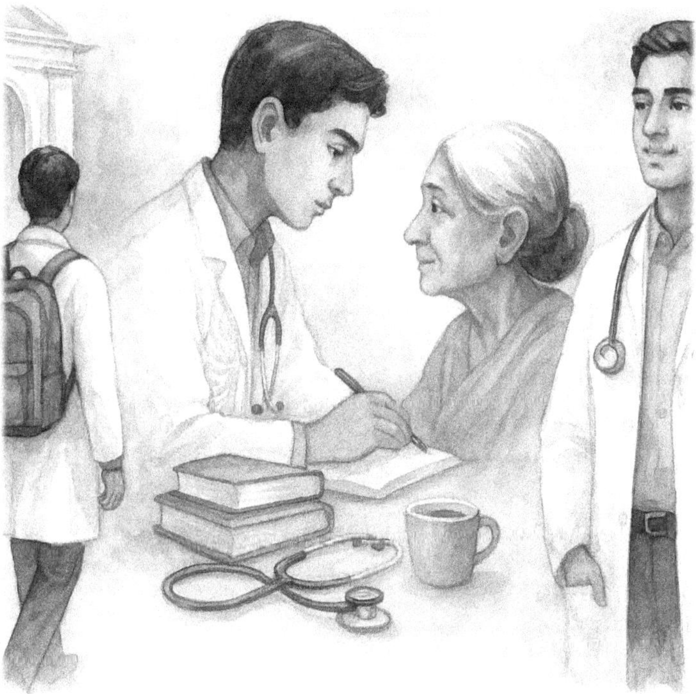

Figure 20.1: Appraisal of Alternative Systems

Ayurveda

Evidence Base: Multiple clinical trials and reviews exist on the use of Ashwagandha, Brahmi, Guduchi, and Triphala for the treatment of chronic health disorders. Studies are available on the use of other herbal medicines for many disorders, like arthritis, type 2 diabetes, and stress. However, the quality of evidence varies greatly due to limited large-scale, multicentric, and blinded RCTs. A significant limitation is the variability in formulations, dosages, and preparation methods of the herbal medicines used.

Challenges in EBM Validation: Isolating the active compound is difficult from polyherbal or herbo-mineral Ayurvedic medicines. Even if the clinical outcome is documented, it is challenging to establish the underlying mechanism. (1)

Standardization: Batch variability affects reproducibility, reliability and regulatory approval.

Toxicity concerns: Some formulations contain metals (*bhasmas*) requiring thorough purification and safety testing.

Evidence Status: Moderately evidence-supported in preventive care and stress modulation. Promising herbal drugs exist, but larger trials, rigorous standardization, and toxicological clarity are needed. There is a vast scope of research and validation.

Yoga

Evidence Base: Yoga is the most studied complementary and alternative medicine practice globally, with numerous studies including RCTs, reviews, and meta-analyses. Substantial evidence supports its use for mental health (anxiety, depression), cardiovascular (hypertension, heart rate variability), respiratory (asthma, chronic obstructive pulmonary disease), musculoskeletal (low back pain, arthritis), and cancer recovery (fatigue, mood, quality of life). Cochrane reviews support yoga for chronic low back pain and anxiety. (2) NIH, Harvard, AIIMS, and Stanford have published yoga-integrated clinical research.

Mechanistic Plausibility: Yoga works via autonomic regulation, improved vagal tone, neuroendocrine effects (e.g., cortisol, serotonin modulation) and musculoskeletal strengthening. All mechanisms are biologically plausible and supported by imaging and biomarker studies. Brain scans show increased grey matter in prefrontal and hippocampal regions in long-term yoga practitioners.

Global Endorsement

- Recognized by the WHO, NIH, NHS (UK), Mayo Clinic, and UNESCO as intangible heritage.
- Integrated into NIMHANS, AIIMS, and Indian medical curricula.
- It is inexpensive, involves no medication, and has few side effects.

Limitations and Gaps

- Different styles are difficult to compare.
- Placebo control is challenging (you can't fake yoga), for blinding. (3)

Evidence Status: There is a strong evidence base and biological plausibility, especially in mental health, lifestyle disorders, and rehabilitation. It may be prescribed as adjunctive therapy in collaboration with AYUSH/Yoga specialists, particularly in chronic conditions. Again, there is a vast scope of research and validation in this field.

Unani Medicine

Evidence Base: Lack of large-scale randomized controlled trials (RCTs). Some preliminary studies have shown symptom relief in musculoskeletal and skin conditions; however, they generally have small sample sizes, are non-blinded or poorly controlled, and have limited replication. Systematic reviews in PubMed/Scopus for Unani remain sparse.

Evidence Status: Lacks substantial evidence; needs trials and standardization before recommendation.

Siddha Medicine

Evidence Base: There are few RCTs and trials available. Some observational or small-scale studies have shown promise in treating arthritis, psoriasis, and metabolic disorders. However, most research is regionally published (Tamil journals, thesis-based work) without peer review or global indexing.

Safety and Rational Use Concerns: Heavy use of herbo-mineral and metallic preparations, including mercury, arsenic, and sulphur, even after purification (suddhi). Toxicology studies and pharmacokinetics are urgently needed. No clear understanding of interactions with allopathic drugs or long-term effects.

Evidence Status: Not evidence-supported for primary therapeutic use under current EBM standards.

Homeopathy

Evidence Base: Over 1000 clinical studies conducted worldwide. Systematic reviews (e.g., Cochrane, NHMRC Australia) conclude there is no strong evidence that homeopathy is more effective than a placebo for any major condition. Some studies indicate modest effects in allergies, migraine, and irritable bowel, but replication and blinding quality are poor. The Swiss and Australian health authorities have removed homeopathy from insurance coverage due to its lack of clinical efficacy.

Evidence Status: Fails to demonstrate biological plausibility and conclusive efficacy. (4) Not advised as a substitute for evidence-based treatments.

A Professional Stand on Traditional Systems

Be a respectful investigator, not a blind believer: uphold cultural sensitivity, but let scientific scrutiny guide your practice.

Respect patient autonomy: Many patients will use traditional therapies, irrespective of your advice. Your role is to understand, not to criticize.

Ask, don't assume: Patients often won't disclose alternative medicine use unless you ask non-judgmentally. This disclosure helps you make an informed decision and protects them from potential drug interactions.

Champion safe science: Promote ethical research on the practice of complementary and alternative medicines. Adapt proven methods but critically examine potential harms.

Student Takeaway: A Scientific Lens

Yoga is well-supported by evidence, with robust global research backing and is already integrated into mainstream healthcare. Ayurveda holds strong promise, with robust research backing its role in prevention and chronic care. To gain broader medical acceptance, more rigorous trials, quality control, and increased transparency are necessary. Unani, Siddha, and Homeopathy reflect cultural trust and experience, but lack scientific validation according to modern evidence-based standards.

☕ Coffee Moment

Evidence is not a tool to dismiss traditions, but a lens to understand what truly helps patients and what may cause harm. As you appraise alternative systems through an evidence-based approach, learn to ask careful questions—about safety, effectiveness, and context. A good doctor remains open-minded yet anchored in data, ethics, and patient welfare. True professionalism lies in balancing curiosity with responsibility, and belief with proof.

References

1. Patwardhan B. Ayurveda and integrative medicine: riding a tiger. J Ayurveda Integr Med. 2011;2(4):165–6.
2. Cramer H, Ward L, Saper R, Fishbein D, Dobos G, Lauche R. The safety of yoga: a systematic review and meta-analysis of randomized controlled trials. Am J Epidemiol. 2015;182(4):281–93.
3. Smith CA, Collins CT, Cyna AM, Crowther CA. Complementary and alternative therapies for pain management in labour. Cochrane Database Syst Rev. 2011;(12):CD009516.
4. Ernst E. Homeopathy: what does the "best" evidence tell us? Med J Aust. 2010;192(8):458–60.

Chapter 21: Integration of Modern and Alternative Medicine

Introduction

Integrated medicine reminds us that healing is not about choosing sides; it's about choosing what works best for the person in front of you. Imagine guiding your patient through breathwork before surgery, or recommending a simple asana to ease their back pain, that's what empowered, 21st-century doctors do. Let us explore the potential of integrative medicine.

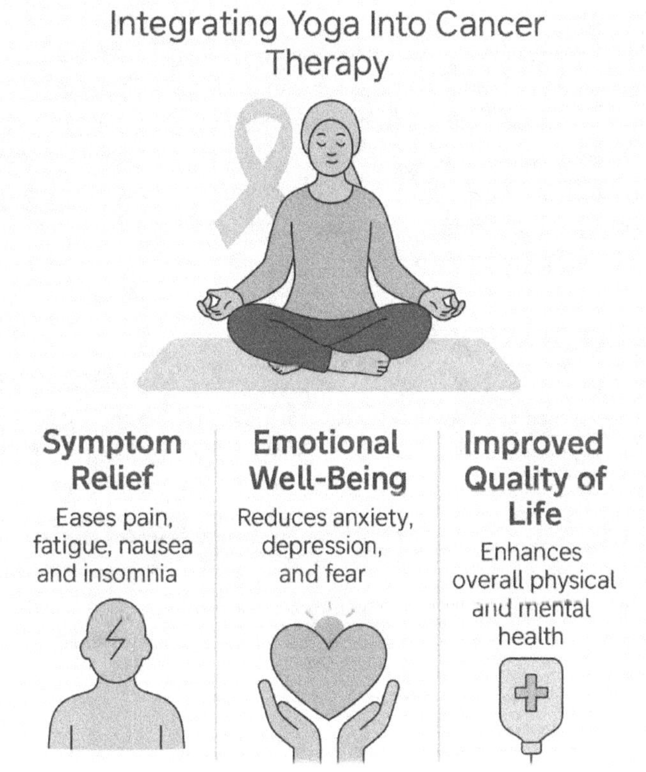

Figure 21.1: Integration of Yoga and Cancer Therapy

Integrated Medicine: Healing Together

Integrated (or integrative) medicine is an approach that combines modern scientific treatments with complementary systems like Ayurveda, Yoga, or Homeopathy to create a holistic, patient-centred healing plan. The goal is not to replace but to enhance, treating the whole person: body, mind, and spirit. (1)

Yoga in Integrated Medicine

Yoga offers evidence-based strategies to prevent, manage, and reverse many conditions. Studies have shown that regular Yoga practice can:

- Lower blood pressure and heart rate.
- Improve glycemic control in diabetes.
- Enhance lung function in asthma and COPD.
- Relieve chronic pain, especially back and neck pain.
- Improve sleep, concentration, and emotional resilience.
- Reduce anxiety, depression, and burnout in students and doctors.

Currently, AIIMS, NIMHANS, PGIMER, and other institutes have ongoing research in Yoga therapy. Yoga now forms part of military training, corporate wellness programs, and astronaut preparation because the discipline of the mind and body transcends all professions. It is no longer confined to the medical classroom; it is integrated into hospitals, ICUs, and clinics. Medical professionals worldwide are exploring Integrative Medicine, where Yoga contributes to cardiac rehabilitation, stroke recovery, anxiety management, chronic pain clinics, palliative care, substance use recovery, and prenatal and postnatal support. (2)

Ayurveda in Integrated Medicine

Ayurveda is increasingly being explored as a complementary system within integrative medical care, particularly for chronic diseases, preventive health, and rehabilitation. Its emphasis on individualised constitution (Prakriti), diet, lifestyle modification, and long-term balance aligns well with modern goals of chronic disease management.

Institutions such as the All India Institute of Medical Sciences (through AYUSH collaboration), the All India Institute of Ayurveda, the Institute of Teaching and Research in Ayurveda, and the Central Council for Research in Ayurvedic Sciences are conducting systematic, outcome-oriented research on Ayurvedic interventions for conditions such as

- Osteoarthritis,
- Metabolic syndrome,
- Gastrointestinal disorders, and
- Stress-related illnesses.

Well-documented integrative models demonstrate benefit when Ayurvedic therapies are used alongside modern medicine such as

- Panchakarma and Rasayana as adjuncts in chronic pain and geriatric care,
- Ayurvedic dietary counselling in diabetes and obesity, and
- selected herbal formulations as supportive care in oncology and palliative

settings.

Long-standing real-world models, such as the Arya Vaidya Sala, further illustrate responsible integration by combining classical Ayurveda with modern diagnostics, safety monitoring, and referral systems. Collectively, these approaches reflect a shift from parallel practice to evidence-guided, patient-centred integration, where Ayurveda contributes to holistic care while modern medicine ensures diagnostic precision and acute management.

Clinical Examples

Diabetes Management

Modern Approach: Oral hypoglycemics, insulin therapy, dietary counselling.

Complementary Addition: Yoga-based stress reduction, Ayurvedic herbs such as *methi* and *karela* under supervision, and personalized diet modifications tailored to the individual's dosha type.

Chronic Pain (Osteoarthritis, Fibromyalgia)

Modern Approach: NSAIDs, physiotherapy, joint protection.

Complementary Addition: Panchakarma detox therapies, acupuncture, turmeric and ashwagandha supplements, and regular yoga for flexibility.

Mental Health (Anxiety, Mild Depression)

Modern Approach: SSRIs, psychotherapy, lifestyle advice.

Complementary Addition: Meditation, pranayama, guided imagery, and Rasayana therapy from Ayurveda.

Palliative Care & Cancer Support

Modern Approach: Chemotherapy, pain management and nutritional support.

Complementary Addition: Homeopathy for symptomatic relief, Reiki, Ayurveda-based immunity boosters and Yoga Nidra for sleep.

Rehabilitation After Stroke or Cardiac Event

Modern Approach: Antiplatelet drugs, physiotherapy, cardiac rehab.

Complementary Addition: Naturopathic diet, breathing exercises, meditation, and gentle yogic postures to restore circulation.

Best Practices for Integrative Medicine

- Always follow evidence-based and safety-first principles.

- Open communication between practitioners of different systems.
- Shared care planning with informed consent from patients.
- Monitoring outcomes and adjusting strategies accordingly. (3)

Student Takeaway

As a future doctor, awareness of these distinctions will:

- Help you guide patients with informed, respectful advice.
- Encourage shared decision-making.
- Avoid harmful interactions between systems.
- Promote interdisciplinary collaboration in integrative health care settings.

Reflect and Write

- Have you seen or experienced any traditional remedies in your home? ------
- What surprised you about AYUSH systems? -----------------------------------
- How might these systems complement your future practice? -----------------
- What challenges do you foresee in integrative medicine? ----------------------

☕ Coffee Moment

In real clinical practice, patients often use more than one system of medicine simultaneously. Your role is not to dismiss or blindly endorse, but to guide safely. Integration in medicine is not about mixing treatments; it is about aligning care with evidence, ensuring safety, and respecting patient values.

References

1. National Institute of Health (NIH). Complementary, Alternative, or Integrative Health: What's In a Name? NCCIH; 2021.
2. Sharma H, Clark C. Contemporary Ayurveda: Medicine and Research in Maharishi Ayur-Veda. London: Churchill Livingstone; 1998.
3. Fønnebø V, Grimsgaard S, Walach H, et al. Researching complementary and alternative treatments—the gatekeepers are not at home. BMC Med Res Methodol. 2007;7:7.

Chapter 22: Principles of Family Practice

Introduction

Family Medicine is a context-based speciality that focuses on the individual behind the disease. It integrates clinical care with the patient's family, environment, beliefs, and lifestyle. Family physicians deliver socially and culturally sensitive care, ensuring prevention, education, and long-term wellness in addition to episodic treatment. Family practice provides comprehensive, continuous and personalized care. A family physician can treat acute and chronic conditions, offer preventive services, manage psychosocial issues, and build long-term therapeutic relationships with patients. Family medicine is a postgraduate speciality that trains family practitioners. (1)

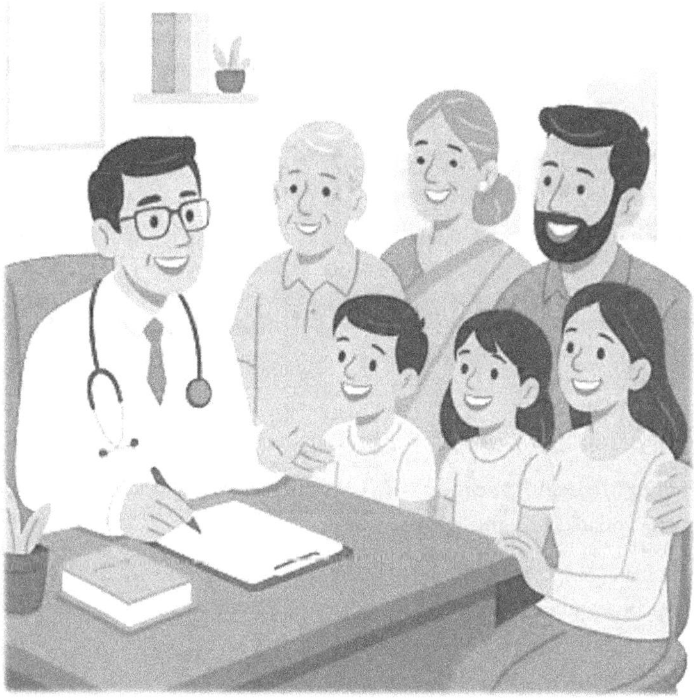

Figure 22.1: Family Physician

Importance of Family Practice in India

India's healthcare landscape presents unique challenges, including a significant rural-urban health divide, a high burden of non-communicable diseases, overburdened tertiary care centres, and limited specialist access in primary care. Family physicians bridge this gap by offering holistic care at the first point of contact and reducing unnecessary referrals. (2) The NMC emphasizes training of family physicians in home-based care, family-oriented clinical reasoning, referral coordination and patient-centred communication.

Core Principles of Family Practice

The NMC outlines the following core principles of family medicine.

Care and compassion: Empathy with patients and their families.

Clinical Competence: Making diagnoses, procedural skills, decision-making, and medical management of common conditions.

Cost-effectiveness: Availability of rational, judicious, and value-based care without over-investigation or over-treatment.

Continuity of Care: Maintaining long-term care in many health conditions.

Comprehensive Care: Managing acute, chronic, preventive, and rehabilitative care within the safe scope and timely referral to dedicated centres if needed. Refer the patient back once they are stable.

Common Problems Management: Skilled in addressing various common conditions at the primary care level.

Coordination of Care: Guiding patients through referrals, back referrals, diagnostics, specialists, and follow-up plans.

Community-based Care and Research: Addressing local health needs, engaging in fieldwork, and contributing to evidence-based interventions.

Communication Skills: Active listening, communication and counselling in emotionally, socially, and ethically complex situations.

Continuing Medical Education (CME): A lifelong commitment to learning skills and staying updated with the best practices.

These domains form the backbone of a family physician's identity, enabling them to care for people, not just patients. The Heart of Family Medicine is continuity and compassion. (3-5)

Training in Family Medicine

India now offers dedicated postgraduate training in Family Medicine through:

DNB in Family Medicine (across accredited hospitals).

MD in Family Medicine (started in select AIIMS and institutions). (2)

Training includes rotations in general medicine, paediatrics, OBG, psychiatry, dermatology, geriatrics, community health, palliative care, and emergency services. These programs focus on broad clinical skills, empathy, and follow-up care, equipping doctors to serve communities efficiently. Christian Medical College

Vellore has pioneered family medicine in India.

Family Practice Around the World

United Kingdom: In the United Kingdom, a General Practitioner (GP) is equivalent to a family physician. GPs act as the first point of contact in the NHS and manage over 90% of healthcare interactions. After medical college, they undergo three years of speciality training in community-based, multi-system, and whole-person care. Gaining global recognition, UK GPs are known for gatekeeping specialist care and coordinating long-term care. They work with electronic health records, evidence-based protocols and participate in research, audits addressing national health priorities. The UK model has inspired reforms in India to position family medicine as a key pillar in the national health strategy.

United States: In the U.S., Family Medicine certification requires a 3-year residency after medical school. Training includes internal medicine, paediatrics, obstetrics and gynaecology, psychiatry, surgery, and geriatrics. Family physicians play a crucial role in primary care. They have opportunities in academics, global health, public health, and integrative medicine.

Australia: Family medicine is known as General Practice, and governed by the Royal Australian College of General Practitioners. Training consists of a 3-to 4-year fellowship that includes preventive care, chronic disease management, Indigenous health, and remote healthcare delivery. GPs are highly respected, well-compensated, and fully integrated into the national healthcare framework.

Middle East: Family medicine is gaining recognition through structured postgraduate programs aligned with international standards. The UAE and Saudi Arabia have also developed family medicine residency programs. Family physicians are in high demand in these regions.

Opportunities in Family Practice

What Family Physicians Do

They provide holistic care across all age groups, manage common illnesses, perform minor procedures, offer antenatal and pediatric care, support elderly health, and guide families on nutrition, hygiene, and mental well-being.

Where They Work

Family physicians are integral across the public and private sectors. They are becoming relevant across different levels of the healthcare system, from PHCs and urban clinics to telemedicine platforms, NGOs, and medical colleges.

Career Growth

Running or joining primary care clinics.
Teaching in DNB and MD programs.
Leading telehealth and digital health initiatives.
Contributing to national missions such as NHM and PM-JAY.
Emerging role in research, policy, or community leadership.
With universal health coverage gaining momentum in India, family physicians will play a key role in healthcare delivery in future.

☕ Coffee Moment

It's Sunday morning, and you're home after weeks in the hostel. Over chai with your parents, your mother shares how the family doctor once stayed late to check on your grandmother, and how he knew the story of every family member.

Reflect and Write

Have you or your family interacted with a family doctor? ----------------------

What qualities make them impactful? --

How do you feel about becoming the first point of contact for a family? -------

References

1. McWhinney IR, Freeman T. Textbook of Family Medicine. 3rd ed. Oxford University Press; 2016.
2. Kumar R. Family medicine at AIIMS and in India: Past, present, and future. Natl Med J India. 2011;24(6):365–7.
3. National Medical Commission. Competency Based Undergraduate Curriculum for the Indian Medical Graduate. Vol. 1. New Delhi: NMC; 2018. (See competencies under Community Medicine and Family Medicine).
4. National Medical Commission. Attitude, Ethics and Communication (AETCOM) Module for the Undergraduate Medical Curriculum. New Delhi: NMC; 2019.
5. Starfield B, Shi L, Macinko J. Contribution of primary care to health systems and health. Milbank Q. 2005;83(3):457–502.

Matrix

A *Matrix* is both a framework and an environment,

the ground in which life takes root, and the structure that holds everything in place.

Here, you will move to understand the larger ecosystem that shapes every patient encounter.

Health in India is not only about doctors and hospitals,

but also about systems, policies, programs, and the interplay between public and private forces and finances.

The Matrix highlights key elements of healthcare,

how healthcare infrastructure is built and stretched, and

why public health programs specifically target certain diseases.

The role of agencies and institutions as unseen support for the nation's health response;

The persistent inequities between rural and urban areas, and rich and poor communities,

challenge us to find solutions.

Matrix represents the living web you join, connecting your stethoscope to the pulse of the nation.

S No.	Matrix: At a Glance
1.	**Chapter 23** Overview: The Living Body of Healthcare The anatomy, physiology, and biochemistry of India's healthcare system: a body with its own pulse, pathways, and blockages.
2.	**Chapter 24** Tiers of the Public Healthcare System in India From sub-centres to AIIMS: the pyramid of care and the promise of reaching the last mile.
3.	**Chapter 25** Health Workforce in India: The Faces Behind the System Doctors, nurses, ASHAs, ANMs, and allied staff: the human engine that keeps the healthcare machine alive.
4.	**Chapter 26** Health Infrastructure in India: Buildings, Beds, and Beyond The hardware of care: hospitals, beds, diagnostics, cold chains, ambulances, telemedicine, and digital bridges.
5.	**Chapter 27** The Indian Healthcare Paradox The uneasy duality: government hospitals as lifelines, private hospitals as powerhouses, and patients caught in between. Other cracks and triumphs.
6.	**Chapter 28** National Health Agencies and Targeted Missions The councils, commissions, and missions that steer India's health battles: from TB to NCDs, from immunization to maternal care.
7.	**Chapter 29** Health Financing in India: Who Pays and How? The invisible bloodstream of healthcare: budgets, insurance, out-of-pocket payments, and the dream of Universal Health Coverage.

Chapter 23: The Living Body of Healthcare

Introduction

Before you master the structure and function of the human body, take a moment to understand the living system that surrounds it: the healthcare system itself. You've stepped into a world where every heartbeat, every breath, and every cry for help must be heard, not only by a doctor, but by a system designed to heal. This system is vast, multilayered, and often invisible in textbooks. But it is the true playground of medicine. Before you open Gray's Anatomy or attend lectures on physiology, explore the structure and function of a different kind of body: the healthcare delivery system. Every doctor, works within a national framework that defines our collective mission. This framework is shaped by India's National Health Policy and Health Goals, which are more than bureaucratic targets; they are promises to the people. If medicine involves understanding the human body, public health involves understanding the body of society. You must know how to treat a patient and how to heal a system. This section is your introduction to that larger, invisible patient, the healthcare system, with its own pulse, needs, and soul.

Drawing the Analogy: Structure, Function, and Flow

Think of this section as your first preclinical subject in public health:

Table 23.1: Anatomy, Physiology and Biochemistry of Public Health

Medical Subject	Public Health Parallel
Anatomy	Structure of the healthcare system
Physiology	Function of how healthcare is delivered
Biochemistry	The forces, reactions, and energy flow in the system, from policies and budgets to care and innovation

Healthcare Anatomy: The Structure

As the human body has bones, muscles, and organs arranged into systems, the healthcare system has its anatomical layers:

- **Subcenters, PHCs, and CHCs** address primary and basic health needs.
- **District hospitals and medical colleges** offer a wide range of clinical care.
- **National institutions and ministries** form the framework that unifies everything through policies, regulations, budgets, and so on.

We will explore the structure of healthcare, including its physical and administrative layout, the roles of individuals, and how patients navigate through the system.

Healthcare Physiology: The Function

Imagine this in motion, as physiology describes how heart beats, and lungs breathe.

- How does a child in a tribal village receive a vaccine?
- How can a stroke patient reach a neurologist?
- How can a distressed newborn find an ICU in a district with few doctors?

This is healthcare physiology: how services are delivered, how systems respond under stress, how referrals are made, and how policies are translated into action. ASHAs and ANMs play a crucial role as healthcare workers (HCWs), reaching every corner of society. As physiology cannot be understood without the context of nutrition, environment, and lifestyle, health systems also depend on what are called the social determinants of health - factors like income, education, sanitation, and gender equity. These shape whether a community stays healthy or falls ill, often more powerfully than medicines or hospitals themselves (1,2).

Healthcare Biochemistry: The Invisible Reactions

Let's explore further. What causes the system to function (or dysfunction)? What drives the movement, the money, the policies, the ethics, the resistance? Biochemistry of healthcare includes:

- Health budgets (the glucose).
- Political will and Insurance schemes (the enzymes and co-enzymes).
- Doctors and HCWs are the ATP - the currency of energy that drives the system.
- Resistance to change or systemic corruption (the metabolic blocks).

Like the human body, a single point of failure, a missing resource, a delay, or a poor policy can cause the system to suffer, with patients and the nation paying the price. As diseases arise when organs fail to coordinate, health systems falter when policies, providers, and individuals lose alignment. (3) Learning about healthcare systems is not extra work. It's your first taste of real-world medicine. (4) You may wonder why you need to learn this as a student. In a few months, you will meet patients not in textbooks, but in real villages, wards, and urban slums.

You need to understand what care is possible, not what is ideal. Understanding the system allows you to navigate, advocate, and innovate, whether you choose to be a rural family doctor, a superspecialist, or a policymaker.

National Health Policy

Every nation's progress is reflected not only in its economy, but in the health and well-being of its people. India's national health policy (NHP) and goals serve as the collective blueprint for achieving this. (5-7)

Framework and Goals

The National Health Policy 2017 serves as the guiding document for health system. It aims to achieve the highest possible level of health and well-being for all, through:

- **Universal access:** Every citizen, regardless of income or geography, can access good-quality healthcare. (universal access)
- **Preventive and promotive care:** The system focuses more on prevention and health promotion rather than only treating disease.
- **Reduction of out-of-pocket expenditure:** Healthcare should not push families into financial distress.
- **Collective responsibility**: Across sectors, including education, sanitation, nutrition, environment, and gender equality.
- **Integration** of traditional Indian medicine systems (AYUSH) in healthcare for promoting healthy lifestyles.

The key objectives of the NHP 2017, with their current status, are as follows.

Table 23.2: NHP 2017- Goals and current status

Indicator	NHP 2017 Goals	Status
Public Health Expenditure	Increase to 2.5% of GDP by 2025.	Expenditure 1.6% of GDP in 2021-22.
Maternal Mortality Ratio (MMR) per lakh live births	Reduce MMR to 100 by 2020 and 90 by 2025.	MMR from 130 (1914-16) to 97 in 2022. SDG target of 70 by 2030.
Infant Mortality Rate (IMR)	28 per 1,000 live births by 2019.	From 39 (2014) to 27 achieved by 2020.
Under-5 Mortality Rate (U5MR)	Reduce U5MR to 23 by 2025.	U5MR dropped to 32 in 2020. Challenge remains.
Total Fertility Rate (TFR)	Achieve and sustain a TFR of 2.1 by 2025.	TFR reached 2.0 by 2020, (replacement level fertility)
Non-Communicable Diseases (NCDs)	Reduce premature mortality from NCDs by 25% by 2025.	Remains challenging despite significant focus.
Disease Elimination	Kala-Azar by 2017 and TB by 2025.	Progress in Kala-Azar; TB remains a challenge.

Digital Health Systems and Innovation for Accessibility

The National Health Mission (NHM) serves as the primary mechanism for implementing India's health policies and is comprised of the National Rural Health Mission (NRHM) and the National Urban Health Mission (NUHM), focusing on healthcare in rural and urban areas, respectively. Ayushman Bharat is another significant initiative aimed at universal health coverage, operating through a "continuum of care" model. It includes the Pradhan Mantri Jan Arogya Yojana (PM-

JAY), a health insurance scheme providing up to ₹5 lakh coverage per family for hospitalization, and the establishment of Health and Wellness Centres (HWCs) to enhance primary healthcare services.

Challenges

Public health spending remains below the target, impacting infrastructure and workforce development. The target of decreasing the proportion of households facing catastrophic health expenditure by 25% by 2025 remains a challenge, despite significant improvements made by the PM-JAY and Ayushman Bharat schemes. The Ayushman Bharat Digital Mission (ABDM) has led to the creation of numerous health accounts; however, we are far behind the target of establishing district-level digital databases by 2020 and an integrated health information architecture by 2025. We will explore the paradoxes and triumphs in the chapters to come.

Coffee Moment

You are posted at a Community Health Centre in a remote part. A pregnant woman arrives in labour. The ANM looks at you and says, "There's no power; the ambulance will take 2 hours." You panic and call your professor. She calmly says, "Use what you have. Remember your referral pathway. Start preparing for a safe delivery." You not only learn medicine, but you also learn the system that holds medicine together.

References

1. World Health Organization. Everybody's business: Strengthening health systems to improve health outcomes. WHO's framework for action. Geneva: WHO; 2007.
2. Frenk J, Gómez-Dantés O. Health systems in transition: The Mexico experiment. Lancet. 2009;374(9707):1788–96.
3. Kruk ME, et al. Building resilient health systems: a proposal for a resilience index. BMJ. 2017;357:j2323.
4. WHO. Monitoring the building blocks of health systems: a handbook of indicators and their measurement strategies. Geneva: WHO; 2010.
5. Ministry of Health and Family Welfare. National Health Policy 2017. Government of India, New Delhi; 2017. Available from: https://main.mohfw.gov.in/sites/default/files/9147562941489753121.pdf
6. National Health Mission. Framework for Implementation – National Health Mission 2025. Ministry of Health and Family Welfare, Government of India; 2022. Available from: https://nhm.gov.in
7. NITI Aayog. SDG India Index and Dashboard 2024–25. New Delhi: NITI Aayog, Government of India; 2024. Available from: https://sdgindiaindex.niti.gov.in

Chapter 24: Tiers of the Public Healthcare System in India

Introduction

From a small village sub-centre to a national referral institute, India's public healthcare is a pyramid built on the promise of reaching the last mile. India's public health delivery system is a structured, tiered network designed to deliver care as close to people as possible and escalate the service as complexity increases. Imagine it like a ladder: Basic prevention and education are at the bottom rung, and critical care, organ transplants and high-end surgeries are at the top. This chapter explores each tier, from the village level to apex institutions.

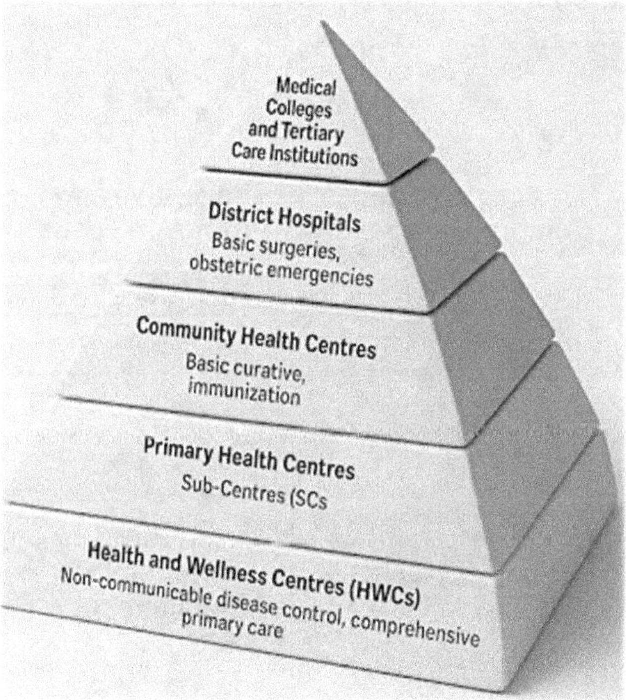

Figure 24.1: Tiers of Public Healthcare System in India

Sub-Centres: The First Footprint

Sub-Centres (SCs) are the most peripheral contact points between the health system and the community. They form the foundation of preventive and promotive healthcare.

- Cover a population of 5,000 in plains and 3,000 in hilly/tribal areas.

- Staffed by Auxiliary Nurse Midwives (ANMs) and occasionally male health workers.

A sub-centre may be small, but it saves lives before they even fall sick. The strength of a pyramid lies in its base; if sub-centres fail, the burden shifts disproportionately upward. (1)

Sub-Centre to Ayushman Aarogya Mandir

In 2018, with the launch of Ayushman Bharat, India began one of the most ambitious reforms in its health system, transforming the traditional sub-centres and primary health centres into Health and Wellness Centres (HWCs), now renamed as 'Ayushman Aarogya Mandirs'. This shift represents a decisive move from limited, selective services to comprehensive primary healthcare for all.

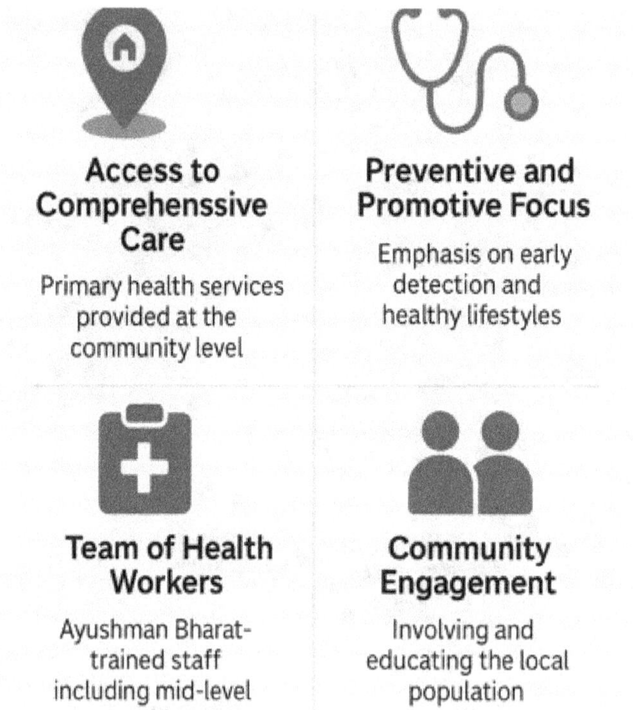
Access to Comprehenssive Care
Primary health services provided at the community level
Preventive and Promotive Focus
Emphasis on early detection and healthy lifestyles
Team of Health Workers
Ayushman Bharat-trained staff including mid-level
Community Engagement
Involving and educating the local population

Figure 24.2: Ayushman Aarogya Mandir

These Ayushman Aarogya Mandirs are designed to be the primary point of contact for families, providing quality healthcare. They deliver a wide range of services, including care for non-communicable diseases, mental health, palliative and rehabilitative care, oral health, ophthalmic and ENT problems, and emergency medical support. (2) Key Features of Ayushman Aarogya Mandirs:

- **Expanded primary care team:** Community Health Officer (CHO), Auxiliary Nurse Midwife (ANM), and Multipurpose Worker (MPW).
- **Free drugs and diagnostics:** Ensuring treatment is not denied because of cost.
- **Screening and early detection:** Hypertension, diabetes, cancers, mental health conditions, and more.
- **Digital integration:** Electronic health records, teleconsultation via *eSanjeevani*, and referral linkages to higher centres.
- **Community outreach:** Health education, awareness drives, and wellness activities, such as yoga sessions.

With a target of 1.5 lakh Ayushman Aarogya Mandirs by 2025, India is building a network where healthcare is closer, broader, and more holistic, a true reflection of health as a public right, not a privilege.

Primary Health Centres: The Basecamp

The PHC is the cornerstone of India's rural health mission, the first formal place where a doctor may be posted.

- Every 5-6 sub-centres report to one Primary Health Centre (PHCs).
- Cover 30,000 population in plains and 20,000 in hilly areas.
- Staffed with a medical officer, nurses, a pharmacist, and a lab technician.
- Provide basic curative care, maternal-child services, disease control, and health promotion.
- Many PHCs, in addition to SCs, are now being upgraded into Health & Wellness Centres under Ayushman Bharat.

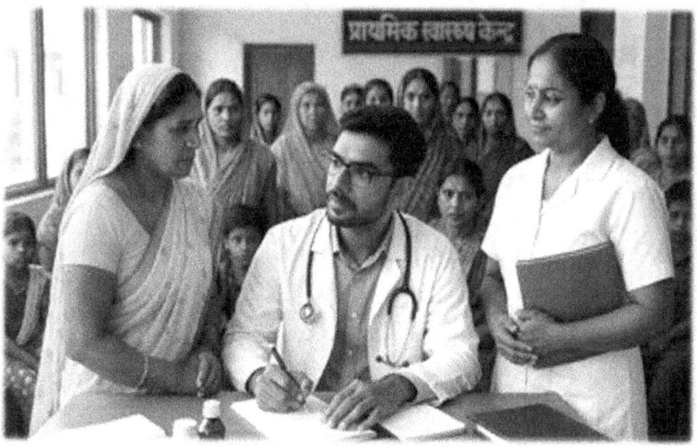

Figure 24.3: Primary Health Centre

Community Health Centre: The First Referral Unit

Every 4 PHCs are linked to a Community Health Centre (CHCs):

- Covers 80,000-1.2 lakh population
- Meant to have four specialists: a surgeon, a physician, an OBGYN, and a paediatrician
- Equipped for basic surgeries, obstetric emergencies, and inpatient care
- Often overburdened and under-resourced, but vital for bridging PHC and district hospitals.

The CHC is the emergency room of rural India - sometimes lifesaving, sometimes overwhelmed.

District Hospitals: The Nerve Centres

Every district should have a District Hospital (DH) as the nodal secondary-level referral centre.

- Offers specialist care, surgery, diagnostics, and inpatient services.
- May have 100–600 beds or more.
- Increasingly upgraded to Medical Colleges under centrally sponsored schemes.
- DHs often also run training programs for paramedics and nurses.

In a well-functioning health system, most patients should be treated up to this level; only the most complex cases need further referral.

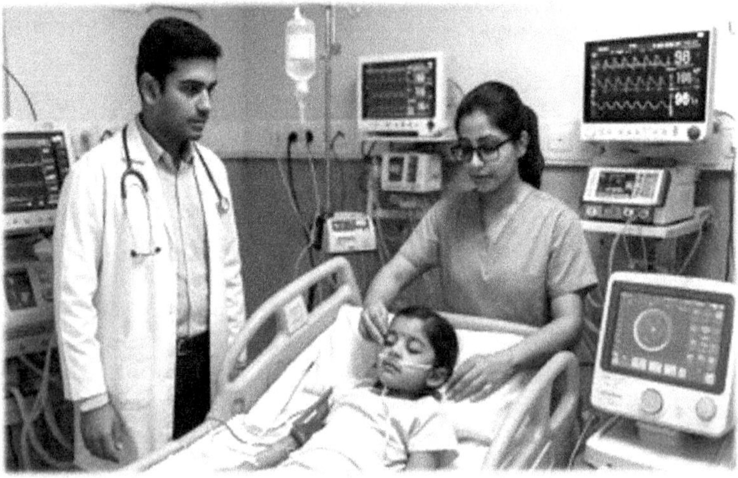

Figure 24.4: Emergency Room of a District or Medical College Hospital

Medical Colleges and Tertiary Care Institutions

This category includes State Medical Colleges and Institutes of national importance, as well as super-speciality hospitals such as AIIMS, PGIMER, JIPMER, SGPGI, and NIMHANS. Primary functions of these centres are to-

- Manage complex cases requiring multispecialty care, advanced procedures and surgeries, critical care, and sophisticated diagnostics and interventions.
- Serve as training centres for advanced medical and paramedical education.
- Conduct research, clinical trials, and develop innovative treatment modalities.
- Often function as referral points for lower-tier healthcare facilities.
- Contribute to or help shape national policies and protocols.

Vertical Programs and Outreach

Beyond the physical pyramid, there are horizontal (community-based) and vertical (disease-specific) initiatives:

- Immunization drives
- Polio campaigns
- Mobile health vans
- TB control, malaria, and HIV programs

These initiatives ensure that healthcare doesn't wait for the patient to arrive; it reaches the people.

Integration and Continuity: A Pyramid or a Puzzle?

Ideally, these tiers work harmoniously, with clear referral pathways and shared patient information. But in reality

- Any patient can bypass the lower levels and head directly to tertiary hospitals.
- PHCs and CHCs are underutilised or non-functional in some regions
- Referral mechanisms are weak or missing.
- Even today, some CHCs run without specialists, highlighting the need for equitable distribution of the workforce. (3)

This leads to a chaotic flow of patients and overburdened tertiary care centres with misplaced priorities, primarily handling crowds of patients who could easily be managed at lower levels. India is now working to rebuild linkages, digitise records, and make the system people-centred through AB-HWCs, Ayushman Bharat Digital Mission, and eSanjeevani telemedicine.

☕ Coffee Moment

You're posted at a PHC. A woman walks in with a labour complication. You stabilize her and refer her to the CHC.
Two days later, her husband returns with sweets.

"She delivered safely, doctor saab… Thank you for sending us on time."

That moment is quiet. No applause. No awards.
A life, safely brought into the world, because the system worked, and you made it work.

References

1. Government of India. Rural Health Statistics 2021-22. Ministry of Health and Family Welfare.
2. Ministry of Health and Family Welfare. Ayushman Bharat – Comprehensive Primary Health Care through Health and Wellness Centres. 2018.
3. Prinja S, et al. Performance of health systems in India: A review of the National Health Mission. Lancet. 2017;389(10065):2437–48.

Chapter 25: Health Workforce – Faces Behind the System

Introduction

In the most high-tech ICU or the quietest village dispensary, the real healthcare engine is not the machines, it's the people. India's health workforce is a diverse, dynamic, and at times overwhelmed community of professionals working to serve over 1.4 billion people. This chapter explores the diverse backgrounds of these individuals, ranging from barefoot workers to cutting-edge surgeons and intensive care specialists, and examines how each contributes to the nation's healthcare fabric.

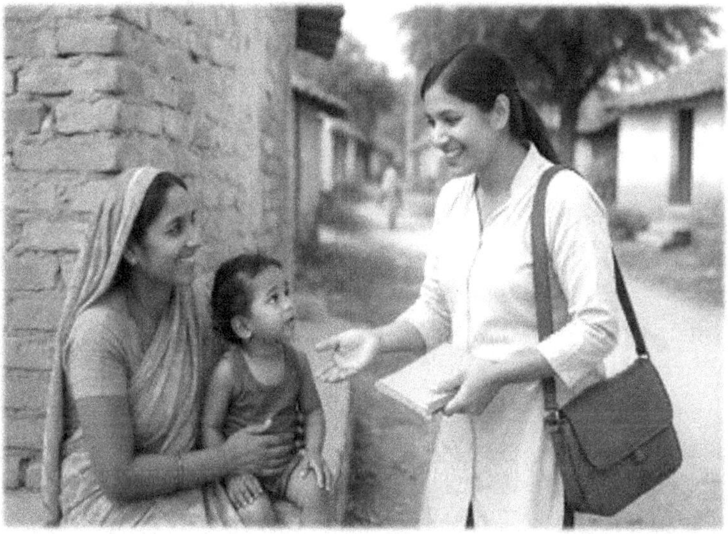

Figure 25.1: ASHA Worker in Field

The Backbone: Doctors, Nurses, and Allied Health Professionals

India has:

- More than 13 lakh registered allopathic doctors
- About 8 lakh AYUSH doctors
- More than 35 lakh nursing personnel

A growing cadre of allied health professionals, including lab technicians, physiotherapists, radiology assistants, and emergency care providers
However, the distribution is highly urban-centric, with a severe shortage in rural and remote regions. (1)

The First Responders: ASHAs, ANMs, and MPWs

They are the unsung heroes of community health:

- **Accredited Social Health Activists (ASHAs):** Every village has one. They mobilize, educate, track pregnant women, follow up on TB and immunizations, and connect the system with the community.
- **Auxiliary Nurse Midwives (ANMs):** Serve at sub-centres, providing antenatal care, facilitating deliveries, offering family planning, and administering vaccinations.
- **Male Multi-Purpose Workers (MPWs):** Often work on vector-borne diseases, sanitation, and response to outbreaks.

Hybrid System

India's health system comprises traditional healers as well as tech-savvy healthcare providers.

- Allopathy.
- AYUSH (Ayurveda, Yoga, Unani, Siddha, and Homeopathy).
- Registered Medical Practitioners (RMPs) in rural areas (some trained, some informal).
- Now, with digital health, new roles are emerging:
- Teleconsultation coordinators.
- Digital health assistants.
- E-health village volunteers.
- This ecosystem is becoming hybrid, holistic, and technology-aided.

Urban-Rural Gap vis-à-vis Public-Private Gap

Recent studies have highlighted several important observations regarding healthcare distribution in India:

- Approximately 70% of medical professionals are concentrated in urban areas, whereas 65% of the population lives in rural regions.
- There is a significant shortage of specialists within Community Health Centres (CHCs) and district hospitals.
- Many medical colleges and Institutes of National Importance (INIs) are experiencing a critical shortage of faculty members. Retention in the government sector, particularly in rural areas, is challenging due to poor incentives and quality of life. (2)

Gender in the Workforce: Strengths and Struggles

- Women dominate roles like nursing, ASHAs, and ANMs.
- Most leadership positions are still predominantly held by men.
- Female healthcare workers face safety issues in fieldwork and work-life balance challenges.

Brain Drain: Achievement or loss

India also faces an outward migration of doctors and nurses, which impacts the availability of healthcare at home while benefiting the host country. (3)

Training, Regulation, and Accountability

Key institutions include

- NMC: Regulates MBBS/MD education and ethics.
- Indian Nursing Council (INC) and State Nursing Councils.
- National Commission for Allied and Healthcare Professions (NCAHP) for allied roles.

Challenges

- Quality gaps between private and public colleges.
- Limited continuing medical education (CME).
- Ethics violations and a lack of accountability mechanisms.
- Competency-Based Medical Education (CBME) is now a step forward in bridging many gaps.

The Road Ahead: Reskilling, Respect, and Reform

To strengthen the workforce:

- More health professionals need training with equitable placement and ethical support.
- Different and innovative career pathways need to be planned for community-level workers.
- Mental health and professionalism need more focus.
- Capacity building using innovative and digital media.

☕ Coffee Moment

It's 5 AM. The PHC is asleep.
You're doing your internship when an ANM walks in, wiping sweat from her brow.
She just helped a tribal woman deliver twins - one breech.

You offer her tea. She waves you off.

"Have to check on another one. She had a fall last night."

You realize: You're not the hero here. She is.

These frontline workers remind us that resilience in health care is not built by machines, but by people. (4)

References

1. World Health Organization. Global Health Workforce Statistics. WHO; 2022.
2. Rao M, Rao KD, Kumar AK, Chatterjee M, Sundararaman T. Human resources for health in India. Lancet. 2011 Feb 12;377(9765):587-98.
3. Sheikh K, Josyula LK, Zhang X, Bigdeli M, Ahmed SM. Governing the mixed health workforce: learning from Asian experiences. BMJ Glob Health. 2017 Apr 7;2(2):e000267.
4. The health workforce in India. World Health Organization (2016). https://iris.who.int/handle/10665/250369

Chapter 26: Health Infrastructure- Buildings, Beds & Beyond

"A doctor needs more than a stethoscope - space, staff, supplies, and systems."

Introduction

Behind every health intervention, whether it is a vaccination, surgery, or delivery, lies a complex infrastructure. It's not just hospitals and beds; it's the cold chains, labs, ambulances, telemedicine kiosks, and even the toilets that together define how care is delivered. As a crucial operator, you need to know all this. This chapter takes you through the hardware of India's healthcare system, its buildings, equipment, and physical reach.

Health Infrastructure

Health infrastructure includes-

System

- Physical Buildings: Sub-centres, PHCs, CHCs, district hospitals, medical colleges, AIIMS.
- ICT Tools: Telemedicine platforms, digital health records.
- Logistics: Ambulances, mobile medical vans, supply chains.

Space

- Beds: Number of beds per 1000 population (India: ~1.3/1000 in 2023).
- Duty rooms, offices, stores and circulation area.

Staff

- Doctor, Nurses, paramedical staff, and security to run the system.
- Administrative hierarchy.

Stuff (Supplies)

- Medical Equipment: oxygen delivery devices, IV fluid and drug delivery, infusion pumps, BiPAP machines, ventilators, X-ray machines, lab analyzers and more.
- Drugs and consumables.
- Sanitation & Utilities: Clean water, power backup, and proper disposal of biomedical waste.

Public Sector Infrastructure: A Tiered Model

India's public health infrastructure is organized as below:

Table 26.1: Public health infrastructure in India

Level	Approx. Numbers (2023)	Typical Services
Sub-Centres	1.6 lakh	Immunization, antenatal care, health education
PHCs	30,000	Outpatient care, minor procedures, NCD screening
CHCs	6,000	30-bed facilities with delivery rooms, labs
District Hospitals	1,200	Specialist services, surgery, blood bank
Medical Colleges & INIs	700+ colleges	Education, research, super-specialty care

Many of these centres are now being upgraded under Ayushman Bharat Health Infrastructure Mission (PM-ASBY).

Private Sector Infrastructure: Growth & Gaps

Private healthcare plays a huge role in India:

- Over 60% of hospital admissions.
- More than 70% of diagnostics and OPD care.

But the private sector is:

- Concentrated in urban areas.
- Highly variable in quality and cost.
- Often unregulated.

It ranges from:

- World-class hospitals (Apollo, Fortis, Medanta).
- To single-doctor nursing homes in towns.
- To informal providers in villages.

Health Infrastructure Gaps: The Missing Pieces

Despite establishing numerous new medical colleges, digital health programs, and expanding insurance coverage, fundamental infrastructure gaps continue to impede frontline healthcare delivery, particularly in rural and underserved areas. India continues to face a shortage of hospital beds and infrastructure compared to global standards. (1) Let's see some of these critical deficiencies:

Shortage of Doctors at the Frontline Health Care Level

Many PHCs and CHCs continue to function without full-time doctors, adequate

ANMs and other staff, especially in remote districts. Vacancies arise from genuine reasons, including the unwillingness of trained doctors to serve in rural areas that lack adequate housing, education for children, and safety.

Broken Chain of Labs and Diagnostic Delays

Functional laboratory services are essential for diagnosing malaria, TB, diabetes, anaemia, and pregnancy complications. But in many PHCs

- There's no technician or equipment.
- Diagnostic delays cause avoidable referrals.
- Patients end up spending time and money on private labs.

Electricity and Water Supply

Many PHCs still lack access to uninterrupted electricity, running water, or clean toilets.

Shortage of Beds and Medicines

- Many PHCs (4-6 beds) and CHCs (30 beds) do not have the mandated inpatient beds.
- Essential drugs, such as antibiotics, iron-folic acid, and anti-diabetic medicines, are frequently out of stock. This increases out-of-pocket expenses.

Missing Emergency and Surgical Services

Many CHCs and district hospitals still lack ICUs, ventilators, surgical facilities, blood storage units, and round-the-clock ambulance availability. Disparities are stark, with rural areas having fewer health facilities and beds than urban centres. (2)

Recent Missions and Initiatives

The government has undertaken numerous initiatives to transform India's healthcare infrastructure. Initiatives such as the National Health Mission and Ayushman Bharat have expanded primary and secondary infrastructure. (3)

- **PM-Ayushman Bharat Health Infrastructure Mission (PM-ABHIM):** Capacity building by strengthening the network of labs, surveillance units, ICU beds and by creating rural and urban health and wellness centres.
- **Comprehensive pediatric care unit for critical care delivery at district hospitals under ECRP-II:** Creating a network of Tele PICU and guided ER management.
- **Emergency and Trauma Care Networks**: Developing regional trauma centres and expansion of ambulance services.
- **Public-Private Partnerships**: Developing dialysis centres, cancer care hubs and

CT scan services.

- **Digital Health Mission**: Creation of unique health IDs and building electronic health record systems.

Telemedicine and Mobile Health

If patients can't reach hospitals, let hospitals reach patients.

- **eSanjeevani** platform: Over 12 crore consultations (as of 2024).
- **Mobile Medical Units (MMUs)**: Vans equipped with basic outpatient department (OPD) services and diagnostics.
- Digital pathology, teleradiology, tele-ICU, and AI-driven triage are expanding.

These solutions are particularly important for hilly, tribal, and underserved regions. Ensuring sustainable financing and investment in infrastructure is critical to achieving Universal Health Coverage. (4)

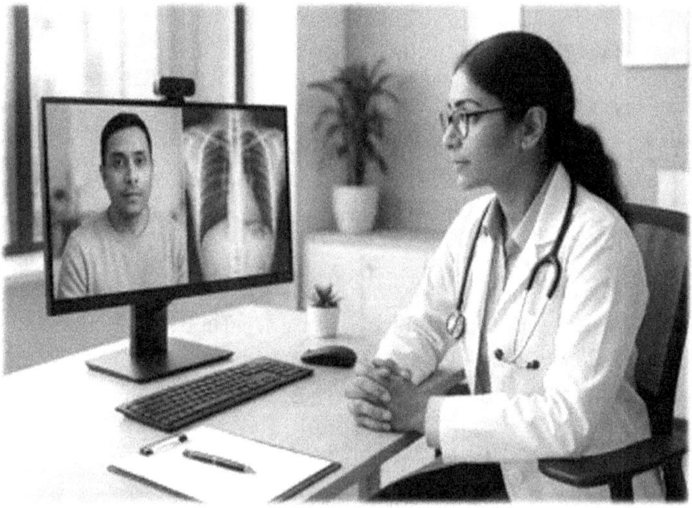

Figure 26.1: Telemedicine

Your Role as a Future Doctor

You'll be expected to:

- Know infrastructure referral pathways (SC → PHC → CHC → DH → Tertiary).
- Make the most of limited resources in rural postings.
- Maintain equipment hygiene and report gaps.
- Utilise digital tools such as ABHA ID, HMIS, Nikshay, and others.

Student Reflection

Fancy buildings are not enough; a real hospital is not only space but a reliable system, staff, supplies, power, and purpose.

Rural India still lacks many of these, yet doctors often do more with less.

If you have the opportunity to work in such a setting, your understanding, empathy, and advocacy will make a significant difference in the lives of the people you serve.

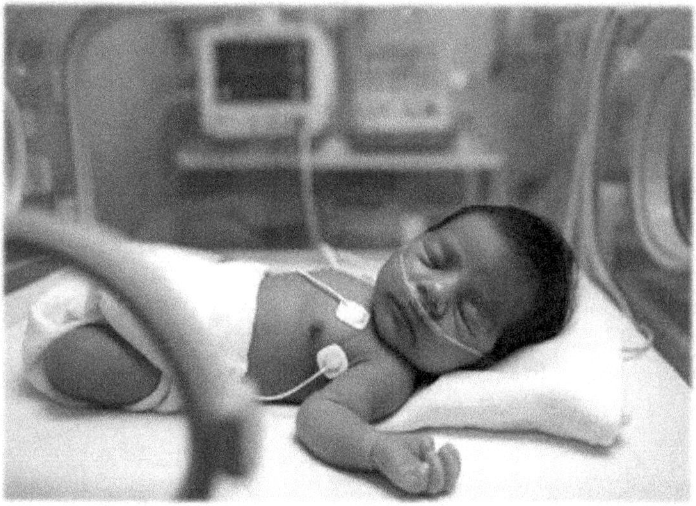

Figure 26.2: A Newborn in SNCU

☕ Coffee Moment

You arrive at your PHC on a stormy day. A pregnant woman walks in, expecting to deliver a premature baby in the next few hours. You quickly evaluate your resources, understand the potential complications, stabilize her with oxygen and IV fluids, arrange for an ambulance with an ANM to escort her, and contact the nearby district hospital to refer her after discussion there.

The telemonitor in the ambulance didn't work, but you stayed in touch with the nurse via WhatsApp video. They reached the district hospital in two hours. Stable! A premature delivery occurred after three hours; the baby needed resuscitation and was admitted to the SNCU.

Two weeks later, the baby's father came with sweets! Thanks, Doctor Saheb. Now the baby is discharged. Mother is healthy!

No ICU. No team. But a timely referral saved two lives!

"You may not fix the system overnight. But you can be the reason someone doesn't have to sleep outside a hospital tonight."

References

V - Matrix ♥ 138

1. World Health Organization. Global Health Observatory: Hospital bed density (per 10,000 population). Geneva: WHO; 2023.
2. National Health Systems Resource Centre. National Health Accounts Estimates for India (2019–20). New Delhi: Ministry of Health and Family Welfare; 2022.
3. Ministry of Health and Family Welfare. National Health Mission: Framework for Implementation. New Delhi: Government of India; 2012.
4. Government of India, NITI Aayog. Health Systems for a New India: Building Blocks. New Delhi: NITI Aayog; 2019

Chapter 27: The Indian Healthcare Paradox

Introduction

India's healthcare is a paradox, underfunded and overburdened, yet inspiring, innovative, and indomitable. It is a system that can perform free heart surgeries in one hospital and run out of paracetamol in another. It produces world-class specialists and still struggles to place a doctor in every PHC. Let's explore the contradictions and courage that characterize Indian healthcare.

Public and Private: The Two Engines of Indian Healthcare

Patients who fall ill face a crucial decision: Where should I go for treatment? Government hospital? Private clinic? Traditional healer? Teleconsultation? India has one of the largest healthcare systems in the world, serving over 1.4 billion people. (1) Welcome to the dynamic, complex, and occasionally chaotic dual system of Indian healthcare: Public vs. Private. Let's explore how it works.

The Public Sector: Care for All, Challenges for Many

Through the network of National Health Mission, PHCs, CHCs, district hospitals and medical colleges, the public sector provides the backbone of health services. (2)

- It is Government-funded (by both state and central governments).
- Designed to offer universal, low-cost or free care.
- Organised in a tiered system: Sub-centres → PHCs → CHCs → District Hospitals → Medical Colleges.
- Handles a large volume of patients.
- Generally, the only system in rural areas
- Provides vital services such as immunization, maternity care, and emergency treatment.
- Integrates National health programs (like TB, malaria, and maternal-child health).

However, challenges include understaffed and overburdened facilities, infrastructure gaps, long waiting times, inadequate equipment, and variable quality. Despite this, public hospitals are often the only lifeline for millions of people.

Utilization Trends (2017–2023)

The shift in utilisation trends reflects the improved public healthcare access and infrastructure that have developed over the last decade, particularly in rural areas.

Table 27.1: Utilization trends of public and private health sectors (2017-23)

Area	Public Sector Use	Private Sector Use
Rural	↑ public sector use from 41.9% → 45.7%	↓ private sector use from 58.1% → 54.3%
Urban	↑ public sector use from 31% → 35.3%	↓ private sector use from 69% → 64.7%

The Private Sector: Diverse and Expanding

The private sector dominates in secondary and tertiary care, accounting for the major share of hospital beds and outpatient visits. (3) The private sector in India encompasses:

- High-end corporate hospitals.
- Small town clinics and charitable hospitals.
- Informal practitioners and quacks at the village level who lack formal degrees.

Key characteristics:

- Often regarded as quicker, cleaner, and more efficient.
- Attracts the majority of urban and middle-class patients.

But there are risks:

- High costs. Nearly 50–60% of health expenditure in India is out-of-pocket, pushing millions into poverty every year. (4)
- Ethical concerns: over-investigation and unnecessary procedures.
- Inconsistent quality, particularly in unregulated small setups.

The Coexistence

India's healthcare system is a dual pulse, side by side yet seldom in sync.

The private sector makes a significant contribution to healthcare, but the public sector serves as the primary safety net.

The lower and middle-income groups primarily seek public healthcare or non-corporate private care.

Government schemes (like PM-JAY) are bridging the gap by engaging private hospitals to provide subsidized care to scheme beneficiaries.

Where They Meet: Public–Private Partnerships

Through the Public–Private Partnership (PPP) models, government schemes like Ayushman Bharat seek to bridge this gap by providing financial protection and engaging both public and private providers. (5)

- Private diagnostics in government hospitals.
- Ambulance services, such as 108 EMRI.
- Government schemes that allow private hospitals to treat public patients.

Your Role: A Doctor in a Diversified System

As a future doctor, you may:

- Work in a government hospital with thousands of patients a day
- Join a private hospital
- Serve in an NGO or telemedicine startup, bridging the two
- Advocate for ethical care in either system

Reflection

Can the government and private sector collaborate, or will profit motives always create conflict?

The Paradox of Priorities

India spends only around 2.1% of its GDP on health (2023 estimate), which is low for a country of its size and ambition. Yet, it runs the world's largest immunization program, substantial health insurance schemes, and significant public health missions like Ayushman Bharat. Why the gap?

- Competing priorities for budget allocation.
- Bureaucratic challenges.
- Political underinvestment in long-term health planning.
- Still, progress continues, sometimes despite the system, not because of it.

Infrastructure & Human Resource Gaps

With the increased number of MBBS seats, the doctor-patient ratio is improving rapidly; however, this is creating a gap in the quality of medical education and training.

- Specialist positions in district hospitals continue to remain vacant.
- Infrastructure in tribal, mountainous, and remote areas is inadequate.

Small Triumphs, Big Ripples

Even in this imperfect system, micro-successes light the way

- Tamil Nadu's supply chain management of essential medicines.
- Kerala's community-based palliative care model.
- Sikkim's achievement of open defecation-free status.

- Odisha's ambulance network (108 service).
- Digital health innovations from states like Andhra Pradesh and Gujarat.

These are lighthouses in the fog, showing what's possible when intent meets innovation.

Global Healer; Local Gaps

India manufactures 60% of the world's vaccines, supplies generic drugs globally, and conducts medical diplomacy through "Pharmacy of the World" campaigns; however, the following is also true.

- In certain villages, patients travel 10 km for essential medicines.
- Mental health care continues to be neglected.
- Out-of-pocket expenses continue to burden people experiencing poverty.

This is the duality you will live and work in.

☕ Coffee Moment

You attended the faculty rounds in the pediatric ICU, with ventilators humming and protocols precise. That evening, you went home to your small town and saw a mother carrying her child on a bike for hours to reach a PHC without a doctor.

Both moments are real.
Both children are yours to care for.
And both sides of this paradox will shape your sense of purpose.

References

1. Ministry of Health and Family Welfare. National Health Profile 2021. New Delhi: MoHFW; 2021.
2. National Health Systems Resource Centre. Indian Public Health Standards: Guidelines for Primary Health Centres and Community Health Centres. New Delhi: NHSRC; 2012.
3. OECD/World Health Organization. Health at a Glance: Asia/Pacific 2022. Paris: OECD Publishing; 2022.
4. National Health Systems Resource Centre. National Health Accounts Estimates for India (2019–20). New Delhi: MoHFW; 2022.
5. Government of India. Ayushman Bharat – Pradhan Mantri Jan Arogya Yojana (PM-JAY): Policy Brief. New Delhi: MoHFW; 2018.

Chapter 28: National Health Agencies and Targeted Missions

Introduction

India's health system is a mosaic of agencies, councils, and missions, each with its own role but united in the goal of protecting health for all. From apex bodies like the National Medical Commission (NMC), which shape education, to implementation agencies such as the National Health Mission (NHM), which bring services to villages, every agency adds a thread to the fabric of care. Alongside them are targeted national programs addressing priority conditions such as tuberculosis, maternal and child health, HIV/AIDS, immunization, non-communicable diseases, and many more. This chapter provides a guided orientation, serving as a roadmap to understand how India organizes its fight against disease and how your future role will align with these structures.

National Health Agencies

Ministry of Health and Family Welfare

Ministry of Health and Family Welfare (MoHFW) is the apex body responsible for formulating national health policies, planning healthcare delivery, and overseeing major health programs. It comprises two departments.

- Department of Health and Family Welfare.
- Department of Health Research (DHR).

Key functions include

- Budget allocation and monitoring.
- Coordination of national programs (like NHM, RNTCP).
- Regulation of medical education through statutory bodies.
- International collaboration with WHO, UNICEF, etc.

National Health Systems Resource Centre

The National Health Systems Resource Centre (NHSRC) provides technical support to strengthen the implementation of the National Health Mission. (1) Established under the NHM, it serves as a think tank and technical support unit. Its major roles are

- Conducting health systems research.
- Capacity building for state health missions.
- Developing public health management guidelines.

- Assisting in health financing and quality assurance.

Indian Council of Medical Research

The Indian Council of Medical Research (ICMR) leads biomedical research in India, supporting disease surveillance, clinical trials, and innovation. (2) It also played a pivotal role during COVID-19 in developing diagnostics, treatment guidelines, and vaccines. Its responsibilities include:

- Medical research on communicable and non-communicable diseases.
- Running research institutes and clinical trials.
- Ethical oversight through institutional review boards.
- Surveillance and data analysis during health emergencies.

National Centre for Disease Control

The National Centre for Disease Control (NCDC) plays a key role in epidemic intelligence, outbreak investigation, and training in field epidemiology. (3) Its functions include

- Monitoring disease outbreaks (e.g., COVID, dengue, chikungunya).
- Training epidemiologists through EIS programs.
- Hosting Integrated Disease Surveillance Program (IDSP).
- Data analytics and public health alerts.

Central Drugs Standard Control Organization

The Central Drugs Standard Control Organization (CDSCO) is a drug regulator operating under the Directorate General of Health Services. Its roles are:

- Licensing and approval of drugs and medical devices.
- Monitoring clinical trials and vaccine development.
- Ensuring drug safety and efficacy.
- Collaborating with the WHO and global regulatory bodies.

National Medical Commission

The Medical Council of India, now replaced by the National Medical Commission, regulates medical education and ethics in India with the following objectives. (4)

- Regulating medical education and training
- Accrediting medical colleges and curricula
- Conducting the National Exit Test (NEXT)
- Maintaining a national medical register

As a student, the NMC's decisions have a significant impact on your learning, exams, internships, and even your career options.

Other Key Institutions

National Institute of Health and Family Welfare (NIHFW)

Functions as an apex teaching, training, and capacity-building institution in public health and family welfare. (5)

Food Safety and Standards Authority of India (FSSAI):

Food regulation and safety.

AYUSH Ministry

Traditional medicine systems including Ayurveda, Yoga, Unani, Siddha, and Homeopathy.

National Health Programs

India's healthcare system doesn't run only hospitals; it also runs missions. These are large-scale, goal-driven programs targeting specific diseases, conditions, or vulnerable populations, such as children, pregnant women, or individuals with TB. National Health Programs (NHPs) are the country's strategic tools to combat widespread health challenges. The WHO, UNICEF, World Bank, and other partners also support various programs. India's health programs started with vertical disease-control missions, such as malaria eradication and family planning, expanded to address significant gaps in the healthcare system. (6)

Why National Health Programs?

India faces significant public health challenges, including: The highest number of tuberculosis cases globally; high prevalence of vector-borne diseases, anaemia, and malnutrition; and high maternal and infant mortality rates, particularly in underserved areas.

Without targeted programs, these issues often go unaddressed. NHPs ensure that necessary resources, such as funding, personnel, and strategic planning, are directed toward solving these public health problems. Programs like RMNCH+A brought reproductive, maternal, newborn, child and adolescent health under a common umbrella, emphasizing that each life stage is connected to the next. It promotes a continuum of care across various life stages and care settings. (7)

Major National Health Programs at a Glance

Snapshot of some of the most impactful programs:

Table 28.1: Major national health programs in India

Program	Focus Area
RMNCH+A **(Reproductive, Maternal, Newborn, Child, and Adolescent Health)**	Entire life-cycle approach to women and child health
National Tuberculosis Elimination Program (NTEP)	TB diagnosis, treatment, and elimination by 2025
Universal Immunization Program (UIP)	Free vaccines for children and pregnant women
National AIDS Control Program (NACP)	HIV/AIDS prevention and ART distribution
National Vector Borne Disease Control Program (NVBDCP)	Malaria, dengue, chikungunya, filariasis, kala-azar
National Mental Health Program (NMHP)	Psychological services in district hospitals
National Programme for Prevention and Control of Cancer, Diabetes, Cardiovascular Diseases and Stroke (NPCDCS)	NCD screening and lifestyle intervention
National Leprosy Eradication Program (NLEP)	Early detection and stigma reduction

Success Stories: What's Working

- Polio Eradication: India was declared polio-free in 2014, thanks to extensive intersectoral efforts and vaccination drives.
- The Janani Suraksha Yojana (JSY) has increased institutional deliveries and improved maternal health and safety.
- Mission Indradhanush: Enhanced immunization coverage in difficult-to-reach areas.
- National TB Elimination Program and National AIDS Control Programme continue to remain flagship efforts.
- TB Notification plays a key role in understanding the actual burden and planning appropriate strategies.

These programs have saved millions of lives through concentrated efforts focused on specific diseases or conditions. (8,9)

Challenges

- **Fragmentation**: Programs often operate as vertical silos instead of integrated services, consuming a significant amount of human resources.
- **Funding gaps**: Delayed or insufficient fund release.

- **Data issues** include underreporting, poor monitoring, and false entries in some districts.
- **Low community engagement**: Without local involvement, programs are at risk of failure.

No mission can work if it doesn't feel like a local cause.

Newer Directions and Integration

The NHM serves as an umbrella framework, integrating multiple vertical programs. (10) Under Ayushman Bharat and NHM, the push is now to:

- Integrate multiple programs at HWCs.
- Use digital health platforms for integration and data tracking (e.g., Nikshay for TB, RCH portal for maternal care).
- Physical integration for comprehensive primary care, not fragmented services.

Your Role as a Future Doctor

You may think these programs are merely government schemes, but they are the system that will influence your work, even if you are not a part of it.

- You'll conduct health camps under RMNCH+A.
- Refer or receive patients for free cataract surgery under NPCDCS.
- Counsel youth under RKSK (Adolescent Health).
- Administer vaccines, assist in mass drug administration, or prepare reports.

Whether in rural internships, urban CHCs, medical college OPDs, or private sector workplaces, you'll be within the NHP ecosystem, even if you don't realize it.

☕ Coffee Moment

You're volunteering at a government immunization drive.
A tribal woman brings her twin girls: one malnourished and the other fearful. You reassure her, assist the ANM in vaccinating the child, connect her with the mid-day meal program at a nearby school, and hand her an ORS packet.

"Ab woh pucca school jaayegi, doctor saab."(Now she will certainly go to school, doctor) She says.

No fancy equipment. No diagnosis. One more life lifted by a national program and your gentle hand.

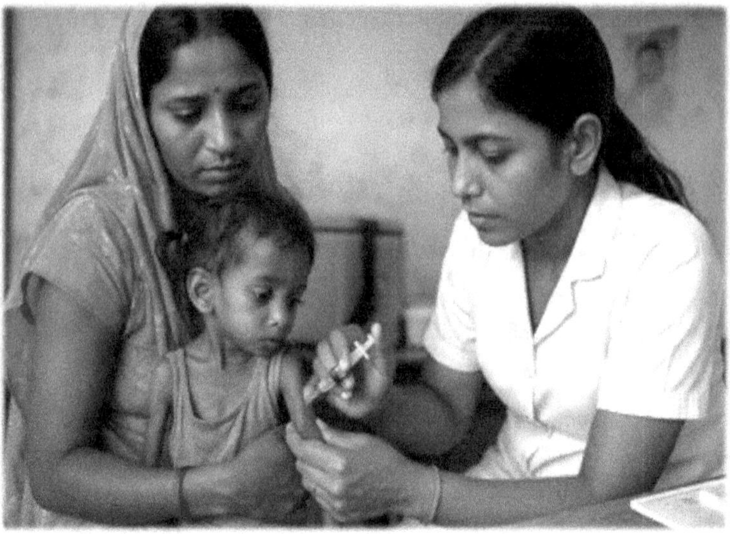

Figure 28.1: A Catch-up Immunization

References

1. National Health Systems Resource Centre. Annual Report 2019–20. New Delhi: NHSRC; 2020.
2. Indian Council of Medical Research. Annual Report 2020–21. New Delhi: ICMR; 2021.
3. National Centre for Disease Control. Annual Report 2021–22. New Delhi: MoHFW; 2022.
4. National Medical Commission. Annual Report 2021–22. New Delhi: NMC; 2022.
5. National Institute of Health and Family Welfare. Annual Report 2021–22. New Delhi: NIHFW; 2022.
6. Ministry of Health and Family Welfare. National Health Programme Compendium. New Delhi: MoHFW; 2017.
7. Ministry of Health and Family Welfare. Reproductive, Maternal, Newborn, Child and Adolescent Health (RMNCH+A) Strategy. New Delhi: MoHFW; 2013.
8. Central TB Division. National Strategic Plan for Tuberculosis Elimination 2017–2025. New Delhi: MoHFW; 2017.
9. National AIDS Control Organisation. Annual Report 2021–22. New Delhi: NACO; 2022.
10. National Health Systems Resource Centre. National Health Mission: Framework for Implementation 2012–2017. New Delhi: NHSRC; 2012.

Chapter 29: Health Financing in India - Who Pays and How?

Introduction

Every injection, every ambulance, every hospital bed- someone, somewhere, pays for it. But who? India's healthcare system is vast, but it runs on something invisible: Money. Every act of care is tied to cost, from a ₹5 ORS packet at an Anganwadi to a ₹5 lakh bypass surgery at an Institute of National Importance (INI) or a corporate hospital. Understanding how healthcare is funded, by individuals, governments, or insurance schemes, is essential. This chapter examines health financing in India, including the sources of funds, their allocation, and who bears the burden. (1) As future clinicians, doctors are not just users of the health system, but translators of policy into practice. Understanding health financing helps you explain entitlements, prevent exploitation, and protect families from financial harm, often as powerfully as a prescription.

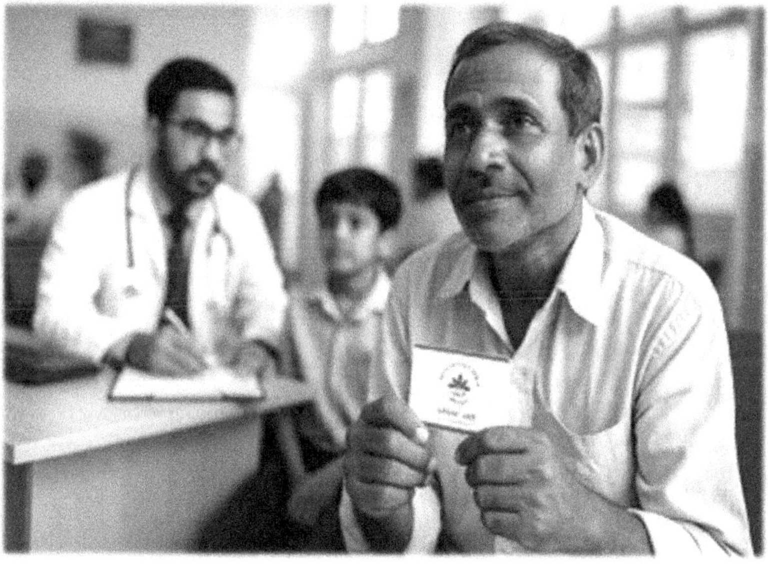

Figure 29.1: Ayushman Bharat Beneficiary

Health Expenditure: The Big Picture

India's Union Budget for 2025–26 has allocated approximately ₹99,859 crore to the Ministry of Health and Family Welfare (MoHFW) and ₹3,901 crore for medical research, totalling around ₹103,760 crore in health-related allocations. This allocation represents an 11% increase over the revised estimate from the previous year. Subsequent increases in Budget 2026–27 have taken the total health-sector allocation to over ₹1.06 lakh crore, marking a sustained upward trend in public health financing. (2,3) Given India's estimated GDP of ₹400 lakh crore, this health allocation represents ~2.5% of total government expenditure, whereas total health expenditure (public + private) is around 3.8% of GDP, which is an improvement from 2020 (2.1%) and aligns with the target set in the National Health Policy (2017). However, this figure is still lower than that of many other countries, such as the UK (9.8%), the USA (16.6%), and Brazil (4%). Healthcare budgeting has real-life consequences.

Where Does the Money Go?

Out of the total allocation:

- ₹37,227 crore (~37%) is allocated for the National Health Mission (NHM), India's flagship program for primary healthcare.
- ₹9,406 crore (approximately 9%) is allocated for Ayushman Bharat – PMJAY, the public health insurance scheme.
- The remaining funds are allocated to support INIs, AIIMS, other apex institutes, medical education, research, and digital health programs.

Health Spending in Context

India's total health expenditure, encompassing public, private, and household sources, accounts for approximately 3.8% of the country's GDP. (1,2)

- The government's contribution to total expenditure is just above 50%.
- The rest is largely out-of-pocket expenditure (OOPE) by households.

Out-of-Pocket Expenditure: The Burden on Families

As per the National Health Accounts (2020)

- 48.2% of health spending was OOPE.
- About 13.6% was through government-run insurance schemes.

Most Indians still pay for healthcare without any formal coverage. Many times, people face debt or experience delays in treatment during a serious illness. (4)

Ayushman Bharat – A Game Changer in Progress

Ayushman Bharat-Pradhan Mantri Jan Arogya Yojana (PM-JAY), launched in 2018, is globally the largest government-funded health assurance scheme aimed at reducing this burden. (5) It offers

- ₹5 lakh per family per year.
- Cashless, paperless treatment in empanelled hospitals (public & private).
- Coverage for secondary and tertiary care, including surgery, ICU, and cancer

care.

While its full effect wasn't reflected in the 2020 data, the 2023–24 data show

- Over 5.7 crore hospital admissions covered.
- Greater involvement of private hospitals.
- Increasing awareness and access, particularly in rural and underserved areas.

PM-JAY is expected to significantly reduce OOPE in the coming years, particularly for major illnesses. Challenges such as limited OPD coverage and issues with inter-state implementation variability still need to be addressed.

Why This Matters to You

You will work in a system funded by public programs and private payments. Understanding schemes such as PM-JAY will enable you to guide patients more effectively. You can serve as an advocate or expert for improved policies and equity, particularly on behalf of rural and low-income families. Budgets reflect priorities. Prioritizing health means prioritizing people.

The Cost of Falling Sick: Out-of-Pocket Expenditure

Out-of-Pocket Expenditure (OOPE) refers to direct payments made by individuals for healthcare services, including doctor consultations, medicines (a significant portion), diagnostics, and hospitalization. (6) For many families, one illness can mean

- Selling livestock or land.
- Pulling children out of school.
- Falling below the poverty line.

A 2021 WHO report estimated that over 63 million Indians are pulled below the poverty line each year due to healthcare costs. PM-JAY is helping to mitigate this burden, particularly for major hospitalisations, though outpatient expenses and medicines remain significant contributors to out-of-pocket spending.

Public Financing: Who Provides, Who Pays?

Public healthcare in India is funded by

- Union Government: Via schemes like Ayushman Bharat, national programs, AIIMS/INIs.
- State Governments: Fund state hospitals, medical colleges, PHCs, etc.
- External aid, CSR, NGOs: for select programs.

Due to limited allocations in certain sectors and underutilization in some states, many facilities remain under-equipped. However, Government health spending is increasing steadily under schemes such as the National Health Mission, and PMJAY.

Insurance in India: Rising but Fragmented

Health insurance is expanding, but remains limited. Challenges are:

- Low awareness.
- Complicated claim processes.
- Charges exceeding coverage capping.

Table 29.1: Different types of health insurance systems in India

Type	Examples	Coverage
Government-sponsored	Ayushman Bharat (PM-JAY), RSBY, CGHS, ESIC	~50 crore beneficiaries
Employer-based	Government/Private sector jobs	~10 crore
Private insurance	Religare, Star Health, etc.	~5 crore (urban elite)
Community schemes	SEWA, cooperative-based	Small but targeted

Despite multiple schemes, coverage remains fragmented, with benefit depth and financial protection varying widely across populations.

Role of Philanthropy

Beyond government and insurance, India's healthcare is supported by

- Charitable hospitals such as the Tata Memorial, Shroff Eye, Aravind Eye Care, and Satya Sai Centres, among others.
- NGOs working in the field of rural clinics, TB and mental health outreach programs.
- Corporate social responsibility (CSR) funding for cancer screening, cardiac disease screening, cleft lip surgeries, ambulance services, etc.

These sources plug gaps, particularly where government reach is limited.

The Way Ahead: Universal Health Coverage

India aims for Universal Health Coverage (UHC): everyone, everywhere, should receive quality healthcare without suffering financial hardship. (7) To achieve this, additional efforts are needed, such as

- Increase health budget to 2.5% + of GDP.
- Improve the efficiency and accountability of spending.
- Strengthen primary care (prevent hospital overload).
- Expand and simplify insurance coverage.
- Invest in digital infrastructure and fraud control.

Financial signals of 2026 budget include:

- Health allocation crossed ₹1.06 lakh crore, the highest ever, reflecting continuity rather than episodic funding
- Ayushman Bharat–PMJAY funding increased, with emphasis on hospital-based care, private sector participation, and faster claim settlement

The PM-ABHIM saw a major boost to support district critical care blocks, public health laboratories and emergency and trauma services. Customs duty exemptions on cancer and rare-disease drugs aim to reduce catastrophic health expenditure for families. Together, these measures suggest a gradual shift from out-of-pocket-driven care toward pooled public financing, though the transition remains incomplete. For a young doctor, this means working in a system that is slowly becoming more protective of patients but still heavily dependent on clinical advocacy at the bedside.

Think Globally, Practice Locally

We will also discuss the healthcare systems employed in various countries in the following chapters. By the end, you will not only understand India's challenges and strengths but also be ready to think about strategic solutions, inspired by the best from around the world, such as

- **The UK**, where every citizen has access to care through the NHS.
- **In the USA**, a broken leg may cost a fortune or be free, depending on your insurance.
- **The UAE (Dubai),** with insurance-driven access.
- **Australia and New Zealand**, where a hybrid system seeks both quality and fairness

Coffee Moment

A man rushes into your OPD, holding his Ayushman card. His eyes are wide, his breath unsteady, but it's not panic; hope trembles on the edge of disbelief.

"Doctor saab... they said my son's heart surgery will be done, and... we don't need to pay anything. Is it true?"

You pause for a moment. Then, you look him in the eye, smile gently, and nod.

"Yes. It's true."

He sits down on the bench, clutching the card like a blessing. His shoulders, once tense with fear, now relaxed. For the first time in months, he exhales.

And in that quiet moment, as the hum of the clinic returns, you realise, you're not just a doctor. You are part of something greater: a safety net that gives a poor man the courage to hope and a child the chance to live without bankrupting her family.

This is what Ayushman Bharat means. Not only health coverage, but dignity. A quiet promise that the right to live doesn't depend on the ability to pay.

References

1. National Health Policy 2017. Ministry of Health and Family Welfare, Government of India. New Delhi: MoHFW; 2017.
2. National Health Accounts Estimates for India (2019–20). Ministry of Health and Family Welfare, Government of India. New Delhi: MoHFW; 2022.
3. Union Budget 2025–26: Demand for Grants, Ministry of Health and Family Welfare. Government of India; 2025.
4. Prinja S, Bahuguna P, Pinto AD, Sharma A, Bharaj G, Kumar V, et al. The cost of universal health care in India: a model-based estimate. *PLoS One.* 2012;7(1):e30362.
5. Lahariya C. Health & wellness centers to strengthen primary health care in India: Concept, progress and ways forward. *Indian J Pediatr.* 2020;87(11):916–29.
6. Karan A, Engelgau M, Mahal A. The household-level economic burden of heart disease in India. *Trop Med Int Health.* 2014;19(5):581–91.
7. World Health Organization. Tracking universal health coverage: 2021 Global Monitoring Report. Geneva: WHO & World Bank; 2021.

Covenant

A covenant is more than a contract; it is a sacred trust.

When you enter medicine, you step into a bond between doctor and patient, between science and conscience, between personal ambition and the greater good.

This bond is fragile yet enduring, invisible yet deeply felt.

It is what sets medicine apart from all other professions.

This section explores the ethical compass to guide your journey.

From constitutional rights and medico-legal dilemmas to fiduciary duty, research integrity, and the delicate balance of collaboration.

These chapters invite you to reflect on what it means to be a trustworthy doctor.

As you cross this threshold, remember:

Knowledge may win admiration,

but it is integrity that earns trust.

Skill may save a life,

but it is compassion that gives healing its true meaning.

And while science can explain disease, it is the covenant of ethics and responsibility that makes you worthy of being called a doctor.

S No.	Covenant: At a Glance
1.	**Chapter 30** Constitutional Roots: Is Health a Right? Constitutional interpretation of right to health; how the judiciary transformed healthcare from a service into a constitutional necessity linked to dignity.
2.	**Chapter 31** Medico-Legal Issues and Ethical Conflicts Doctors often navigate grey zones where law, ethics, and patient care intersect. Explore ethical challenges of balancing patient welfare with legal frameworks.
3.	**Chapter 32** The Edge of Life and Ethics End-of-life care and organ transplantation bring some of the toughest decisions a doctor may face. See how law, ethics, and compassion converge in such moments.
4.	**Chapter 33** Professionalism and Fiduciary Duty Patients entrust their lives to doctors. Explore professionalism, trustworthiness, and the duty to always act in the patient's best interests.
5.	**Chapter 34** Good Clinical Practice and Ethics in Research Integrity and ethics in medical research, patient protection, respect for colleagues, and responsibilities of investigators.
6.	**Chapter 35** Doctor–Industry Relationship Healthcare industry, conflicts of interest and ethical ways to collaborate without compromising integrity.
7.	**Chapter 36** Balancing Collaboration and Integrity Collaboration with ethics. Sharing credit, managing conflicts of interest, and maintaining integrity while working across teams, institutions, and industries.

Chapter 30: Constitutional Roots- Is Health a Right?

Introduction

A nation's constitution reflects not only its laws but also its love for its people, care for people experiencing poverty, and shaping of the future. When you read the Indian Constitution, you will not find "Right to Health" listed with the right to life, liberty, or speech. And yet, health is everywhere, like the bloodstream beneath the skin of our laws. The Indian Constitution does not explicitly mention health as a fundamental right; however, it addresses people's health through the directive principles of state policy. (1)

Health as a Directive Dream

In India's federal structure, health is a state subject under the Constitution. This means that state governments bear the primary responsibility for delivering health services. However, the Directive Principles of State Policy (Part IV) says that public health is not only a legal obligation but a moral commitment. It mandates that the State prioritise improvingf nutrition, living standards, and public health for its citizens. Article 39(e) protects the health of workers, while Article 41 guarantees public assistance in cases of illness, disability, and ageing. These principles are not enforceable by courts but guide governance and law-making with ethical force.

Judicial Interpretations

Article 21, which guarantees the right to life and personal liberty, has been interpreted by the Supreme Court to include the right to health. (2) In Paschim Banga Khet Mazdoor Samity vs. West Bengal State (1996), the Supreme Court ruled that "The government has a constitutional obligation to provide adequate medical services." (3) Since then, numerous other cases have reaffirmed that health is not a luxury but a constitutional necessity for living with dignity. This judicial interpretation broadened the meaning of life to include living with dignity and access to healthcare.

The Central–State Puzzle

Although states are primarily responsible for healthcare delivery, the central government plays a crucial role, particularly in:

- Funding and designing national programs, such as NHM and PM-JAY.
- Regulation of drugs, medical education, and public health emergencies.
- Providing direct healthcare through Institutes of National Importance (INIs), including AIIMS, PGIMER, JIPMER, and others.

The AIIMS Act and Central Healthcare Delivery

Despite health being a state subject, the central government establishes direct patient-care institutions to ensure uniform standards of tertiary care and academic excellence across regions. A notable example is the All India Institute of Medical Sciences (AIIMS), which is governed by the AIIMS Act of 1956. Other INIs, like PGIMER Chandigarh, JIPMER Puducherry, and NIMHANS Bengaluru, operate similarly, under their own Acts or administrative orders.

- These institutes are established and funded directly by the Union government.
- These institutes are referral centres for patient care, research hubs for innovation, and training centres for healthcare professionals.
- These institutions act as the central nervous system of India's health education and super-speciality care.

Role of the People: From Panchayats to Patients

"Healthcare is not something that happens to the people; it happens *with* the people." India is a signatory to international treaties such as the International Covenant on Economic, Social and Cultural Rights (ICESCR), which recognize the right to health as a fundamental human right. (4)

When we think about healthcare, we often imagine hospitals, medical professionals, and various medical equipment. However, in a vast and diverse country like India, the true essence of health is rooted in individual citizens, families, and communities. From village health workers to gram panchayats, and from school teachers to ASHAs, India's healthcare delivery system is a massive jigsaw puzzle that comes alive when we visualise the people as part of the picture.

The Role of the Panchayat

India's Constitution empowers villages through Panchayati Raj Institutions (PRIs), and health is one of their core responsibilities. Local leadership can make or break health delivery in rural areas. Ayushman Bharat attempt to operationalize this vision by expanding access to primary care and financial protection to citizens of India. (5)

Village-level bodies frequently oversee health sub-centres, monitor nutrition programs, and support sanitation initiatives.

PRIs serve as the local arm of community-based health planning and currently partner in implementing programs such as Ayushman Bharat – Health & Wellness Centres (HWCs).

ASHAs

Every village in India features a woman who walks miles, talks endlessly, and carries her community's health in her hands. She is an ASHA, Accredited Social Health Activist, the foot soldiers of public health.

- Introduced through the National Health Mission (NHM).
- Serves as a connection between the community and health services.
- Mobilizes pregnant women, tracks immunizations, distributes ORS, and educates about TB, sanitation, family planning, and other health topics.
- Plays a critical role in health surveillance, awareness, and vaccine campaigns.

An ASHA is not only a health worker; she is the system's heartbeat.

Mothers, Grandparents, and Traditional Wisdom

Healthcare in India has traditionally been a home-grown phenomenon. A grandmother's tip for fever, a mother's pulse on nutrition, and traditional midwives (dais) have all existed and influenced healthcare more than the formal system. Recognizing these roles with respect builds cultural sensitivity in modern healthcare. Community trust can often override a prescription. What your textbook teaches you, their lived experience confirms or questions. Listen.

Patient as a Partner

Empowered patients are equal partners in care. In the era of health literacy, patients are:

- Asking questions.
- Googling symptoms.
- Demanding dignity and clarity.
- Filing lawsuits when care fails.

Your ability to communicate, engage, and respect others will define your success more than your stethoscope ever will.

Your Role in the Constitutional Dream

As an MBBS student at a state or private medical college or at one of the AIIMS, you are shaped by a system that reflects federal cooperation and constitutional compassion.

- When you care for a sick child in a PHC, you fulfil Article 47.
- Conducting community education in health camps, you strengthen Article 39.
- When you advocate for equitable care and system change, you embody the spirit of Article 21.

☕Coffee Moment

You're posted in a rural PHC. You're the only doctor.
An elderly woman brings in a child with diarrhoea. She's already given ORS, knows about handwashing, and is part of a Self-Help Group.
You realize, you're not saving this village. They're keeping themselves.
Sometimes, all you have to do is honour their effort, guide their journey, and not get in the way.

Reflection

Should India formally declare "Right to Health" as a Fundamental Right?

What role can central institutions like AIIMS play in making that a reality, especially in underserved regions?

References

1. Bhattacharya D. The Right to Health: A Constitutional Perspective. Indian J Med Ethics. 2013;10(4):244-7.
2. Bandhua Mukti Morcha vs Union of India, AIR 1984 SC 802.
3. Paschim Banga Khet Mazdoor Samity vs State of West Bengal, AIR 1996 SC 2426.
4. United Nations. International Covenant on Economic, Social and Cultural Rights. UN General Assembly Resolution 2200A (XXI). 1966.
5. Ministry of Health and Family Welfare. Ayushman Bharat: Comprehensive Primary Health Care through HWCs. New Delhi: MoHFW; 2018.

Chapter 31: Medico-Legal Issues and Ethical Conflicts

Introduction

Clinical practice operates within a legal framework to protect patients and physicians. Medical errors, negligence cases, conflicts over reproductive rights, and organ transplantation highlight the intersection of law and ethics. Doctors often face dilemmas where legal requirements and ethical duties seem to clash. (1) This chapter examines medicolegal dilemmas and emphasises accountability, transparency, and empathy. Let's understand the *why*, *how*, and *real-life relevance* of clinical documentation first.

Documentation in Patient Care

In medicine, what isn't written often isn't remembered or legally recognized. Documentation transforms patient encounters into an accurate record to guide diagnosis, continuity of care, audits, research, and legal protection. (2-4)

Why Documentation Matters

- **Continuity of Care:** Ensures that every healthcare worker, from nurse to consultant, knows what has been done and what's next.
- **Safety & Accuracy:** Reduces medical errors, test duplication, and missed diagnoses.
- **Communication:** A well-documented note speaks clearly across shifts, departments, and disciplines.
- **Legal Record:** Protects both patient and doctor; in court, what is written is what counts.
- **Ethical Practice:** Reflects professionalism, accountability, and respect for patient rights.
- **Research & Education:** Case records serve as learning material and data for clinical research.

What Good Documentation Includes

- **Patient identifiers:** Name, age, hospital identification number, date, and time.
- **History & examination findings:** Objective, clear, chronological.
- **Investigations & results:** With relevant interpretations.
- **Diagnosis & differential diagnoses:** Logical and evidence-based.
- **Treatment plan:** Drugs, doses, timings, and procedures performed.
- **Progress notes:** Daily updates, patient response, and changes in plan.

- **Signature and designation:** Always end with your name and role.

Golden Rules

- Be accurate, legible, timed, and signed.
- Never alter or erase entries; use a single line to strike out errors.
- Avoid subjective comments or blame.
- Respect confidentiality: no social media posts or photos of patient data.

Medical Errors, Negligence, and Malpractice

Medical Errors

A medical error is an unintended act (or omission) that harms or can potentially harm a patient. Errors may be due to misdiagnosis, wrong medication, poor communication, or system failures. Not all errors are indicative of negligence, but every error presents a learning opportunity. For example, administering the wrong drug dose due to misreading handwriting is an error, even if caught early, before causing harm.

Negligence

Negligence occurs when a doctor fails to provide the standard of care that a reasonable and prudent peer would offer in similar circumstances, resulting in harm. (5) It goes beyond error; it implies a lapse in diligence. For instance, ignoring critical lab results or failing to monitor a patient after surgery may constitute negligence.

Medical malpractice

It refers to negligence that results in injury or death, potentially leading to legal action. Courts often ask:

- Was there a duty of care?
- Was that duty breached?
- Did it directly cause harm?
- Did measurable damage occur?

When all four conditions are met, malpractice is established. The Consumer Protection Act (CPA) brought doctors under the purview of consumer law, increasing litigation risks. (6)

Why It Matters for Students

- Patient Safety: Being aware of errors and negligence fosters a culture of vigilance and accountability.
- Professionalism: Transparency and honesty in reporting errors build trust.

- Legal Protection: Proper documentation and communication safeguard both patients and doctors.

Imagine you prescribed the right drug but forgot to explain its side effects. The patient stops taking the medicine due to dizziness, worsening their illness. Error may be human, but negligence is avoidable.

Disclosure of Medical Errors

Doctors are human, and errors occur in clinical practice. When an error is identified, it must be disclosed to the patient and reported to the institute. Failure to disclose may lead to medico-legal claims, loss of trust and ethical breaches.

- **Ethical Obligation**: Transparency is essential for building trust. Patients have a right to know about errors that could affect their health.
- **Remediation**: Providing an honest explanation of corrective steps can help mitigate harm and legal consequences.
- **Institutional learning**: Reporting errors helps organisations identify systemic problems and prevent recurrence.

Case Scenario: Medical Error

A 5-year-old girl, Mansi, arrives with her mother at a busy clinic for a follow-up. She has asthma, and you adjust her medications. Her mother reminds you about her booster shots. In the rush, you tell the nurse to prepare the injection and leave it in the adjoining room. Later, you give it to Mansi, assuming it was the vaccine, but the nurse informs you it was gentamicin for another patient.

Core Concepts

Medical Errors in Clinical Care: Medical errors, such as giving the wrong medication, can seriously impact patient safety and trust. It can occur due to a combination of factors.

- **Systemic Issues**: Attention and communication lapses in a busy clinic.
- **Human Factors**: Assumed the syringe was correct without verification.
- **Practice:** Lack of clear medication labelling and tracking protocols.

Addressing these issues requires implementing standardised procedures, enhancing communication among staff, and cultivating a safety culture.

Disclosure of Medical Errors: Transparency is crucial when disclosing medical errors. The ethical guidelines suggest:

- **Honesty**: Inform the patient and family about the error with genuine regret.
- **Explanation**: Outlines how the error happened and the steps to fix it.

- **Action Plan**: Outlining measures to prevent similar errors in the future.

Not disclosing medical errors can have several adverse outcomes:

- **Medico-Legal Implications**: Concealing negligence carries the legal risk.
- **Social Consequences**: Patients and their families may feel betrayed, which can damage relationships and reputations.
- **Loss of Trust**: Nondisclosure damages trust in the doctor-patient relationship.

Decision-Making Process

- **Immediate Action**: Upon realizing the error, assess Mansi for any immediate adverse reactions to the gentamicin.
- **Informing the Patient and Family**: Communicate the error to Mansi's mother, explaining what happened and the potential implications.
- **Medical Management**: Monitor Mansi for any side effects of gentamicin, such as nephrotoxicity or ototoxicity, and provide appropriate care.
- **Reporting the Incident**: Document the error in the medical record and report it to the hospital's quality assurance team.
- **Implementing Preventive Measures**: Review and revise clinic protocols to include medication double-checking, clear labelling, and improved communication among staff.

Outcome

Mansi was monitored closely for any adverse effects of gentamicin. Fortunately, she did not exhibit any signs of toxicity. Her mother appreciated the transparency and the steps taken to rectify the situation. The clinic implemented new protocols, including a medication verification system, to prevent future errors.

Adolescent Abortion and Reproductive Rights

Medicine frequently overlaps with ethics, law, and social norms, particularly in areas like reproductive rights and organ transplants, leading to debates on autonomy, dignity, exploitation, and the dual role of doctors as caregivers and law enforcers. Reproductive health care is sensitive and contested, especially for minors seeking abortion. The 2021 Indian Medical Termination of Pregnancy (MTP) Act specifies gestational limits, medical indications, and consent. Adults can terminate pregnancies under statutory conditions and medical advice. For adolescents below 18, guardian consent is required, raising concerns about autonomy and confidentiality. (7) Doctors must also be aware of reporting obligations under the Protection of Children from Sexual Offences (POCSO) Act, since sexual activity involving minors may require legal reporting. Thus, every decision must weigh medical care, legal compliance, and patient dignity. Here, the following principles must be balanced:

- **Autonomy**: respecting the adolescent's voice and confidentiality.
- **Beneficence**: ensuring medical safety and psychological support.
- **Justice**: following the law to prevent misuse or coercion.
- **Legal responsibility**: Mandatory reporting to law enforcement agencies under the POSCO and MTP Acts.

Case: A Family in Dilemma

Dr Mehra has been the trusted family doctor of Mr and Mrs Sharif for over a decade. One evening, the couple arrives at his clinic with their 16-year-old daughter, Sara. Unlike their usual warmth, the atmosphere is tense. After a brief silence, Mr Sharif gestures to his wife, who, with tears in her eyes, explains that Sara has missed her period for four months. An ultrasound revealed a 16-week pregnancy. The parents requested a Medical Termination of Pregnancy (MTP), but Sara refused. She insists that the foetus represents her love and that terminating it would be murder. Her parents are distraught, fearing societal stigma and harm to Sara's future. They believe, as guardians, they have the right to decide. Sara, however, argues that she is old enough to make her own choices. The couple turn to Dr Mehra for guidance through this nightmare.

Core Concepts

- **MTP Act (2021 amendment):** Termination up to 24 weeks is permitted conditionally. For minors (<18 years), guardian consent is mandatory.
- **POCSO Act (2012):** Any sexual intercourse with a girl under 18 years is rape, regardless of consent. Doctors must mandatorily report such cases.
- **Adolescent Autonomy:** Ethically, the adolescent's voice matters. Practically, legal constraints limit her authority.
- **Male Counterpart:** If the partner is a minor, he is treated as a "child in conflict with law" under the Juvenile Justice Act. Major faces charges of statutory rape (IPC 376), with imprisonment ranging from 10 years to life.

Decision-Making Process

- **Medical Safety:** Assess gestational age, health risks, and a safe termination.
- **Consent:** As Sara is a minor, legal guardian consent is required. Her refusal must still be respected as part of the counselling process.
- **Mandatory Reporting:** Inform authorities under the POCSO Act, irrespective of family preference.
- **Male Counterpart's Liability:** If the minor is involved, the proceedings are referred to the Juvenile Justice Board. If an adult, he faces statutory rape charges.
- **Counselling:** Provide Sara with emotional support, ensure her dignity, and

involve the Child Welfare Committee to safeguard her rights.

Outcome

The doctor explains to the family that, by law, the pregnancy must be reported under POCSO. Guardian consent is required for MTP. With court/Child Welfare Committee intervention, safe termination is allowed per the MTP Act. Meanwhile, an investigation begins against the male counterpart. Sara receives not only medical care but also psychological counselling to cope with trauma.

Learning Points

- MTP requires guardian consent for minors and cannot proceed solely based on adolescent preference.
- Every adolescent pregnancy is a POCSO case, mandating legal reporting.
- The male partner, whether a minor or an adult, faces legal consequences.
- Doctors must balance empathy and confidentiality with legal obligations.
- Child Welfare Committees play a vital role in safeguarding minor's rights.

☕ Coffee Moment

Dr Mehra sat with a coffee that night, reflecting: "I wanted to listen to Sara's voice and fear. But the law demanded more: mandatory reporting, guardian consent, and legal action." Medicine is not only about healing bodies; sometimes it means standing at the difficult crossroads of empathy, law, and ethics.

References

1. Beauchamp TL, Childress JF. Principles of Biomedical Ethics. 8th ed. New York: Oxford University Press; 2019.
2. Medical Council of India. Competency-Based Undergraduate Curriculum for the Indian Medical Graduate. Vol 1. New Delhi: MCI; 2018.
3. World Health Organization. Patient Safety Curriculum Guide: Multi-professional Edition. WHO Press; 2011.
4. General Medical Council (UK). Good Medical Practice. London: GMC; 2020.
5. Jacob A. Medical negligence and the law in India. Indian J Urol. 2008;24(2):161-7.
6. Indian Medical Association vs VP Shantha, AIR 1996 SC 550.
7. Ministry of Health and Family Welfare. Medical Termination of Pregnancy (Amendment) Act, 2021. New Delhi: MoHFW; 2021.
8. Gillon R. Medical ethics: four principles plus attention to scope. BMJ. 1994;309(6948):184–8.

Chapter 32: Ethics at the Edge of Life

Introduction

There are moments in medicine when science and humanity meet at their most fragile boundaries — when life is fading, and choices are weighty. At such edges, doctors are called not only to treat but to guide, comfort, and uphold dignity. In the context of organ transplantation, doctors address both the technical aspects of the procedure and the ethical considerations of fairness and scarcity. Similarly, in end-of-life care, doctors provide compassionate care that respects the patient's wishes, even when a cure is no longer possible. (1)

For young medical students and doctors, these are not abstract debates but living realities you will one day encounter — in ICUs, in quiet wards, in conversations with grieving families. This chapter discusses some delicate moments where medicine is less about heroic intervention and more about listening with empathy and respecting their choices at their most vulnerable moments. These experiences have the potential to transform you as a person and a professional.

Organ Transplantation and the Ethics of Scarcity

Organ transplantation is a field marked by numerous ethical and legal conflicts. The shortage of available organs often tempts desperate patients to consider commercial solutions, despite clear prohibitions against such practices. Organ donation is one of the greatest acts of altruism, yet it requires robust systems to ensure fairness, consent, and transparency. (2) In India, the Transplantation of Human Organs and Tissues Act (THOTA), 1994 (amended in 2011), strictly forbids the sale or purchase of human organs. Donations are permitted only from close relatives or through voluntary altruism, subject to the scrutiny of an authorization committee. (3) This conflict highlights several lessons:

- **Fiduciary duty** requires doctors to protect vulnerable individuals from coercion, even if it angers the patient.
- **Transparency** is crucial: explaining the laws, the rationale behind them, and possible legal avenues for transplantation.
- **Health economics** must be acknowledged: scarcity of resources demands fair allocation, which commercial markets distort.

Case Scenario

Mr Rajshekhar, a 48-year-old industrialist, storms into the outpatient clinic. He suffers from end-stage kidney disease and has been on dialysis for months. Frustrated with the waiting list for deceased donor kidneys, he demands, "Doctor, I have money. Why can't I buy a kidney? Find me a poor worker willing to sell, and I will pay whatever it takes." When told that organ trade is illegal, his voice rises in anger: 'So my money is useless? My life has no value? Why should I wait when I can solve this immediately?'

Core Concept

- **Organ Transplantation Ethics and Law:** The Transplantation of Human Organs and Tissues Act (THOTA, 1994; amended 2011) in India prohibits the trade of organs and commercial transplantation. Organs may only be donated voluntarily, either by close relatives or altruistic donors approved by an Authorization Committee. Ethical principles include:
- **Non-exploitation:** Preventing people with low incomes from being coerced into selling organs.
- **Justice:** Ensuring equitable allocation of scarce resources.
- **Fiduciary duty:** The doctor must act in the patient's best interest while upholding the law and ethics.

Decision-Making Process

- **Medical Discussion:** Explain Mr Rajshekhar's prognosis, options for dialysis, and transplant pathways.
- **Legal Explanation:** Clarify that organ purchase is prohibited, and engaging in such activity could lead to prosecution under the THOTA.
- **Ethical Clarification:** Emphasize that commercial trade exploits vulnerable populations and undermines fairness and equity.
- **Alternative Pathways:** Counsel him on registering with the state transplant registry, potential deceased donor waiting lists, and promoting organ donation awareness.
- **Supportive Care:** Provide psychosocial counselling to manage frustration and offer support networks for patients awaiting transplant.

Outcome

Though initially angry, Mr Rajshekhar nderstood that purchasing a kidney was not an option. He is placed on the state transplant registry, continues dialysis, and is encouraged to join an advocacy group. With time, he shifts from anger to acceptance, becoming an advocate for legal organ donation awareness in his community.

Learning Points

- Organ trade is illegal and unethical; doctors must refuse such requests.
- Scarcity of organs must be addressed through policy, awareness, and voluntary donation.
- Doctors must combine firm legal clarity with compassionate communication to

guide patients who are frustrated.

- Upholding justice protects both individual patients and vulnerable communities.

☕ Coffee Moment

That evening, the doctor reflected over a quiet cup of coffee: "Mr Rajshekhar's anger came from fear of death, not greed. My job was not just to say no, but to help him see dignity in waiting and hope in the possibility of life through lawful means."

Non-Abandonment and End-of-Life Care

Medicine is often equated with a cure, but the reality is that not all illnesses can be cured. The physician's duty does not end at such times; it changes. Patients and families need compassion, presence, and guidance as much as they once sought treatment. The ethical principle of non-abandonment requires doctors to continue supporting patients, even when medical interventions cannot halt the progression of the disease.

The Concept of Non-Abandonment

Non-abandonment is the assurance that "I will not desert you, even when cure is no longer possible." It emphasizes continuity of care, emotional support, and presence. According to Quill and Cassell (1995), non-abandonment is "a promise of ongoing care through the patient's illness trajectory, especially at its most vulnerable stage." (4) When a physician withdraws, avoiding visits, delegating symptom control, or distancing themselves emotionally, patients and families feel abandoned, which deepens suffering.

Empathy During Failure

Patients nearing the end of life are not seeking miracle cures but a human connection. A physician's willingness to listen, hold a hand, or acknowledge suffering affirms the patient's dignity. Empathy in these moments demonstrates that the patient is still valued, despite the inevitable decline. Studies demonstrate that communication with empathy reduces anxiety, builds trust, and enhances quality of life (5)

Communication and Closure

End-of-life communication requires honesty, sensitivity, and respect. Discuss prognosis honestly while providing hope to maintain comfort and dignity. Guide families to consider palliative or hospice services when curative therapy is no longer effective. Provide closure with compassionate dialogue, helping patients and families prepare for the journey ahead.

Avoiding these conversations deprives patients of reassurance and families of guidance. Professionalism requires presence, even when outcomes are poor. End-of-life care encompasses not only clinical decisions but also ethical, emotional, and legal considerations, particularly in the context of withholding or withdrawing life-sustaining treatment. (6)

Principles to Learn

- **Presence matters more than cure:** Being there, listening, and accompanying the patient.
- **Empathy:** Patients value kindness as much as medicine.
- **Communication is care:** Honest, transparent, and compassionate dialogue is part of treatment.
- **Continuity of care:** Do not delegate the patient to someone else when hope for a cure fades.
- **Respect dignity:** Dying is a profound life phase that deserves respect and support.

Reflection:

In the words of Eric Cassell, "The goal of medicine is to relieve human suffering." Even when we cannot add days to life, we can add life to days - through presence, empathy, and communication. (4)

Case Scenario

Mr Ramesh, a widower, writes to Dr Iyer, his late wife's oncologist, two months after her passing. His wife, Meena, had battled breast cancer for five years.

Dear Doctor,

It has been three months since my wife, Mrs Meena, passed away. I write not in anger but in hope that lessons from her care may help other patients receive the compassion she was denied.

Five years ago, when Meena was diagnosed with breast cancer, we sought you for your reputation and were not disappointed. Your skill and aggressive treatment gave us two disease-free years, for which we remain grateful. But when the cancer returned and eventually overwhelmed her, things changed. When we needed you most, you seemed unable to face failure. Though you prescribed pain medication and arranged for nursing support, you avoided seeing Meena. Your office often redirected us to our family doctor, and when we did meet, you spoke briefly, without eye contact or comfort. In her final admission, despite our many requests, you never came to see her. She longed for a word or a touch of reassurance that never came.

Doctor, patients do not always expect a cure, but they always expect care. Compassion and presence matter even when medicine cannot succeed. Meena and I felt abandoned when we were most vulnerable. I bear you no ill will; your skills allowed us to spend years together, for which I am thankful. But knowledge alone is not enough. True healing comes with empathy, compassion, and non-abandonment. I hope Meena's experience reminds you that every patient, cured or not, deserves your presence. With empathy, all patients become your successes, irrespective of outcome.

Sincerely,
A grieving husband

Core Concept

Non-abandonment: The role of the physician extends beyond medical interventions. Healing includes empathy, compassion, presence, and guiding families through suffering, especially when a cure is impossible. Abandonment, even if unintended, fractures trust and deprives patients of dignity at life's end.

Decision-Making Process

Dr Iyer's choice: He withdrew emotionally when treatment failed, focusing on technical care but avoiding presence.

Alternative approach: Honest communication about prognosis, involvement in hospice transition, and simple acts of presence, such as holding a hand or offering words of comfort, would have honoured both patient and family.

Outcome

While Meena's physical pain was managed, the emotional and relational needs of both patient and family went unmet. The family carried grief compounded by feelings of abandonment. The letter served as a painful but powerful reminder to the doctor that patients remember presence more than prescriptions.

Learning Points

- The physician's role is to be a healer, not a technician.
- Failure of treatment does not end responsibility; non-abandonment is key.
- Honest prognosis discussions and hospice care demonstrate professionalism.
- Empathy and presence can bring peace, even when a cure is impossible.

Balancing Ethics and Law

Case scenarios illustrate how personal values, patient expectations, and legal frameworks can intersect. Physicians may sympathize with a frightened adolescent or a desperate patient awaiting a kidney, but cannot disregard the law. At the same time, they must avoid being seen as cold enforcers of rules. Balancing patient autonomy, beneficence, and legal obligations requires constant reflection. The task is to remain a compassionate guide, explaining limitations, advocating alternatives, and respecting patient dignity while ensuring compliance.

Imagine sitting with your peers in the canteen after a heavy ethics lecture. Someone asks, "If you were the doctor in the 'adolescent abortion' case, would you follow the law strictly, or secretly respect the minor's wish?" Another replies, "And what if your own relative needed a kidney, would you still defend the ban on organ sales?" The steaming cup in your hand reminds you: these aren't hypothetical puzzles, you will face them.

Conflicts are unavoidable and will arise when personal values clash with statutory law.

Legal literacy. Doctors must be aware of acts like the MTP Act, POCSO Act, and THOTA.

Patient-centred communication: It reduces anger, fear, or distrust, even when the law prevents specific actions.

Advocacy role: Beyond individual care, doctors should support systemic reforms, better sex education, improved access to contraception, organ donation awareness, and transparent waiting lists. The challenge is not choosing between law and empathy, but blending both with integrity.

☕ Coffee Moment

Later, while reflecting with a colleague over coffee, Dr Iyer admitted softly, "I thought withdrawing spared me pain, but in doing so, I left my patient alone in hers." The pause hung heavy, reminding him that being present in failure is as important as being celebrated in success.

References

1. Beauchamp TL, Childress JF. Principles of Biomedical Ethics. 8th ed. New York: Oxford University Press; 2019.
2. Global Observatory on Donation and Transplantation. Organ Donation and Transplantation Activities 2020. World Health Organization; 2021.
3. Ministry of Health and Family Welfare. The Transplantation of Human Organs and Tissues Act, 1994 (as amended in 2011). New Delhi: MoHFW; 2011.
4. Quill, T.E., & Cassell, J. (1995). Nonabandonment: A central obligation for physicians. Annals of Internal Medicine, 122(5), 368–374.
5. Back, A.L., Arnold, R.M., Tulsky, J.A. (2009). Mastering Communication with Seriously Ill Patients. Cambridge University Press.
6. Indian Council of Medical Research. Definition of Terms Used in Limitation of Treatment and Providing Palliative Care at the End of Life. New Delhi: ICMR; 2018.

Chapter 33: Professionalism, Altruism and Fiduciary Duty

Introduction

Professionalism is the commitment to carrying out one's duties with excellence, empathy, and accountability in one's profession. It encompasses more than technical competence; it demands teamwork, honesty, integrity, confidentiality, respect for patients and colleagues, and awareness of potential conflicts of interest in their work. (1) This chapter explores teamwork in performing professional and fiduciary duties.

Teamwork and Fiduciary Duty

Healthcare is never a solo act but a coordinated team effort. While doctors are the most visible decision makers, proper patient care depends on the harmony of frontline doctors, nurses, technicians, physiotherapists, assisting staff, pharmacists, and administrators working together. As medical students or doctors, it is vital to see yourself not as a lone hero, but as part of a collective team, united by a single purpose: the patient's well-being.

Hospitals function as complex ecosystems, with teams working across shifts to ensure continuity of care. Effective teamwork makes this seamless, even as responsibilities shift from one professional to another. At its core, teamwork relies on clarity of roles, closed-loop communication, mutual respect, constructive intervention and knowledge sharing through respectful communication. This is clearly visible in high-stakes moments such as a code blue or resuscitation, where seconds matter and compliance with principles of effective team dynamics and calm professionalism directly influences survival. Yet these same principles, when practiced daily in ward rounds and clinics, foster a culture of safety, accountability, and trust. Teamwork, therefore, is not only critical in emergencies, but it is also the everyday expression of professionalism and fiduciary duty in medicine.

The Physician as Fiduciary

A physician is more than a healer; they are a fiduciary, a trustee of the patient's health and dignity. A fiduciary duty means that a doctor must always act in the best interest of the patient, prioritizing their welfare over personal or institutional gain. (2) Patients place their lives in the hands of doctors, relying on their expertise and honesty. This creates a responsibility to act in the patient's best interest, even when inconvenient or challenging. However, no doctor can function like a machine; continuous care is ensured through teamwork, systems, and shared accountability. No doctor can provide effective care in isolation; professionalism also extends to collaboration within teams. (3)

Key Principles

Teamwork and Collaboration: Each healthcare professional contributes unique skills. Observe and engage with nurses, technicians, social workers, and allied health staff. This will broaden your understanding of holistic patient care and teach humility.

Respect and Communication: Respect is the foundation of team culture. Whether you are a student or a senior consultant, communicate openly, listen actively, and create a safe space where colleagues can raise concerns or ask questions without fear of blame.

Setting Boundaries and Systems: Doctors must strike a balance between their duty to patients and their own well-being. Systems such as duty rosters, on-call schedules, and handovers ensure patient safety while preventing physician burnout. By embracing teamwork and fiduciary duty, you honour your patients and the invisible network of professionals who share the responsibility with you. Professionalism is not limited to grand gestures but is tested daily in small decisions, keeping confidences, being honest, and respecting boundaries. (4)

Altruism in Medicine

Altruism is the selfless concern for the well-being of others. For doctors, it means placing the patient's interest above personal gain, sometimes at the cost of comfort, time, or recognition. It is not about neglecting yourself, but about holding patient welfare.

Why Altruism Matters in Medicine

- **Trust:** Patients trust doctors because they believe decisions are made in their best interest, not for personal gain.
- **Professional Identity:** Altruism distinguishes medicine from many other professions.
- **Resilience:** Serving others often gives meaning that sustains doctors through long hours and stress.
- **Ethics:** Altruism aligns with the principles of beneficence and non-maleficence.

Examples of Altruism in Practice

- A resident doctor stayed an extra hour to comfort an anxious child before surgery.
- A physician guiding a low-income family toward free government schemes, instead of expensive tests.
- Sharing knowledge freely with juniors and colleagues, knowing it improves patient care.

The Balance

True altruism is not about self-sacrifice to the point of exhaustion. Doctors must also care for their own well-being. The idea is not “me or you” but “me and you”: finding ways to heal others without losing oneself. This balance keeps altruism sustainable.

☕ Coffee Moment

Late at night, you’re finishing rounds when a patient’s family timidly asks if you could explain the treatment plan again. You’re tired, your coffee is cold, and yet you pause, sit with them, and explain gently. Their anxious eyes soften with relief. That moment of service — unseen, unrecorded — is altruism. It is what makes medicine not just a job, but a calling.

Case Scenario: Shadow duty

Ashish, a second-year medical student, is assigned to shadow Sister Mary, a senior nurse in the medical ward. Throughout the day, he observes her monitoring vital signs, administering medications, comforting anxious patients, and coordinating with other staff. During rounds, she corrects a medication dose for a patient with kidney disease, reminding a junior doctor to adjust it. Patients greet her warmly, clearly trusting her presence. Ashish realizes that her role is much broader than he initially thought.

Core Concept

Teamwork in Healthcare: Teamwork is the coordinated effort of multiple healthcare professionals, doctors, nurses, technicians, and support staff, each contributing unique expertise to patient care. Effective teamwork requires respect, open communication, and recognition that no single professional can provide complete care in isolation.

Decision-Making Process: Ashish noticed that Sister Mary’s intervention prevented potential errors and improved patient safety. He understands that good clinical decisions often emerge from collaboration, where input from every team member is valued and respected. Instead of seeing himself as “above” nurses, he treats their knowledge and observations as integral to clinical care.

Outcome: By the end of the day, Ashish gained new respect for nurses’ critical role. He resolves to communicate more openly with nursing staff, seek their perspectives during patient management, and foster humility in teamwork.

Learning Points

- Nurses are not just assistants but vital partners in healthcare delivery.
- Hierarchical attitudes can obstruct communication and harm patients.

- Effective teamwork enhances safety, efficiency, and patient satisfaction.
- Medical students should learn to value and integrate the expertise of every team member.

Coffee Moment

Later that evening, over a quiet coffee in the hostel canteen, Ashish tells his friends, "I thought doctors led everything in a hospital. However, today I realised that the system wouldn't function without nurses. From now on, I will listen more carefully when a nurse speaks up." With this newfound humility, the coffee tastes warmer.

References

1. Cruess RL, Cruess SR, Steinert Y. Teaching Medical Professionalism. 2nd ed. Cambridge: Cambridge University Press; 2016.
2. Hall MA. The legal and historical foundations of patients as fiduciaries of physicians. Yale J Health Policy Law Ethics. 2002;2(1):1–36.
3. West MA, Lyubovnikova J. Illusions of team working in health care. J Health Organ Manag. 2013;27(1):134–42.
4. Swick HM. Toward a normative definition of medical professionalism. Acad Med. 2000;75(6):612–6.

Chapter 34: Good Clinical Practice & Ethics in Research

Introduction

Research in medicine is not only about clever ideas and clean statistics; it is about protecting people while seeking better answers. Good Clinical Practice (GCP) is the international standard for designing, conducting, recording, and reporting studies involving human participants. Ethics give GCP its core: respect for persons, beneficence, and justice. Clinical research must strike a balance between generating knowledge and protecting the rights and welfare of human participants. (1) This chapter shows you how to turn those values into everyday actions, whether you are doing a simple survey, a case series, or a clinical trial.

Core Principles

- **Respect for Persons:** Voluntary, informed consent; extra safeguards for children, pregnant women, the cognitively impaired, and the economically or socially vulnerable.
- **Beneficence & Non-maleficence:** Maintain a favourable risk–benefit balance; promptly identify and address harms.
- **Justice:** Fair selection of participants; no group bears risks disproportionately or is excluded from potential benefits without reason.
- **Scientific Validity:** A poorly designed study is unethical because it risks exposing participants without providing a reliable opportunity to obtain knowledge.
- **Transparency & Accountability:** Register trials prospectively, follow the approved protocol, and report results honestly, whether they are positive or negative. (2)

Good Clinical Practice

GCP provides a universal benchmark for designing, conducting, and reporting clinical trials. (3) Every research should follow GCP as below

Ethics Approval & Registration: Obtain approval from the Institutional Ethics Committee or IRB **before** beginning. Prospectively register clinical trials in national trial registries.

Protocol & SOPs: A clear, feasible protocol with predefined outcomes, eligibility, safety plan, monitoring, and analysis. Standard Operating Procedures minimize errors.

Informed Consent and Assent: Focus on the process, explain the purpose, procedures, risks, benefits, alternatives, the right to withdraw, data use, and compensation or medical care for injury. Use the participant's language; for minors, obtain guardian consent plus age-appropriate assent.

Data Integrity: Records must be Attributable, Legible, Contemporaneous, Original, Accurate, and also Complete, Consistent, Enduring, and Available. Keep source documents; ensure audit trails for electronic data.

Safety Reporting: Define and report serious adverse events (SAEs) within mandated timelines; maintain a continuous chain of communication from detection to the IEC, sponsor, and regulator.

Monitoring & Quality by Design: Prevent problems (training, pilot testing, checklists) rather than merely detecting them—Independent oversight (e.g., Data Safety Monitoring Board) for interventional studies with material risk.

Confidentiality & Privacy: Collect the minimum necessary data; code/de-identify; store securely; restrict access; disclose only as permitted in consent/ethics approval.

Compensation & Care: Provide free medical care for study-related injury and compensate as per applicable rules. Insurance/contingency plans should be in place **before** enrolment.

Conflict of Interest (COI): Declare financial and academic COIs; separate clinical care decisions from research incentives.

Authorship & Publication Ethics: Follow ICMJE authorship criteria; avoid ghost, gift, or guest authorship. No plagiarism, data fabrication, or selective reporting. (3)

Mandatory trial registration and informed consent are safeguards to uphold transparency and participant rights. (4) In India, research ethics is governed by the ICMR National Ethical Guidelines and CDSCO's Good Clinical Practice standards. (5) Indian regulatory bodies continue to align with international GCP while addressing local ethical challenges. (6)

Professionalism in Research

Respect in research extends not only to patients but also to colleagues and peers. If you are recruiting patients from another clinician's unit, using laboratory services, or relying on specialized software developed by a peer, ethical practice requires transparency. This includes obtaining written permission, formally acknowledging their contribution, and, where appropriate, offering authorship or collaborator status. Such practices foster trust, prevent disputes, and promote a collaborative spirit. Academic integrity is not only about avoiding plagiarism; it is also about recognizing the ecosystem of people and resources that make your work possible. (7)

Practical Steps for Students

- Frame a meaningful, minimal-risk question.
- Speak to a mentor early. Draft a 2–3 page protocol: background, objectives, design, eligibility, sample size, outcomes, consent, data sheet, analysis, timelines.
- Seek IEC approval (yes, even for surveys or audits if identifiable human data are involved).
- Write your consent in simple local and English language.
- Protect data. Lock cabinets; password-protect files; remove identifiers when analysing.
- Track safety. Define what you will consider an adverse event and outline the process for escalating it.
- Report honestly. Register and analyse as per plan, document deviations, and share results, even if "negative."

Case Snapshot: The Shortcut That Backfired

An enthusiastic team starts a "routine" prospective case series on post-operative infections. To save time, they begin collecting identifiable data before receiving IEC approval, planning to "submit soon." A patient later complains about the unauthorised use of her photographs. The IEC halts the project; data already collected cannot be used; the team must retrain, redo consent, and issue an apology.

Lessons: Do not collect data without prior approval; consent must be specific to the research use; quality and ethics are inseparable.

Coffee Moment

One young researcher sighed: "I never realised how many invisible hands shape a study - the nurse who helps with follow-up calls, the statistician who checks my analysis, the senior who gives me access to their patients. Research is never a solo act. The more I acknowledged them, the more I felt at peace with my work - and the more my colleagues trusted me."

References

1. World Medical Association. Declaration of Helsinki: Ethical principles for medical research involving human subjects. JAMA. 2013;310(20):2191–4.
2. National Commission for the Protection of Human Subjects of Biomedical and Behavioral Research. The Belmont Report. Washington, DC: US Government Printing Office; 1979.
3. International Council for Harmonisation of Technical Requirements for Pharmaceuticals for Human Use. ICH Harmonised Guideline: Integrated Addendum to ICH E6(R1): Guideline for Good Clinical Practice E6(R2). Geneva: ICH; 2016.

4. Viergever RF, Li K. Trends in global clinical trial registration: an analysis of numbers of registered clinical trials in different parts of the world from 2004 to 2013. BMJ Open. 2015;5(9):e008932.
5. Indian Council of Medical Research. National Ethical Guidelines for Biomedical and Health Research Involving Human Participants. New Delhi: ICMR; 2017.
6. Central Drugs Standard Control Organization. Good Clinical Practice Guidelines for Clinical Trials on Pharmaceutical Products in India. New Delhi: Ministry of Health and Family Welfare; 2001.
7. International Committee of Medical Journal Editors. Defining the Role of Authors and Contributors [Internet]. ICMJE; 2024 [cited 2025 Feb 20]. Available from: http://www.icmje.org/recommendations/

Chapter 35: Doctor - Industry Relationship

Introduction

Modern medicine relies heavily on innovation. New medicines, diagnostic tools, and medical devices are continually changing the way doctors treat patients. The industry plays a significant role in driving this innovation, with pharmaceutical companies, device manufacturers, and biotech firms leading the charge. As a result, doctors and industry intersect in various ways, including clinical trials, research partnerships, medical conferences, and ongoing education. (1)

Doctor-industry relationship

Although collaboration is vital, it also poses significant ethical issues. Doctors are entrusted to act solely in their patients' best interests. In contrast, the industry's primary accountability is to its shareholders and profits. When these two worlds intersect, tensions can emerge. The key ethical question is: How can doctors collaborate with the industry to further scientific progress without undermining patient trust or their own professional integrity? (2) The following key principles govern doctor-industry relationship

1. Primacy of Patient Welfare

Always put the patient's best interest first. It is unethical to enter into a relationship with the industry that may compromise a doctor's judgment and harm the patient's well-being.

2. Transparency

Disclosure is essential. Doctors should openly declare financial ties, research funding, or gifts from industry when presenting findings, publishing research, or advising patients. Transparency fosters trust and enables others to evaluate potential bias. (3)

3. Professional Independence

Doctors must maintain independence of thought and decision-making. Gifts, incentives, or marketing materials should never influence prescriptions, referrals, or device choices. Independence protects the doctor's role as a trusted adviser rather than a commercial agent.

4. Accountability

Doctors are accountable to patients, professional bodies, regulators, and society. Ethics codes, policies, and guidelines (e.g., NMC, AMA, ICMJE) ensure accountability. (2,3)

5. Proportionality in Engagement

Engagement with industry should be proportionate and justifiable. For example, receiving research grants for scientifically valid trials is appropriate; accepting costly vacations disguised as "educational meetings" is not.

Forms of Interaction and Ethical Challenges

1. Gifts and Hospitality

Small tokens, such as pens, diaries, or stethoscopes, may seem harmless, but research shows that even minor gifts can influence decisions. Large gifts or luxury hospitality may cross ethical boundaries and serve as inducements. Many professional bodies now restrict or prohibit the acceptance of gifts. (1)

2. Sponsored Conferences and Continuing Medical Education (CME)

Pharmaceutical companies frequently sponsor conferences, sometimes covering travel, accommodation, and registration costs. While CME is vital for doctors, the funding source can lead to conflicts of interest. Independent, peer-reviewed CME without commercial influence is the highest standard.

3. Clinical Trials and Research Funding

The industry funds numerous clinical trials. While this partnership can advance scientific progress, risks arise if commercial interests influence trial design, data analysis, or the reporting of results. Selective reporting of positive results or suppression of negative findings is a well-documented phenomenon. Ethical practice requires independent oversight, informed consent, and the publication of all results. (4)

4. Consultancy and Advisory Roles

Doctors may serve on advisory boards or as industry consultants. This is legitimate if based on expertise, but should be disclosed and compensated fairly. Conflicts occur when advisory roles intersect with prescribing decisions or policy-making.

5. Medical Education and Curriculum Influence

The industry sometimes tries to influence medical education by subtly emphasizing products or therapies. Educators need to protect curricula from commercial bias, ensuring a balanced, evidence-based training.

6. Direct-to-Consumer Influence

In some countries, drug advertisements target the public, pressuring doctors to prescribe branded drugs. Doctors must rely on their professional judgment, resisting undue influence from both the industry and patient demand driven by advertising.

Case Scenario: "The Sponsored Conference"

A young cardiologist, Dr Radhika, is finishing a busy outpatient session when a pharmaceutical representative approaches her. With a warm smile, he says, "Doctor, we are organizing an international cardiology conference in Dubai. We'd love for you to attend. The company will sponsor your flight and five-star accommodation for four nights. Your registration fee will also be waived. You'll only need to attend a two-hour product session, after which you can enjoy the city. To appreciate your valuable time, we'll also provide you with an honorarium."

Dr Radhika is tempted. She has always wanted to attend an international event and visit Dubai, but she wonders: Is this an educational opportunity or a marketing ploy that might influence her prescribing patterns?

Core Concept

Conflict of Interest in Doctor-Industry Relationships: A conflict of interest (COI) arises when professional judgment regarding patient welfare may be influenced, or appears to be influenced, by secondary interests such as gifts, travel, or financial benefits. Even if decisions remain clinically sound, the perception of bias can erode patient trust. Medical codes of ethics (e.g., the NMC in India, the AMA internationally) restrict the acceptance of hospitality or gifts that could compromise independence. (2,5)

Decision-Making Process

- **Evaluate the Offer:** Is this an independent academic conference or an industry-sponsored promotional event?
- **Ethical Reflection:** Would accepting this benefit influence or appear to influence her prescribing decisions?
- **Professional Guidelines:** The NMC Code discourages acceptance of foreign hospitality, luxury travel, or cash honoraria from pharma companies.
- **Alternatives:** She could attend the same conference independently, paying her own way, thereby preserving professional integrity.
- **Decision:** Dr Radhika declined the sponsorship and instead applied for institutional CME funding to attend another conference where her paper was accepted for presentation.

Outcome

Though she foregoes the luxury offer, Dr Radhika maintains her professional independence and credibility. Later, she attends the conference with partial institutional support and feels reassured that her decisions are guided by patient interest, not industry incentives.

Learning Points

- Doctors must remain vigilant to conflicts of interest in their interactions with the industry.
- Even if intentions are good, perception of bias can harm trust.
- National and institutional ethical codes provide clear boundaries against undue influence.
- True professional growth comes from independent, unbiased learning.

☕ Coffee Moment

That evening, over coffee with a colleague, Dr Radhika admitted, "It would have been so easy to say yes. But I asked myself whether it is justified and ethical? That question gave me my answer." Her coffee tasted lighter, knowing she had chosen integrity over indulgence.

References

1. Wazana A. Physicians and the pharmaceutical industry: is a gift ever just a gift? JAMA. 2000 Jan 19;283(3):373-80.
2. Medical Council of India. Code of Ethics Regulations, 2002 (amended 2016). New Delhi: MCI; 2016.
3. International Committee of Medical Journal Editors. Defining the Role of Authors and Contributors [Internet]. ICMJE; 2024 [cited 2025 Feb 20]. Available from: http://www.icmje.org/recommendations/
4. Bekelman JE, Li Y, Gross CP. Scope and impact of financial conflicts of interest in biomedical research: a systematic review. JAMA. 2003 Jan 22;289(4):454-65.
5. Institute of Medicine (US) Committee on Conflict of Interest in Medical Research, Education, and Practice. Conflict of Interest in Medical Research, Education, and Practice. Washington (DC): National Academies Press; 2009.

Chapter 36: Balancing Collaboration and Integrity

Introduction

The doctor–industry relationship is a double-edged sword. At its best, it fosters innovation, research, and improved care. At its worst, it risks eroding patient trust and corrupting medical judgment. Ethical practice requires vigilance, transparency, and integrity. As future doctors, you must know that even small influences can shape choices. Doctors cannot and should not avoid industry entirely. Innovation relies on collaboration, and the ethical task is to engage responsibly. (1) The safeguard is a simple compass: always ask whether this serves the patient first. If the answer is unclear, caution is wise.

- Pursue partnerships that promote genuine research or patient care.
- Reject benefits that might bias judgment.
- Learn about the subtle influences of marketing psychology.
- Advocate for system-wide policies that encourage transparency and fairness.

Why This Matters

For medical students, the doctor–industry relationship might seem distant. But these pressures are real from the very first prescription pad. Pharmaceutical representatives may visit clinics, invite doctors to dinners, or sponsor student events. Recognizing ethical boundaries early helps safeguard future practice. Students and doctors should learn to ask:

- Am I upholding the dignity of the profession and the primacy of patient welfare?
- Would I be comfortable if my patient were aware of this gift or relationship?
- Could this influence my decision-making, even unconsciously?

Conflicts of Interest

A conflict of interest (COI) occurs when a doctor's personal or financial interests might influence or seem to influence their professional judgment. Notably, the mere appearance of a conflict can be as detrimental as an actual conflict, as it damages trust. (2) Common types of COI include:

- **Financial COI**: receiving payments, shares, or royalties.
- **Academic COI**: pressure to publish favourable results for industry sponsors.
- **Institutional COI**: When hospitals or universities benefit financially from industry contracts.

Managing COI requires:

- Full disclosure to patients, peers, and journals.
- Recusing oneself from decision-making when a conflict of interest exists.
- Independent oversight by ethics committees or regulators.

Ethical Frameworks and Guidelines

NMC Code of Ethics (India): Prohibits accepting gifts, hospitality, and paid travel from the industry. Promotes transparency in research and forbids endorsement of commercial products. (3)

American Medical Association (AMA) Codes: Emphasize patient primacy, independence, and disclosure. (4)

ICMJE Guidelines: Conflicts are required to be disclosed when publishing research. (5)

Institutional Ethics Committees (IECs): Oversee industry-sponsored trials, ensuring participant protection and data integrity.

Referral Bonuses and Ethical Concerns

Referral bonuses, also known as "fee-splitting" arrangements, where doctors receive financial incentives for directing patients to specific hospitals, laboratories, or diagnostic centres, pose significant ethical and legal challenges. The following are core ethical issues in this-

- **Conflict of Interest**: Such arrangements risk shifting the doctor's priority from patient welfare to financial gain. Decisions about where to admit a patient, what tests to order, or which treatments to recommend may be subconsciously biased by monetary incentives.
- **Erosion of Trust**: The doctor–patient relationship is built on fiduciary duty and trust. If patients learn that referrals are influenced by hidden commissions, it undermines confidence in medical advice.
- **Professional Integrity**: Medical codes of ethics (e.g., the NMC in India) explicitly prohibit fee splitting. Doctors must act independently, with clinical decisions based solely on what is best for the patient.
- **Legal Implications**: In India, arrangements involving referral bonuses may violate the provisions of the Prevention of Corruption Act and the professional misconduct provisions under the NMC regulations.
- **Entrepreneurial vs. Ethical Balance**: Doctors may legally own or operate diagnostic centres or pharmacies, but such relationships must be transparent. Profit cannot override patient autonomy, informed consent, and best interests.

Case Scenario: "The Bonus Offer"

Dr. Sameer, a physician, is approached by a corporate hospital manager with a lucrative proposal: "For every patient you refer to our hospital, we'll pay you 20% of hospital charges. For outpatient referrals, you'll get 30% of billed collections. In return, you'll be part of our extended family and can set your own consultation fees."Dr Sameer is torn. The arrangement promises financial security, but he wonders if he can remain unbiased when advising patients where to go.

Core Concept

Referral Bonuses and Fee-Splitting: Fee-splitting is an unethical practice in which doctors accept financial rewards for directing patients. It creates a conflict of interest, risks exploitation, and is prohibited by medical ethical codes.

Decision-Making Process

- **Temptation:** Dr Sameer recognizes the financial appeal but reflects on its impact on patient trust.
- **Ethics:** He considers whether he could honestly tell patients about the arrangement.
- **Professional Guidance:** NMC regulations prohibit fee splitting, categorizing it as professional misconduct.
- **Alternative:** Instead of accepting bonuses, Dr Sameer advocates for transparent collaborations where patients are referred based on facilities, quality, and affordability, rather than commissions.

Outcome

Dr Sameer declines the offer, choosing to protect his independence and reputation. His patients continue to trust his recommendations, and he remains respected in his community.

Learning Points

- Referral bonuses compromise fiduciary duty and professional independence.
- Patients deserve transparency. Decisions must be clinically driven, not financially driven.
- Fee-splitting is prohibited under ethical codes and may have legal consequences.
- Doctors can engage in entrepreneurship, but integrity and transparency must guide every step they take.

☕ Coffee Moment

Later, over a coffee with his colleague, Dr Sameer said, "The money was tempting. But I asked myself, if my own child were sick, would I want the doctor's advice swayed by a hidden deal? The answer was enough." The coffee felt warmer, knowing he had chosen trust over temptation.

References

1. World Health Organization. Framework for Action on Interprofessional Education and Collaborative Practice. Geneva: WHO; 2010.
2. Lo B, Field MJ, editors. Conflict of Interest in Medical Research, Education, and Practice. Washington (DC): National Academies Press; 2009.
3. Medical Council of India. Code of Ethics Regulations, 2002 (amended 2016). New Delhi: MCI; 2016.
4. American Medical Association. Code of Medical Ethics. Chicago: AMA; 2021.
5. International Committee of Medical Journal Editors. Defining the Role of Authors and Contributors [Internet]. ICMJE; 2024 [cited 2025 Feb 20]. Available from: http://www.icmje.org/recommendations/

Crossroads

A Crossroads is where paths meet and

choices must be made - often quickly,

sometimes with lasting consequences.

In medicine, ethical and medicolegal dilemmas are such crossroads.

A decision may balance life and law,

compassion and protocol,

duty and conscience.

This section does not give you formulas but presents real cases that distil these tensions,

helping you practice the art of decision-making.

Each dilemma is a mirror, asking you:

What kind of doctor will you be when the decision is yours to make?

Here, you learn that being a doctor is not only about knowledge, but about judgment —

the courage to choose wisely when no option is simple and ethics is in the grey zones

S No.	Crossroads: At a Glance
1.	**Chapter 37** – Beneficence: Explores beneficence in context of public health and individual responsibility.
2.	**Chapter 38** - Non-maleficence: "Do no harm". A well-intended treatment can cause harm and doctors must constantly weigh risks.
3.	**Chapter 39** - Confidentiality: Here, you learn how confidentiality protects trust and where its limits lie.
4.	**Chapter 40** - Justice and Triage: When resources are scarce, who gets priority? This dilemma explores fairness, triage, and the ethics of resource allocation in emergencies.
5.	**Chapter 41** - Consent for OPD Examination of a Female Patient: Sensitive examinations require more than skill - dignity, consent, and protection against abuse of power.
6.	**Chapter 42** - Informed Consent for Elective Surgery: Consent is not a signature, but a process for autonomy.
7.	**Chapter 43** - Emergency Care Without Patient Capacity: Can life-saving care be given without consent? Emergency room where urgency tests both law and ethics.
8.	**Chapter 44** - Accurate Medical Documentation: Patient file is not only clinical note - it is evidence, accountability, and a legal record.
9.	**Chapter 45** - Fiduciary Duty vs Fatigue: Doctors are human too. When exhaustion strikes, how do you balance self-care with duty to patients?
10.	**Chapter 46** - Sponsored Workshop & Conflict of Interest: Industry sponsorship can open doors or cloud judgment. Transparency, influence, and professional independence.
11.	**Chapter 47** - Reproductive Rights in Adolescents: Consent, confidentiality, and law intersect in cases of adolescent abortion. Rights, duties, and social context.
12.	**Chapter 48** - Parental Refusal vs Child's Best Interests: When parents decline care for a child, doctors must decide whether to respect wishes or override them to protect life.
13.	**Chapter 49** - Organ Donation: Organ transplantation saves lives but raises deep questions about consent, ownership, and ethics of scarcity.
14.	**Chapter 50** - Life on a Machine: End-of-life decisions, advance directives, and autonomy are at the heart of this dilemma, where medicine meets human dignity.
15.	**Chapter 51** - Irreversible Brain Injury: Withdrawal of support and the possibility of organ donation in brain-dead patients brings the sharpest test of law, ethics, and compassion.

Chapter 37: Dilemma in Beneficence

Arjun, a 7-year-old boy, is brought to the pediatric outpatient clinic with severe anaemia. His parents are poor daily-wage workers and have been giving him home remedies, but his condition has worsened. On examination, he is pale, underweight, and fatigued. Investigations reveal iron deficiency anaemia with borderline cardiac strain, and timely treatment could prevent progression to heart failure.

Core Concept

Beneficence is the ethical obligation of healthcare providers to actively act in the best interest of the patient, with the intent of maximising benefit and improving overall well-being. It goes beyond merely avoiding harm and requires positive action to promote health, prevent disease progression, and relieve suffering.

In clinical practice, beneficence involves:

- Timely medical intervention to prevent foreseeable complications.
- Anticipation of future harm, not just treatment of current symptoms.
- Consideration of the patient's social, economic, and familial context, especially when these factors directly affect health outcomes.

In children, beneficence carries an added responsibility, as they depend on adults and healthcare systems to advocate for their long-term physical, emotional, and developmental well-being. (1)

Approach

Immediate Care: Start iron and nutritional supplementation promptly and arrange hospital admission for monitoring due to his cardiac strain.

Address Barriers: Link the family to government nutrition schemes (e.g., Mid-Day Meal, Poshan Abhiyaan) and hospital welfare programs.

Holistic Benefit: Educate the parents about nutrition and the prevention of recurrence. Arrange follow-up to ensure continuity of care. (2,3)

Outcome

Within weeks, Arjun improved, his haemoglobin levels rose, and his growth parameters improved. The family expressed gratitude for the kindness and practical help they received.

Learning Points

- Beneficence requires active steps to improve a patient's well-being, not only avoiding harm.

- Practical problem-solving is often as important as medical treatment.
- Acting in the best interest of the patient may include addressing social determinants of health.

☕ Coffee Moment

Later that evening, as the clinic quietened and the day's charts were finally closed, the pediatrician sat with his coffee and reflected. 'Treating anaemia was straightforward; treating poverty was not'. Yet, in that small act of arranging support and guidance, a child's future had shifted course. He realised that beneficence is not only about prescribing the right medicine, but about recognising when a family needs a hand to hold the ladder, so they can climb out of illness themselves.

References

1. National Medical Commission. AETCOM module for undergraduate medical education. New Delhi: NMC; 2018 (rev. 2019).
2. Government of India. POSHAN Abhiyaan: Guidelines. New Delhi: Ministry of Women & Child Development; 2018.
3. World Health Organization. Closing the gap in a generation: health equity through action on the social determinants of health. Geneva: WHO; 2008.

Chapter 38: Dilemma in Non-Maleficence

Mr Ramesh, a 45-year-old man from a rural area, presents to the outpatient department with a chronic cough and breathlessness. He has been receiving treatment from an unqualified local practitioner ("quack") who prescribed him repeated courses of high-dose oral steroids for months without monitoring. On examination, Ramesh has signs of uncontrolled diabetes, thin skin with bruising, and early cataracts, side effects of prolonged steroid misuse. After a proper evaluation, the MBBS doctor diagnoses him with moderate COPD and poorly controlled diabetes secondary to steroid overuse. The doctor now faces an important decision: how to reverse the damage, provide effective treatment, and prevent further harm, while addressing the past inappropriate care.

Core Concept

Non-maleficence is the ethical principle that obliges healthcare providers to avoid causing harm, whether through action or inaction. It extends beyond avoiding overt mistakes and includes the responsibility to recognise, prevent, and stop ongoing or foreseeable harm, even when such harm has arisen from prior treatment given with good intentions.

In clinical practice, non-maleficence requires doctors to:

- Critically evaluate existing therapies, rather than blindly continuing them.
- Withdraw or modify harmful interventions safely, balancing the risks of stopping treatment against the risks of continuing it.
- Protect patients from unsafe medical practices, including irrational prescriptions and unmonitored therapies.
- Educate patients compassionately, without blame, to prevent future harm.

Non-maleficence is therefore not passive restraint, but an active ethical commitment to patient safety and rational care, especially when correcting the consequences of inappropriate treatment. (1)

Approach

Immediate Harm Control: Discontinue inappropriate steroid regimen, initiate tapering plan to avoid adrenal crisis, treat hyperglycemia promptly.

Evidence-Based Management: Prescribe inhaled bronchodilators and corticosteroids. Optimize diabetes management through lifestyle modifications and safe pharmacotherapy. (2)

Patient Education: Explain the risks associated with unsupervised medication use and encourage follow-up care in a healthcare facility. Report harmful practices to the appropriate health authorities.

Shared Responsibility: Emphasize that while the doctor ensures safe, evidence-based treatment, the patient must communicate symptoms, understand instructions, and return for review if symptoms worsen. (3)

Outcome

Within weeks, Ramesh's blood sugar improved, and his breathing stabilized. He expressed gratitude. The doctor's adherence to non-maleficence prevented further harm and corrected the unsafe trajectory set by prior care.

Learning Points

Sometimes, the most important intervention is to stop a harmful practice. Patient education is crucial in preventing future harm.

☕ Coffee Moment

Over evening coffee, the doctor reflected, "Medicine is not only about adding treatments, but often about removing the wrong ones. Sometimes, healing begins with subtraction." He realised that non-maleficence is not about doing less medicine, but about doing only what is safe, necessary, and justifiable.

References

1. Beauchamp TL, Childress JF. Principles of biomedical ethics. 8th ed. New York: Oxford University Press; 2019.
2. Global Initiative for Chronic Obstructive Lung Disease (GOLD). Global strategy for the diagnosis, management, and prevention of COPD—2024 report. Fontana, WI: GOLD; 2024.
3. World Health Organization. Patient safety curriculum guide. Geneva: WHO; 2011.

Chapter 39: Dilemma in Confidentiality in Patient Care

A 20-year-old college student visits the psychiatry clinic with anxiety and panic attacks. She discloses sexual harassment by a family member during a private consultation and requests that her parents not be informed, fearing conflict and stigma. Later, her father visits and asks for details of her condition. The physician must choose between respecting her confidentiality and the cultural expectations of family involvement. (1)

Core Concept

Confidentiality is the ethical and legal duty of healthcare professionals to protect a patient's personal and medical information from unauthorised disclosure. Respecting confidentiality is fundamental to the doctor–patient relationship, as trust allows patients to share sensitive information honestly, enabling accurate diagnosis and effective care. (1,2)

From a medico-legal perspective, patient information may be disclosed only with the patient's informed consent, or under specific legal and ethical exceptions:

- When required by law (e.g., notifiable diseases, court orders),
- When disclosure is necessary to prevent serious harm to the patient or others,
- When permitted under professional guidelines and public health obligations.

Unauthorised disclosure without valid justification can result in disciplinary action, loss of professional credibility, and legal liability.

In the Indian **socio-cultural context**, families often play a central role in healthcare decisions and may expect to be informed, particularly for adolescents and young adults. However, cultural sensitivity does not override patient autonomy or confidentiality. Doctors must navigate this balance carefully by:

- Assessing the patient's capacity and preferences,
- Seeking explicit consent before sharing information,
- Encouraging, but not forcing, family involvement where it benefits care.

Confidentiality, therefore, is not secrecy at all costs, but a thoughtful, patient-centred commitment to privacy, trust, and ethical judgement.

Approach

The doctor explains confidentiality boundaries, assesses immediate risks, encourages voluntary disclosure to a trusted person, and documents the reasoning. To the father, the doctor politely cites professional and legal obligations. (3)

Outcome

The patient continues therapy and later shares her situation with a supportive cousin. Trust is preserved, and family support is gained without violating her wishes.

Learning Points

- Confidentiality is fundamental to patient trust and care.
- Cultural norms must be balanced with ethical and legal duties.
- Clear communication and documentation protect both patient and physician.

☕ Coffee Moment

The young psychiatrist reflected on the patient's trembling voice and the whispered plea. She understood that confidentiality is about more than rules; it creates a safe space in a world. She thought, "Sometimes silence is also a form of healing." With that sip, she felt the weight of trust, heavier than any prescription.

References

1. National Medical Commission. AETCOM module for undergraduate medical education. New Delhi: NMC; 2018 (rev. 2019).
2. National Medical Commission. Indian Medical Council (Professional Conduct, Etiquette and Ethics) Regulations, 2002 (amended 2016). New Delhi: NMC; 2016.
3. Government of India. The Mental Healthcare Act, 2017. New Delhi: MoHFW; 2017.

Chapter 40: Dilemma on A Question of Justice

At a small district hospital, Dr Pathak faces an ethical dilemma when two patients arrive simultaneously: a 70-year-old woman with severe pneumonia needing ventilatory support and a 25-year-old accident victim with head trauma. With only one ventilator, the team must make a critical choice.

Core Concept

Justice in Healthcare: Justice in healthcare refers to the ethical obligation to ensure fairness and equity in the distribution of healthcare resources, particularly when resources are limited. It requires that decisions be based on morally relevant clinical criteria, rather than personal bias, social status, age, gender, or perceived social worth. (1) In situations of scarcity, such as limited ICU beds, ventilators, or emergency services, justice demands that healthcare providers:

- Treat similar clinical situations similarly, using objective medical assessment.
- Prioritise patients based on likelihood of benefit, urgency, and potential for recovery, rather than on emotion or external pressure.
- Follow transparent, consistent, and institutionally supported decision-making processes, rather than individual discretion alone.
- Document and communicate decisions clearly, recognising the emotional burden such choices place on both families and healthcare teams.

Justice does not mean providing the same treatment to everyone, but rather allocating resources in a way that is ethically defensible, clinically sound, and socially responsible, especially in resource-constrained settings.

Approach

Dr Pathak reviews clinical details with his team. The older woman has significant comorbidities and a poor prognosis; the younger man has a higher chance of meaningful recovery. After consulting both families, the team decides to allocate the ventilator to the younger patient (beneficence) while arranging high-flow oxygen and rapid transfer for the older patient (justice with compassion). Every step, including reasoning, was documented to maintain medico-legal transparency. Emotional support was provided to the woman's family to acknowledge their loss and grief. (1,2)

Outcome

The younger man stabilised with ventilatory support and was prepared for neurosurgical referral. The older woman was managed with alternative measures during transfer, though her condition remained guarded.

Learning Points

- Justice requires balancing fairness, beneficence, and respect for all patients.
- Transparency in decision-making, involving families, and proper documentation reduces conflicts.
- Policies and triage protocols are crucial for guiding clinicians during periods of resource scarcity.
- Emotional support and communication are as important as medical action in such crises.

☕ Coffee Moment

Later, as the team sat together over evening tea, they reflected on the weight of their choice. The silence spoke of the emotional burden of triage. They realised that fairness in medicine is not about easy answers, but about compassionate, ethically sound decisions made in the best interest of all patients.

References

1. World Health Organization. Ethics and COVID-19: resource allocation and priority-setting. Geneva: WHO; 2020.
2. Beauchamp TL, Childress JF. Principles of biomedical ethics. 8th ed. New York: Oxford University Press; 2019.

Chapter 41: Dilemma on Consent for OPD Examination

A 26-year-old married woman visits the gynaecology outpatient department complaining of lower abdominal pain and irregular menstrual cycles. The attending resident suggests a pelvic examination to aid diagnosis. The patient appears hesitant, and her mother, who accompanied her, insists that the doctor proceed quickly without "unnecessary questions."

Core Concept

Consent: A voluntary, informed agreement by a patient to allow a healthcare professional to perform an examination, procedure, or treatment. (1)

Informed Consent in OPD: Even for routine outpatient procedures like a pelvic exam, consent, preferably written for intimate examinations, is essential, especially for female patients.

Medico-Legal Considerations

Under Indian law and the Medical Council of India (now NMC) regulations, any examination of a female patient involving the genital, breast, or rectal areas must be conducted with her informed consent and in the presence of a female attendant/chaperone. Forcible or non-consensual examination can amount to assault under Section 354 of the IPC. (1,2)

Approach

- The doctor explains the purpose, nature, and steps of the pelvic examination, including the use of a chaperone.
- The patient is reassured that she may decline or request postponement.
- After understanding, she gives her verbal and written consent.
- The examination is then conducted with a female nurse present, maintaining privacy and dignity throughout. (3)

Outcome

The findings point toward pelvic inflammatory disease. The patient appreciates the respectful communication and privacy.

Learning Points

- Always obtain explicit informed consent before intimate examinations.
- The presence of a female attendant is mandatory for examining female patients.
- Good communication preserves trust and reduces medico-legal risk.

☕ Coffee Moment

Later, as the resident sipped her evening coffee, she recalled the patient's anxious eyes before the examination. A simple pause to explain why the exam was needed, how privacy would be protected, and that she could refuse had transformed fear into cooperation. "Consent isn't just a signature, it's about restoring dignity when patients feel most vulnerable." The coffee tasted warmer.

References

1. National Medical Commission. Indian Medical Council (Professional Conduct, Etiquette and Ethics) Regulations, 2002 (amended 2016). New Delhi: NMC; 2016.
2. General Medical Council. Intimate examinations and chaperones. London: GMC; 2013 (updated 2019).
3. Royal College of Obstetricians and Gynaecologists. Maintaining standards: guidelines for good practice—chaperones. London: RCOG; 2015.

Chapter 42: Dilemma in Consent for Elective Surgery

A 52-year-old woman is diagnosed with gallstones and advised a laparoscopic cholecystectomy. She understands the recommendation but expresses worry about anaesthesia, recalling a neighbour's complications. Her husband, however, insists on signing the consent form himself, telling her, Doctor knows best. The surgical team is ready to proceed the next day.

Core Concept

Informed Consent in Surgery

Medico-Legal Aspect: In India, valid consent must be informed, voluntary, and given by the patient if the patient is an adult with decision-making capacity. (1) The surgeon must clearly explain the surgery, its benefits, risks (including anaesthesia), alternatives, and consequences of refusal. Pre-printed blanket forms and consent signed only by a relative can be challenged. (1,2)

Socio-Cultural Factors: In some families, male relatives often dominate health decisions, even for capable women. Cultural respect for authority can silence patient concerns. Fear of appearing weak may stop patients from voicing anxieties.

Professional Responsibility: Ensuring the patient's autonomy is essential. Proper documentation of the discussion is as necessary as obtaining the signature. (2)

Decision-Making Process

Private Discussion: The surgeon arranges a meeting with the patient alone, allowing her to express concerns without family pressure. The procedure, risks, benefits, alternatives, and anaesthesia details are explained in simple language.

Addressing Concerns: The patient's fears about anaesthesia are acknowledged, and reassurance is provided with safety protocols.

Voluntary Decision: Adequate time is given to decide, ensuring her choice is free of coercion. (3)

Outcome

The next day, the patient signed the consent form after clarifying her doubts. She undergoes surgery confidently, and the documentation reflects a legally valid and ethically sound consent.

Learning Points

- Consent is a communication process, not just a formality; substitute consent is invalid.
- Cultural barriers must be navigated sensitively, without undermining patient autonomy.
- Documentation of the conversation is crucial for both patient trust and legal protection.
- Adult patients with decision-making capacity must provide their own consent.

☕Coffee Moment

That evening, the surgeon reflected over coffee: "Her husband thought he was protecting her. But in truth, she only needed to be heard. A signature matters less than the dignity of choice."

References

1. National Medical Commission. Indian Medical Council (Professional Conduct, Etiquette and Ethics) Regulations, 2002 (amended 2016). New Delhi: NMC; 2016.
2. Supreme Court of India. Samira Kohli v. Dr Prabha Manchanda (2008) 2 SCC 1.
3. National Medical Commission. AETCOM module for undergraduate medical education. New Delhi: NMC; 2018 (rev. 2019).

Chapter 43: Dilemma on Patient Without Capacity

A 45-year-old man is brought to the emergency department (ED) after a road traffic accident. He is unconscious, has multiple fractures, and is bleeding profusely. His blood pressure is dangerously low, indicating hemorrhagic shock. No family members or acquaintances are present, and no identifying documents are found immediately.

Core Concepts

Incapacity

When a patient lacks the ability to understand, evaluate, and communicate decisions about their own healthcare. (1)

Emergency Consent Principle

In life-threatening situations where the patient cannot consent, healthcare providers are ethically and legally permitted to proceed with necessary interventions to save life or prevent serious harm. (1) Under Indian law and global norms (e.g., WHO, GMC UK, AMA), consent is implied in emergencies when delay risks life. The Indian Supreme Court affirms doctors' duty to provide immediate care without waiting for consent. Documenting findings, urgency, and actions is vital for medico-legal defence. (2,3)

Approach

The ED team immediately initiates resuscitation, secures the airway, controls bleeding, and arranges urgent surgery. Efforts to identify the patient and contact relatives continue in parallel. All steps are documented, including the rationale for proceeding without formal consent.

Outcome

The patient stabilizes after surgery. Six hours later, the family is located and informed of the interventions. They express gratitude for the timely, life-saving actions.

Learning Points

- Emergency care takes precedence over consent when a delay risks life.
- Documentation is crucial for maintaining transparency and ensuring legal safety.
- Parallel efforts should be made to identify and contact the next of kin.

Coffee Moment

That night, as the casualty team took a coffee break, the junior doctor recalled an unconscious patient who arrived without attendants. There was no time for consent or family signatures, only to act or watch life slip away. A senior responded, "Our duty is to save lives in emergencies. One day, if we were on that stretcher, we'd hope someone acts first and explains later." The strong coffee reflected the realization that urgency sometimes is the voice of consent.

References

1. National Medical Commission. Indian Medical Council (Professional Conduct, Etiquette and Ethics) Regulations, 2002 (amended 2016). New Delhi: NMC; 2016.
2. Supreme Court of India. Paschim Banga Khet Mazdoor Samity v. State of West Bengal (1996) AIR 2426.
3. World Health Organization. Emergency care systems framework. Geneva: WHO; 2018.

Chapter 44: Dilemma on Accurate Medical Documentation

Dr Siddharth, a junior resident in medicine, attends to a 52-year-old male with uncontrolled diabetes and foot infection. He prescribes IV antibiotics and wound care, but due to a busy night shift, he forgets to update the treatment chart and daily progress note. The next morning, the consultant notices no record of antibiotic administration, wound assessment, or the patient's consent for planned surgical debridement. The nursing notes and vital signs are incomplete for two shifts.

Core Concepts

Professional Responsibilities: Maintaining a good record-keeping system ensures continuity of understanding, supports research, and facilitates accurate claims. Standards require legible, factual, and timely entries, including the date, time, and signature. (1)

Medico-Legal Aspects: In India, medical records are considered legal documents, as mandated by guidelines such as the Clinical Establishments Act and the MCI/NMC Code of Ethics. Inaccurate or incomplete records can harm patient safety and lead to litigation. Lack of proper documentation may be seen as negligence if an adverse event occurs, even if care was given. (1-3)

Decision-Making Process

Identify Lapse: Consultant highlights missing records and educates Dr Siddharth.

Corrective Action: The patient's current status is reassessed, and missing details are reconstructed as accurately as possible.

System Strengthening: The unit implements a checklist and handover template to ensure continuity of care and real-time EMR updates.

Outcome

Dr Siddharth receives feedback, undergoes brief record-keeping training, and adopts a habit of real-time documentation, ensuring patient safety and legal protection.

Learning Points

- Medical records are legal and clinical documents; poor documentation equates with negligence.
- Continuity of care between shifts depends on the accuracy, legibility, and timeliness of notes.
- Documentation fosters trust, transparency, and accountability.

☕ Coffee Moment

That evening, as Dr Siddharth sipped his coffee in the canteen, a senior resident remarked: "The pen can protect you as much as the stethoscope." Siddharth smiled, realizing that writing notes was not a clerical burden but part of medical treatment, an invisible bridge between care, safety, and trust.

References

1. Government of India. Clinical Establishments (Central Government) Rules, 2012—medical records. New Delhi: MoHFW; 2012.
2. National Medical Commission. Indian Medical Council (Professional Conduct, Etiquette and Ethics) Regulations, 2002 (amended 2016). New Delhi: NMC; 2016.
3. World Health Organization. Patient safety: implementation manual—communication & documentation. Geneva: WHO; 2011.

Chapter 45: Dilemma on Fiduciary Duty vs Fatigue

Dr Singh, a general surgeon in a small town completed a gruelling 16-hour day, handling multiple emergency surgeries and outpatient visits. Barely able to keep his eyes open, he collapsed into bed, hoping for uninterrupted rest. At 1 AM, urgent knocking woke him. Villagers stood at his door, carrying a teenage girl bitten by a snake. His spouse, concerned for his health, reminded him that another hospital, 5 km away, was operational and that he had already requested not to be disturbed. Yet, the villagers insisted: the local nursing home advertised 24-hour emergency services, and they trusted him. Dr Singh faced a dilemma between his exhaustion and his duty to the patient.

Core Concept

Fiduciary Duty

In medicine, fiduciary duty refers to a physician's responsibility to act in the patient's best interest, prioritising patient welfare over personal convenience. It also acknowledges the need for safe systems that protect both patients and healthcare providers from undue risk or burnout. (1,2)

Decision-Making Process

Dr Singh paused to weigh his options. On one hand, he was terribly fatigued, and proceeding could compromise his own health and judgment. On the other hand, refusal to act might endanger the girl's life, given the time-sensitive nature of snake envenomation.

Considering the urgency and lack of immediate alternatives, he attended to the patient. He stabilized her, administered antivenom, and arranged follow-up care. Meanwhile, the situation highlighted the inadequacy of relying on a single exhausted physician without supportive systems in place.

Outcome

The girl survived and recovered, grateful for Dr Singh's intervention. The villagers praised his dedication, though his spouse and colleagues remained concerned about his well-being. The case prompted discussion at the hospital about recruiting an on-call night duty doctor to ensure continuity of care without overburdening a single individual. (3,4)

Learning Points

- Physicians hold a fiduciary role, prioritizing patient welfare, but this must be balanced against their personal limitations.

- Systemic solutions (night shifts, cross-coverage, staffing policies) are essential to reduce reliance on one individual.

☕ Coffee Moment

Dr Singh sat with his spouse the next morning over tea. She gently said, "You saved a life last night, but who will save you if you collapse one day?" He smiled, realizing the truth in her words, and decided to hire one more medical officer to ensure continuity of services. Medicine is not about individual heroism, but about building systems.

References

1. National Medical Commission. AETCOM module for undergraduate medical education. New Delhi: NMC; 2018 (rev. 2019).
2. Swick HM. Toward a normative definition of medical professionalism. Acad Med. 2000;75(6):612–6.
3. Accreditation Council for Graduate Medical Education. Common program requirements (duty hours). Chicago: ACGME; 2020.

Chapter 46: Dilemma on The Sponsored Workshop

A device company invites Dr Arvind, an orthopaedic surgeon, to attend a "training workshop" on a new knee implant system at a luxury hill resort. The company covers travel, accommodation, and meals and also provides him with an honorarium. Dr Arvind attends, enjoys the hospitality, and begins to favour the company's implants in his practice. Some months later, a report appeared in the newspaper about regulatory scrutiny of "conflict of interest" in orthopaedic implant use, naming a few surgeons, including Dr Arvind. Patient advocacy groups questioned whether patients were treated in their best interest. Soon, the hospital administration opens an internal inquiry. Dr Arvind realizes that what once felt like harmless sponsorship has damaged his reputation and strained patient trust.

Core Concept

Professional Independence and Transparency

Doctors are fiduciaries; they must act in the best interest of patients. Accepting hospitality or financial support that appears to influence decisions undermines professional independence. Even if choices remain clinically sound, the perception of bias erodes public confidence. (1-3)

Decision-Making Process

Temptation: Dr Arvind saw the workshop as an educational and networking opportunity, without reflecting on its commercial bias.

Action: By accepting lavish hospitality, he blurred the line between professional learning and promotional marketing.

Consequence: His motives were publicly questioned, and an institutional inquiry threatened to undermine his credibility.

Alternative: Attending such workshops independently or through hospital CME funds would have preserved transparency and trust.

Outcome

Though no malpractice was proven, Dr Arvind's reputation suffered. He became more cautious about industry interactions, learning that credibility, once lost, is difficult to regain.

Learning Points

- There is no free lunch.

- Accepting industry sponsorship creates a real or perceived conflict of interest.
- Patient trust is fragile and can be lost even without wrongdoing.
- Institutions monitor doctor–industry interactions to ensure compliance with ethical codes.
- Professional independence and transparency safeguard both patient care and the physician's reputation.

Coffee Moment

Dr Arvind sighed over coffee with a colleague, "I thought it was just a workshop. I didn't realize the real cost would be a question of my integrity and loss of trust." His colleague nodded, "Sometimes the price of a free trip is higher than we think."

References

1. Medical Council of India. Indian Medical Council (Professional Conduct, Etiquette and Ethics) Regulations, 2002 (amended 2016). New Delhi: MCI; 2016.
2. Institute of Medicine (US). Conflict of interest in medical research, education, and practice. Washington (DC): National Academies Press; 2009.
3. Wazana A. Physicians and the pharmaceutical industry: is a gift ever just a gift? JAMA. 2000;283(3):373–80.

Chapter 47: Dilemma on Reproductive Rights

Dr Ananya, a first-year resident in Obstetrics & Gynaecology, attends to Meera, a 17-year-old unmarried college student who is 14 weeks pregnant. She requests a medical termination of pregnancy (MTP), stating that the relationship was consensual, but she cannot continue the pregnancy due to social stigma and economic constraints. Her parents are unaware. The senior consultant explains that under Indian law, termination up to 20 weeks is permissible under certain conditions. However, since Meera is a minor, her consent alone is not legally valid. Guardian consent and mandatory reporting are required under the POCSO Act. Meera is distressed, fearing police involvement and the social humiliation that may follow.

Core Concepts

Medical Termination of Pregnancy (MTP)

Regulated under the MTP Act, allowing abortion within specified gestational limits and conditions. (1,2)

Reproductive Rights

Every individual has the right to safe, legal reproductive health services, but these rights intersect with age-of-consent laws.

Medico-Legal Issues: Overlap of the MTP Act with the POCSO Act complicates care, as all sexual activity with a minor (<18 years) is treated as statutory rape. (1,3)

Socioeconomic Issues: Stigma, financial hardship, and gender inequality hinder access to safe abortion.

Ethical Issues: Balancing autonomy (Meera's wishes), beneficence (acting in her best interest), non-maleficence (avoiding harm), and justice (complying with law).

Decision-Making Process

Clinical Assessment: Ultrasound confirms gestational age at 14 weeks; no contraindications for MTP. (2)

Counselling: Procedure, risks, alternatives, and legal requirements (reporting under the POCSO Act) are explained. Psychological support is provided. (3)

Consent Process: Since Meera is 17, consent from a legal guardian is mandatory.

Reporting: A police intimation is filed as per the POCSO. Confidentiality is maintained to protect Meera's dignity.

Male Counterpart's Responsibility:

If **minor (<18 years):** He is considered a "child in conflict with law" under the Juvenile Justice Act. The Juvenile Justice Board decides the course, with potential reformative measures. If **adult (≥18 years):** He faces statutory rape charges with imprisonment from 10 years to life, regardless of consensual claim. (1,3)

Procedure: Safe abortion is carried out as per guidelines with post-abortion care including contraceptive counselling, STI screening, and mental health support.

Documentation: MTP forms, consent papers, and police intimation are recorded.

Outcome

Meera undergoes a safe MTP after obtaining guardian consent. She receives privacy-respecting care, contraceptive advice, and referral to a counsellor. The case is reported under the POCSO Act, and the male counterpart is being investigated in accordance with the law. Dr Ananya learns to balance empathy, confidentiality, and strict legal compliance.

Learning Points

- Doctors must be well-versed in the MTP Act and the POCSO Act, as both directly affect adolescent pregnancies, and reporting is mandatory.
- Consent from a minor is insufficient; consent from a guardian is mandatory.
- The male counterpart faces legal consequences irrespective of "consent" due to statutory rape laws.
- Socioeconomic barriers and stigma must be addressed sensitively.
- Professionalism means acting with compassion within the law while safeguarding patient dignity.

☕ Coffee Moment

Later, sipping tea in the hospital canteen, Dr Ananya replayed Meera's fearful words in her mind. "Was I helping her, or punishing her with the law?" she wondered. A senior reassured her: "You did both, protected her health and upheld the law. Sometimes, compassion means walking the narrow path between two truths."

References

1. Government of India. The Medical Termination of Pregnancy (Amendment) Act, 2021. New Delhi: MoHFW; 2021.
2. MoHFW. Comprehensive abortion care—training and service delivery guidelines. New Delhi: MoHFW; 2018 (updated 2022).
3. Government of India. The Protection of Children from Sexual Offences Act, 2012. New Delhi: MWCD; 2012.

Chapter 48: Dilemma on Parental Right to Refuse Treatment

A 5-year-old boy is brought to the pediatric emergency department with severe respiratory distress due to pneumonia. The treating team recommends immediate hospitalization, intravenous antibiotics, and oxygen therapy. The child's parents, who follow a faith-based healing practice, refuse hospital admission and request only outpatient treatment.

Core Concepts

Parental Rights

Parents generally hold the legal authority to make healthcare decisions for their minor children. (1)

Best Interests Principle

Healthcare decisions for children should prioritize the child's life, health, and well-being over parental preferences.

Medico-Legal Context: In India, while parents have rights, the state assumes a *parens patriae* role to protect children from neglect. Under the Juvenile Justice Act, refusal of life-saving treatment may constitute medical neglect. Doctors are ethically and legally obliged to intervene in emergencies, even against parental refusal, and may seek judicial or welfare authority intervention if needed. (1-3)

Decision-Making Process

Counselling: The doctor explains the seriousness of pneumonia, risks of deterioration, and the likelihood of recovery with prompt treatment.

Parental Refusal: Despite explanations, the parents continue to refuse admission.

Escalation: The treating team involves hospital administration and informs child welfare authorities.

Emergency Intervention: Under implied consent for life-threatening conditions, oxygen and antibiotics are initiated immediately to stabilize the child.

Legal & Ethical Balance: Documentation is made of parental refusal, discussions, and steps taken.

Outcome

The child receives timely treatment and recovers after a week of hospital care. The parents, initially resistant, later express gratitude upon seeing the improvement.

Hospital administration and child welfare authorities support the medical team's actions, affirming that the intervention was in the child's best interests.

Learning Points

- A child's right to life and health supersedes parental refusal in emergencies.
- Cultural and faith-based beliefs should be respected, but not at the cost of safety or survival.
- Indian law (Juvenile Justice Act, parens patriae doctrine) protects doctors who act in the best interest of the child.
- Proper documentation and escalation through appropriate authorities are essential.

☕ Coffee Moment

That evening, a resident reflected over coffee: "The parents thought faith alone could save their child. But in choosing to act, we honoured not only the law, but the boy's chance to live and breathe again. Sometimes protecting a child means being firm, even when hearts are heavy."

References

1. Government of India. The Juvenile Justice (Care and Protection of Children) Act, 2015. New Delhi: MWCD; 2015.
2. Indian Academy of Pediatrics. Ethics guidelines for pediatric practice. Mumbai: IAP; 2017.
3. United Nations. Convention on the Rights of the Child. New York: UN; 1989.

Chapter 49: Dilemma on Organ Donation

Ravi, a 28-year-old man, is declared brain-dead in a tertiary hospital after a road traffic accident. The hospital's transplant coordinator approaches his grieving parents about the possibility of donating his organs to save other lives. The father is supportive, but the mother is hesitant; she fears religious disapproval and doubts whether her son's body will be treated respectfully. Meanwhile, the ICU team faces the challenge of meeting legal consent requirements under the Transplantation of Human Organs and Tissues Act (THOTA), ensuring ethical conduct, and addressing the family's concerns in a sensitive manner. (1)

Core Concepts

Organ Donation

The act of giving one's organ or tissue, either during life (living donation) or after death (deceased/cadaveric donation), for transplantation into another person in need, with legal, ethical, and medical safeguards. (1)

Medico-Legal Framework in India

The Transplantation of Human Organs and Tissues Act (THOTA) regulates the removal, storage, and transplantation of human organs and tissues.

- Defines brain death criteria (two sets of tests by independent doctors).
- Requires written informed consent from the donor (if living) or next of kin (if deceased).
- Prohibits organ trade; penalties for commercial dealings.
- Establishes Authorization Committees for living donations (esp. unrelated donors).
- Mandates NOTTO (National Organ and Tissue Transplant Organization) registry for equitable allocation.

Medico-legal obligations: Accurate certification of brain death. Proper documentation (Form 8 for consent, Form 10 for brain death) and transplant allocation according to registry priority. (1-3)

Approach in Practice

Early, Sensitive Communication: Trained transplant coordinators should approach families privately, after explaining brain death clearly. Use culturally appropriate language.

Legal Compliance: Strictly follow THOTA guidelines and maintain transparency in documentation and allocation. (1)

Addressing Myths & Concerns: Explain that organ retrieval is done with dignity and does not interfere with religious rituals. (3)

Socioeconomic Support: Link financially vulnerable recipients to government schemes.

Logical Outcome of the Case

In Ravi's case, after compassionate counselling, both parents agreed to the donation. His heart, kidneys, and corneas were allocated through the state registry, saving four lives. The hospital honoured the donor's memory in a small ceremony with the family's consent, reinforcing public trust.

Learning Points

- Organ donation requires strict adherence to legal provisions to ensure ethical practice and public trust.
- Sensitivity to cultural, religious, and emotional concerns is crucial for obtaining informed family consent.
- Doctors must advocate for equitable access to transplantation and combat the commercialisation of this vital resource.

☕ Coffee Moment

During a night shift, a young intern stood quietly as the transplant coordinator handed a thank-you card to Ravi's parents after the donation. The mother, still in tears, said softly, "My son couldn't live, but he will still breathe somewhere in this world." Over that cup of coffee later, the intern realized, medicine is not only about saving lives, but also about giving life a second chance.

References

1. Ministry of Health & Family Welfare. The Transplantation of Human Organs and Tissues Act, 1994 (as amended 2011). New Delhi: MoHFW; 2011.
2. National Organ and Tissue Transplant Organization (NOTTO). Operational guidelines. New Delhi: MoHFW; 2019.
3. World Health Organization. WHO guiding principles on human cell, tissue and organ transplantation. Geneva: WHO; 2010.

Chapter 50: Dilemma in Life on a Machine

Mrs Jayanti, a 78-year-old woman, had often told her doctor, after witnessing her husband's prolonged suffering on a ventilator, "Promise me you won't put me on a machine." Months later, she was admitted with severe pneumonia and hyponatraemia. In the emergency room, she was hypoxic and required intubation. Her consciousness fluctuated - sometimes gesturing to remove the tube, sometimes confused. Hours later, her son arrived and pleaded, "Do everything possible."

Core Concept

Autonomy versus Beneficence

Autonomy refers to a patient's right to make informed decisions about their own medical care, including the right to accept or refuse life-sustaining treatment. Beneficence, in contrast, obliges doctors to act in the patient's best medical interest, especially in emergencies. Ethical dilemmas arise when these two principles appear to conflict.

Advance directives, whether written or clearly expressed oral statements, are expressions of patient autonomy regarding future medical treatment in situations where the patient may lose decision-making capacity. They guide clinicians in respecting the patient's previously stated values and preferences. However, for advance directives to be ethically and legally actionable, they must be:

- Clear and specific, avoiding ambiguity about circumstances and interventions,
- Made when the patient had decisional capacity,
- Documented and communicated, wherever possible,
- Interpreted within the prevailing legal framework.

In emergency settings, when capacity fluctuates and documentation is absent or incomplete, clinicians must carefully balance:

- The known or reasonably inferred wishes of the patient,
- The immediate duty to preserve life and relieve suffering, and
- The role of surrogate decision-makers, whose authority is to represent the patient's values, not substitute their own.

Thus, ethical decision-making in such cases lies not in choosing autonomy *or* beneficence, but in integrating both through thoughtful, patient-centred judgement, guided by prior wishes, clinical urgency, and ethical proportionality. (1,2)

Approach

The team first stabilized Mrs Jayanti with intubation, antibiotics, IV fluids, and correction of hyponatraemia. They debated the validity of her prior statement versus her son's surrogate decision. An ethics discussion focused on balancing autonomy with beneficence, assessing her decision-making capacity, and the absence of a written directive. The team also explained the situation compassionately to her son, ensuring he is part of the decision-making process. (1,3)

Outcome

Mrs Jayanti was managed on a ventilator in the ICU. Over two days, her condition improved, and she was extubated. To her relief, she had no memory of distress during ventilation. She expressed gratitude to both her son and the medical team for preserving her life while respecting her dignity.

Learning Points

- Autonomy and advance directives serve as guides, but must be evaluated for clarity and legal weight.
- Capacity assessment is essential when patients are confused.
- Surrogate decision-making should reflect the patient's values, not only family preferences.
- Shared decision-making and documentation are vital in ethically complex cases.

☕ Coffee Moment

Over coffee, students reflected: "Sometimes saving a life and respecting wishes seem contradictory, but empathy, dialogue, and ethics can bridge that gap."

References

1. Indian Council of Medical Research. Definition of terms & guidance for limitation of treatment & palliative care at end of life. New Delhi: ICMR; 2018.
2. Supreme Court of India. Common Cause v. Union of India (2018) 5 SCC 1.
3. Indian Society of Critical Care Medicine. End-of-life care policy: consensus statement. Indian J Crit Care Med. 2014;18(9):615–35.

Chapter 51: Dilemma on Irreversible Brain Injury

Mr Arun, a 65-year-old male, was admitted to the ICU following a severe stroke that resulted in significant brain damage. Despite aggressive medical interventions, his neurological status remained unchanged, and he was diagnosed with a persistent vegetative state. His family was informed of the prognosis and the likelihood of no meaningful recovery.

Core Concept

Advance Directives and Family Wishes

Mr Arun had previously expressed to his family that he would not want to be kept alive on a ventilator. However, he did not have a formal advance directive documenting these wishes. His family, while aware of his preferences, was divided on the decision to withdraw life support. (1,2)

Decision-Making Process

Medical Assessment: The medical team conducted thorough evaluations, including neurological assessments, to confirm the extent of the brain injury and rule out reversible causes. The prognosis was deemed poor, with no meaningful recovery. (1,3)

Family Discussions: The medical team facilitated multiple discussions with the family to understand Mr Arun's values and preferences as a surrogate decision-maker.

Ethics and Legal Consultation: Consultation with the ethics committee and legal counsel ensured that the decision to withdraw life support was in accordance with ethics, applicable laws and regulations.

Outcome

After careful consideration and consensus among the family, the decision was made to withdraw life support. Mr Arun passed away peacefully. His family decided to honour his wishes by donating his organs, providing the gift of life to several recipients.

Learning Points

- Advance directives provide clarity but are often absent; in such cases, families become surrogates guided by the patient's best interests.
- Ethical and legal consultation supports families and doctors during sensitive end-of-life decisions.

- Withdrawing life support is not abandonment; it is a recognition of medicine's limits, combined with respect for dignity.
- Organ donation at the end of life can transform grief into a meaningful and hopeful legacy for others.
- Honest, compassionate communication is central to navigating such conflicts.

☕ Coffee Moment

Later, over coffee in the hospital lounge, a young resident asked, "Wasn't it hard to stop treatment?" The senior physician replied gently, "Sometimes healing is not about prolonging life, but honouring it. In giving dignity to Mr Arun, and in donating his organs, his family showed us that endings can also be beginnings." The room fell quiet, and the coffee tasted more soulful than ever.

References

1. Indian Society of Critical Care Medicine & Indian Association of Palliative Care. Joint position statement on end-of-life care and palliative care. Indian J Crit Care Med. 2020;24(Suppl 6):S1–S36.
2. Supreme Court of India. Common Cause v. Union of India (2018) 5 SCC 1.
3. Ministry of Health & Family Welfare. The Transplantation of Human Organs and Tissues Act, 1994 (as amended 2011). New Delhi: MoHFW; 2011.

Part 2: Foundations of Living Medicine

Revive

Where Every Second Counts

There comes a time in every doctor's journey when knowledge alone is not enough.
A collapsing child, a breathless grandmother, a stranger whose heart has suddenly stopped - in these moments, you cannot turn the page or wait for a lecture. You must act, and you must act now.

This is the spirit of Revive.
Here, you will step into the world of emergencies, where seconds are precious and hesitation can cost a life. These chapters will prepare you to see clearly, decide swiftly, and move courageously when it matters most.

In *Revive*, you will learn the cognitive science of

CPR and first aid,

the psychomotor skills to perform them and

the affective strength to lead, comfort, and support

a team through crisis.

Carry this section with reverence.

Read and practice it often, revisit it always. Because these are not skills for exams; these are skills for life, someone else's life, placed in your hands.

Your training from *Revive* will become someone's heartbeat, someone's breath, someone's tomorrow.

S No.	Revive: At a Glance
1.	**Chapter 52** Skills to Save a Life: Introduction to Sanjeevani Vidya From books to bedside: how knowledge becomes action. Simulation, mastery, and the journey from "knowing" to "doing."
2.	**Chapter 53** Cardiopulmonary Resuscitation: Cognitive Domain The science of CPR — what it is, why it matters, and the golden window where survival is decided.
3.	**Chapter 54** Cardiopulmonary Resuscitation: Psychomotor Domain Hands-on: recognizing arrest, compressions, breaths, AED use. Step-by-step skills that make the difference.
4.	**Chapter 55** Cardiopulmonary Resuscitation: Affective Domain The heart behind the hands: courage, teamwork, communication, and debriefing after the storm.
5.	**Chapter 56** Choking and Foreign Body Airway Obstruction When airway is blocked: swift steps to free the breath in infants, children, and adults.
6.	**Chapter 57** CPR in Special Circumstances Beyond algorithms: drowning, trauma, pregnancy, lightning, pandemics, and prone CPR.
7.	**Chapter 58** CPR Awareness, Community Readiness & Certification From the classroom to the community: creating a culture of lifesaving through training, certification, and outreach.

Chapter 52: Skills to Save a Life-Sanjeevani Vidhya

Introduction

Imagine you witness a child who has collapsed in front of you, or helping a breathless grandmother with a metered dose inhaler. In such situations, only knowledge is insufficient; you need to act swiftly with high precision. MBBS is a call to learn what saves lives and perform it at the right time when it matters most. In this section, you will go through the journey from knowledge to action and learn those skills that are the very essence of becoming a doctor.

As you embark on your medical journey, you will encounter new terms in these pages. Don't be daunted. Most explanations are in plain language, and when we use precise medical words, it's to help you build the professional vocabulary you'll need during MBBS. Let the unfamiliar words pass by once or twice, and return to them as your learning deepens. Revisit these chapters before skills sessions, ward postings, OSCEs, and throughout your career, because CPR and first aid are lifetime skills, not merely first-year topics. Each reread will bring more clarity, and the exact steps you practice now can save a life at any point in your medical journey. Mastery comes with practice and repetition, so don't hesitate to revisit these chapters as often as you need.

From Knowing to Doing: Books to Bedside

During school days, learning was often synonymous with acquiring knowledge, typically based on information and assessed through marks and multiple-choice questions.

Four dimensions of knowledge

- **Factual**: basic elements (terminology, details).
- **Conceptual**: interrelationships of elements (theories, models),
- **Procedural**: how to perform something (methods, techniques).
- **Metacognitive**: self-awareness of cognition.

You will need to apply all these dimensions in your journey ahead.

Three Domains of Learning

- **Cognitive domain**: Acquiring and applying medical knowledge.
- **Psychomotor domain**: Mastering practical skills and procedures.
- **Affective domain**: Application, communication, professional behaviour, ethics, and patient-centred care.

Four Levels of Clinical Competence

You need to transform the knowledge into clinical competence. Miller's Pyramid of Clinical Competence nicely captures this transformation. (1) The four levels of clinical competence are:

- **Knows**: Understands the facts, like what CPR is.
- **Knows How**: Understands the procedure, like when and how CPR is performed.
- **Shows How**: Demonstrate the skill safely, like CPR, in a simulation lab.
- **Does**: Performs the skill in real life, under pressure, like performing CPR on a patient in the ER.

Bloom's taxonomy focuses on the cognitive learning process. You will see that learning goes from remembering to creating. (2)

- **Remember**: recall basic concepts and information.
- **Understand**: ability to explain concepts.
- **Apply**: situational application of information.
- **Analyze**: draw connections among ideas.
- **Evaluate**: being able to justify a decision.
- **Create**: produce an original work or new concept.

Learning Pyramid

The Learning Pyramid represents the average retention rate of information after 24 hours, depending on the teaching or learning method used. Teaching is the most powerful learning. The learning journey that begins with a lecture, reading a book, or watching a video should extend to demonstrate, discuss, practice, and teach others to gain mastery and confidence. As you become proficient, you will be able to teach complex concepts to your peers, nurses, patients, and even schoolchildren. When you teach CPR to a 10-year-old schoolboy or explain handwashing to a patient's family members, you don't only pass on a skill; you amplify its power and you multiply lives saved.

Table 52.1: Retention rates of different systems of learning

Method	Retention	Explanation
Lecture	~5%	Passive listening
Reading	~10%	Slightly better, still passive.
Audiovisual	~20%	Combines hearing and seeing
Demonstration	~30%	Seeing a skilled act boosts memory.
Discussion	~50%	Interactive dialogue for understanding.
Practice Doing	~75%	Hands-on activities anchor skills deeply.
Teaching	~90%	Explaining concepts tbrings mastery.

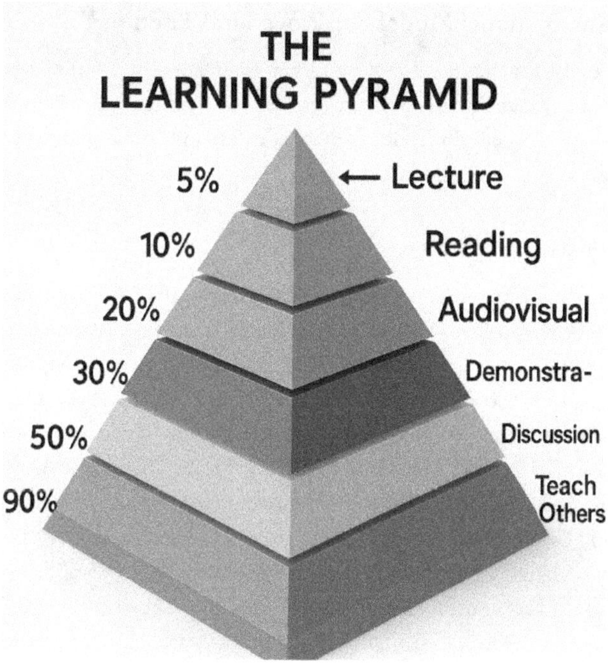

Figure 52.1: The Learning Pyramid

Simulation: The Power of Practice

Can you learn how to fly a plane by simply reading books or attending lectures? Not for sure! Like aviation, medicine is a high-stakes and time-sensitive field. Simulation-based learning is a cornerstone for skill modules. (3) You will practice these skills through skills labs, mannequins, practice while watching videos, and structured feedback. You need to set your biological clock to certain rhythms and train your hands and head to work as a unit to deliver action in a time-sensitive manner. Simulation allows you to make mistakes (safely), build your muscle memory, learn team dynamics and coordination and gain confidence in certain skills before facing real-life patients

Mastery Over Mediocrity: 84% is the New Pass

In school, 33% or 50% marks were sufficient for you to pass an exam. In medicine, if you get a skill only half-right, there is a chance that someone might not go home alive just because a caregiver was proficient only up to 50% of a life-saving skill. That's why we set a high benchmark. For every skill, be it donning gloves, providing CPR or giving first aid, you must aim for mastery, not familiarity. Often, this will mean a passing criterion of 80–84% or higher in certain skill sets or examinations, and that's not pressure; it's preparation. Each practice session is a rehearsal for someone's survival.

Six-Step Instructional Model For Procedural Training

Learn → See → Practice → Prove → Do → Maintain—to promote retention and confidence. For training of healthcare workers and community awareness, spaced 'low-dose–high-frequency' refresher sessions, community drills, and integration with local systems are strongly encouraged. (3)

CPR Updates 2025

The International Liaison Committee on Resuscitation (ILCOR) updates CPR and First Aid recommendations annually and undertakes an extensive review every five years. Through its continuous Consensus on Science with Treatment Recommendations (CoSTR) process, ILCOR experts systematically analyze clinical trials and new evidence to inform their recommendations. These scientific statements provide a basis for regional councils and scientific bodies, such as the American Heart Association (AHA), the European Resuscitation Council (ERC), the Indian Resuscitation Council Federation (IRCF), and the Indian Academy of Pediatrics, to periodically update their guidelines. This book contains the 2025 updates across the CPR and first aid sections, to align with the latest global evidence and consensus. A few key take-home messages from the 2025 guidelines are summarised below, in case you have already learned them from previous sources, to bring to your attention important changes. (4)

1. In adult cardiac arrest, resuscitation should generally start on-site where the patient is found, if it is possible to safely and effectively perform high-quality CPR. (5)
2. Position the patient's torso approximately at the rescuer's knee level to deliver chest compressions effectively. (5)
3. Chest compressions and ventilations should both be performed by healthcare workers for all adult and pediatric patients in cardiac arrest, irrespective of the cause of cardiac arrest. (5)
4. Mechanical CPR devices are not recommended for routine use.
5. For patients not breathing but having a pulse, or those receiving CPR with an advanced airway in place, deliver 10 breaths per minute (one breath every 6 seconds) in adults and 20-30 breaths per minute (one breath every 2-3 seconds) in infants and children. (5,7)
6. CPR for patients with obesity should be provided by using the same techniques, adjusting force to achieve the recommended compression depth.
7. In case of severe foreign-body airway obstruction (FBAO), give cycles of five back blows (slaps) alternating with five abdominal thrusts in adults and children above one year of age, while cycles of five back blows (slaps) alternating with five chest thrusts in infants until the object is out or the patient becomes unresponsive. Abdominal thrusts are not recommended in infants. (5-7)
8. Rescuers are required to use personal protective equipment (PPE) when

performing CPR under specific circumstances. (5)

9. Ventilation and oxygenation should be initiated quickly in infants and children, as they have respiratory conditions as a major cause of cardiac arrest. (7)
10. Lay rescuers should provide breaths if able and willing for out-of-hospital cardiac arrest (OHCA) in infants and children. In adults with OHCA, compression-only CPR may be initiated as an alternative. (4-7)
11. High-quality CPR is the foundation of resuscitation. It includes ensuring push hard (adequate chest compression depth), push fast (compression rate 100-120/min), allowing complete chest recoil between compressions, avoiding excessive ventilation and minimizing interruptions in CPR.
12. Alternative CPR techniques: Interposed abdominal compression remains investigational and not routinely recommended; Cough-CPR is a short bridge in a conscious, monitored adult, never a public instruction; Avoid precordial thump. (8)
13. For infant chest compression, use either the single-hand technique or the two-thumb encircling hands technique. The Two-fingers technique, recommended earlier, is ineffective in achieving proper depth. (7)
14. Prompt defibrillation for shockable rhythms, i.e. ventricular fibrillation (VF) and pulseless ventricular tachycardia (pVT), is critical. Peri-shock pauses should be minimal. (7)

Coffee Moment

While sipping coffee, Ajay thinks, I didn't choose medicine to memorise textbooks. His senior says, You chose it for deeper reasons.

It is going to be rigorous. You may feel uncomfortable at times. But it will be worth every drop of sweat and every moment of reflection. Someday, you will stand somewhere between life and death with the armour of your life-saving knowledge and skills for someone you don't know. Here, the transformation begins. You can call it **Sanjeevani Vidya**!

References

1. Miller GE. The assessment of clinical skills/competence/performance. Acad Med. 1990;65(9):S63–7.
2. Bloom BS. Taxonomy of educational objectives: The classification of educational goals. New York: David McKay; 1956.
3. Hewett Brumberg EK, Douma MJ, Alibertis K, Charlton NP, Goldman MP, Harper-Kirksey K, et al. 2024 American Heart Association and American Red Cross Guidelines for First Aid. Circulation. 2024;150:e519–e579.
4. Bray JE, Smyth MA, Perkins GD, Cash RE, Chung SP, Considine J, et al. Basic Life Support: 2025 International Liaison Committee on Resuscitation Consensus on Science With Treatment Recommendations. Circulation. 2025 Oct 21;152(16_suppl_1):S34-S71.

5. Kleinman ME, Buick JE, Huber N, Idris AH, Levy M, Morgan SG, et al. Part 7: adult basic life support: 2025 American Heart Association Guidelines for Cardiopulmonary Resuscitation and Emergency cardiovascular Care. Circulation. 2025;152(suppl 2):S448–S478.
6. Joyner BL, Dewan M, Bavare A, de Caen A, DiMaria K, Donofrio-Odmann J, et al. Part 6: pediatric basic life support: 2025 American Heart Association and American Academy of Pediatrics Guidelines for Cardiopulmonary Resuscitation and Emergency Cardiovascular Care. Circulation. 2025;152(suppl 2):S424–S447.
7. Cao D, Arens AM, Chow SL, Easter SR, Hoffman RS, Lagina AT III, et al. Part 10: adult and pediatric special circumstances of resuscitation: 2025 American Heart Association Guidelines for Cardiopulmonary Resuscitation and Emergency Cardiovascular Care. Circulation. 2025;152(suppl 2):S578–S672.

Chapter 53: CPR - Cognitive Domain

In medical science, some moments demand much more than knowledge; they demand action. When the human heart stops beating, you do not have hours or even minutes. You have seconds to act. In those seconds, a hand placed right to push fast at the rate of 100-120 chest compressions per min, the correct technique to push hard with adequate chest recoil, and the ability to deliver a rescue breath with minimal interruption to the rhythm of chest compressions will mean the difference between a life lost and a life saved. In this chapter, we will focus on the cognitive domains of cardiopulmonary resuscitation (CPR). Further, we will discuss psychomotor (skills in sequence) and affective (teamwork and communication) domains.

Use of Uniform Terminology

Standardized terminology helps improve communication and accuracy in emergency response, training and education. The 2025 AHA Guidelines further standardize resuscitation terminologies for global consistency, replacing 'rescue breaths' with 'breaths,' promoting 'lay rescuer' over 'bystander,' and differentiating between ROSC and ROC recovery of circulation. (1) Interpret carefully if you encounter these terminologies in literature with overlapping or different meanings.

Cardiac Arrest: A sudden and complete cessation of heartbeat. It's an electrical failure where the heart abruptly stops pumping blood. The person collapses, becomes unresponsive and stops breathing. Every second matters, and every minute without action drastically reduces chances of survival. This medical emergency requires immediate CPR and defibrillation without waiting for professional help or reaching the hospital. In such a situation, any 'bystander' becomes a lifesaver 'lay rescuer' if correct sequence of actions is started immediately. Identify the cardiac arrest, call for help, start CPR by pushing hard and pushing fast, placing hands in the centre of the chest, use an AED as soon as available and continue until professional help arrives or the person revives.

Cardiopulmonary Resuscitation: CPR is an emergency lifesaving procedure used in cardiac arrest when the heart stops beating. It combines chest compressions by bare hands to maintain blood circulation and breaths (or ventilation) to provide oxygen, thereby sustaining vital organs until advanced care is available. CPR is the essential link to survival, bridging the critical minutes between cardiac arrest and definitive treatment. It requires no equipment, medicine, or major expertise. It is also known as Basic Life Support (BLS), or Basic Cardiac Life Support (BCLS). In conditions when ventilation is not possible, even compression-only life support is vital, also known as hands-only CPR.

Breaths vs. Ventilations

Breaths: In reference to CPR, 'breaths' are given when a person is in cardiac arrest (unresponsive, not breathing, no pulse) or has a pulse but is not breathing. Breaths can be given using a pocket mask, a face shield, or mouth-to-mouth breaths. The term "rescue breaths" is no longer used.

Ventilations: Used when health care professionals provide assisted breathing through a mechanical device, such as a bag and mask device or an advanced airway.

Lay Rescuer vs. Bystander

Lay Rescuer: Preferred term for a non–health care professional who provides emergency care, replacing "layperson" or "lay responder." This term emphasizes active participation and encourages prompt lifesaving response by the public.

Bystander: It represents someone just present rather than taking action.

ROC vs. ROSC

Return of Circulation (ROC): Used when circulation is restored mechanically, such as by extracorporeal membrane oxygenation (ECMO) or other mechanical support systems.

Return of Spontaneous Circulation (ROSC): Used when circulation returns spontaneously, through recovery of native cardiac function without mechanical intervention.

Cardiac arrest can strike anyone, anywhere, in a hospital bed, at home, on a busy street or even at school. CPR must begin immediately, without waiting for assistance. You are the only help until further help arrives. The ability to perform CPR empowers every citizen and healthcare provider to be the first responder in someone's most critical moment by initiating bystander CPR. Whether it's in-hospital cardiac arrest (IHCA) or out-of-hospital cardiac arrest (OHCA), timely CPR can mean the difference between life and death. (2) When we teach BLS, we create a circle of protection. We turn bystanders into lifesavers. 'Because God couldn't be everywhere, He created mother.' In the same spirit, we train lifesavers because a doctor can't be everywhere.

What is the Survival Window?

Without immediate intervention in cardiac arrest, irreversible brain damage begins within 4–6 minutes, and death is almost certain within 10 minutes. The "golden minutes" after cardiac arrest are the most vital:

Table 53.1: Time-senstive injuries after cardiac arrest

Time After Arrest	Injury
0–1 min	Brain injury begins
3–4 min	Irreversible brain damage possible
6–10 min	Very low survival chances

CAB: Compressions-Airway Breathing Sequence in CPR

Historically, resuscitation training followed the ABC sequence (Airway–Breathing–Circulation). However, current evidence emphasises the importance of chest compressions as the first step, leading to a new mnemonic: C-A-B. (3, 4) This means that while starting CPR for cardiac arrest, start with chest compression followed by maintenance of airway and delivery of breaths (bag and mask, mouth to mask or mouth to mouth).

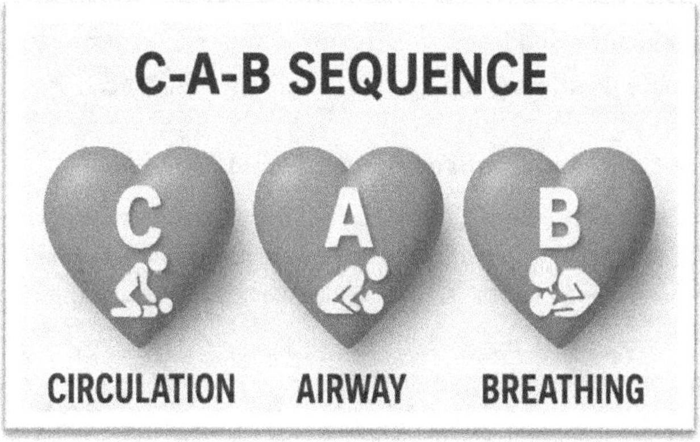

Figure 53.1: Sequence in CPR

Cardiac Arrest vs. Heart Attack

Cardiac arrest is a sudden and complete cessation of heartbeat, while a heart attack or myocardial infarction (MI) is a circulatory problem due to a blockage in the arteries, leading to reduced blood flow to some areas of the heart muscle. The person usually complains of chest pain or tightness, pain radiating to the jaw, arm, or back, nausea, sweating, or breathlessness, but remains conscious and keeps breathing. If not treated immediately, a heart attack may lead to cardiac arrest. In such a situation, one should immediately call for emergency medical support, assist the patient to a seated position, and remain calm. If not allergic or contraindicated, administer aspirin (300 mg) to chew while medical help arrives, or take the patient to a nearby healthcare facility. A heart attack is a warning; cardiac arrest is complete collapse. You will learn how to provide first aid for a heart attack in the coming section.

Why Does Cardiac Arrest Occur?

Common causes of cardiac arrest in different age groups are as below-

Table 53.2: Common causes of cardiac arrest in different age groups

Cause	Description
Arrhythmias like ventricular fibrillation (VF) and ventricular tachycardia (VT)	Chaotic heart rhythm causes ineffective pumping. Major cause in adults.
Respiratory failure due to airway obstruction, severe pneumonia, drowning etc.	Hypoxia (oxygen deprivation), major cause in infants and children.
Birth asphyxia and congenital heart disease	In newborns
Severe electrolyte imbalance	Potassium or calcium disturbance
Myocardial infarction (MI)	Heart muscle damage during 'heart attack'
Severe trauma or blood loss	Hypovolemia leading to heart failure
Sudden infant death syndrome	Common in small infants

Reversible Causes of Cardiac Arrest: "The Hs and Ts"

In-hospitals, cardiac arrest may be preceded by signs of deterioration such as hypoxia, bradycardia, and hypotension, offering a chance for prevention if monitored closely. You must remember some Hs and Ts as reversible causes of cardiac arrest.

Table 53.3: Reversible causes of cardiac arrest: "the Hs and Ts"

Category	Cause
H	Hypovolemia, Hypoxia, Hydrogen ion (acidosis), Hyper or Hypokalemia, Hypothermia, Hypoglycemia
T	Tension pneumothorax, Tamponade (cardiac), Toxins, Thrombosis (pulmonary or coronary), Trauma

Activating Emergency Response System

The emergency medical system (EMS) in India is not well-structured to respond to cardiac arrest. Emergency medical ambulance services can be reached through uniform numbers such as 102, 108, and 112 in different states; however, their response time does not match the response time required to manage out-of-hospital cardiac arrest (OHCA) in most community settings. However, these services are good for transportation to the hospital, so the first lay rescuer should shout for help from nearby bystanders to quickly compose a team of two or more lay rescuers and ask the second lay rescuer to activate the ambulance system and get practically quickest available medical transport service without delaying CPR for the victim. In specific settings, such as airports, malls, office complexes, and certain residential colonies where public access AEDs and first-aid/emergency response kits are available, first lay rescuers should instruct the second lay rescuer to retrieve it immediately without delaying CPR for the victim. A 3rd lay rescuer should be recruited if available, who should assist the 1st rescuer in providing CPR. The 2nd rescuer should join back as soon as possible.

For in-hospital cardiac arrest (IHCA), health care providers should shout for help from nearby healthcare providers to assist and activate the code blue or rapid response teams available in the hospital without delaying CPR. If such a uniform dialling or announcement system does not exist in the hospital, delegate the second rescuer the responsibility of obtaining an AED/manual defibrillator and an emergency trolley from the nearest ICU/ward or ER while continuing CPR with the help of the 3rd healthcare providers or a lay rescuers onsite, until further help arrives.

Adult, Child, Infant and CPR

In CPR, classifying a person as an adult, child, or infant helps determine the correct compression depth, hand technique, breath volume, and AED usage. Children and infants have smaller, more fragile bodies and different heart and lung dynamics. Applying adult techniques to a younger child may cause harm; using pediatric techniques on an adult may be insufficient. (5)

Conventional Definitions

- **Newborn/Neonate**: Birth to 28 days of life.
- **Infant**: One month to one year.
- **Child**: 1-18 years. Some hospitals consider pediatric age (children) to be up to 12 or 15 years.
- **Adult**: Older than the cutoff age for a child

Definitions for CPR Purpose

In resuscitation, the *functional* definition often differs slightly because physical development is more important than chronological age:

- **Adult CPR** is recommended for anyone showing clear signs of puberty (axillary hair in boys, breast development in girls) or ≥8 years old.
- **Child CPR** for victims older than 1 year but who have not reached puberty.
- **Infant CPR** is used for children under 1 year (excluding newborns).
- **Newborn/Neonatal Resuscitation** follows separate guidelines (e.g., NRP), which cover immediate care at birth and during the NICU stay.

This distinction is important so that the rescuer applies the right compression depth, hand/finger technique, ventilation ratio, and AED use.

How Cardiac Arrest is Different in Adults and Children?

Table 53.4: Adult versus pediatric cardiac arrest

Feature	Adults	Children & Infants
Common cause of cardiac arrest	Cardiac (arrhythmias)	Respiratory (asphyxia, airway)
Priority in treatment	Early defibrillation (Use AED with CPR)	Early ventilation and oxygenation with CPR
Event	Arrest is often sudden	Often preceded by signs of poor breathing or shock

What is High-Quality CPR?

To be effective, every element of CPR must meet specific benchmarks. You will learn the skill and technique of providing CPR in the next chapter. Once you have learned this, you are advised to revisit the elements of high-quality chest compression for a better understanding. Here are key quality metrics:

Table 53.5: Components of high-quality chest compression

Parameter	Recommended Standard
Compression depth	5–6 cm in adults; at least 1/3 chest depth in children and infants.
Compression rate	100–120 per minute.
Chest recoil	Full recoil between compressions, do not lean on chest.
Minimize interruptions	Aim for <10 seconds break for chest compression during rhythm checks or AED use.
Avoid excessive ventilation	1 breath every 6 sec for adults and every 2–3 sec for children.
Compression fraction	≥ 80% i.e., hands on chest for 80% of resuscitation time.

Automated External Defibrillator and Manual Defibrillator

Arrhythmia (VF and pVT) is the most common cause of cardiac arrest in adults. To revert VF or pVT, the calculated delivery of an electric shock is needed through an AED or a manual defibrillator. AED is an easy-to-use, portable device that can be operated by even laypersons. When attached to the patient via leads and pads and switched on, it automatically analyses heart rhythm and guides the rescuer with voice prompts such as "Attach pads… Stand clear… Shock advised… Press the button to deliver shock." To make them easily accessible to the public, AEDs are strategically placed in common areas of hospitals, airports, malls, and gyms. There is a need to develop the network of public access AEDs in India.

Manual defibrillators are advanced equipment to deliver a manually calculated dose of shock. It is used by trained healthcare providers in hospital settings. It requires the rescuer to interpret the rhythm (VF, pulseless VT, asystole, PEA) and understand the indication before selecting the energy dose for shock delivery.

Post-CPR Debriefing: Learn from Every Code

After every resuscitation event or code blue, irrespective of outcome, team members should sit down briefly and analyze key points-

- What went well and where were the delays?
- Whether communication was effective.
- Were drugs administered appropriately and on time?
- What did we miss?
- How can we do better next time?

Immediate (hot) and delayed (cold) debriefing play a key role in system improvement, turning every code into a learning opportunity. (1)

Chain of Survival: From Prevention to Recovery and Survivorship

In high-stakes resuscitation scenarios, every action is part of a systematic chain. This is known as the "Chain of Survival", and it connects every link in the resuscitation process, from prevention and early detection to recovery and survivorship. This term is a globally recognized resuscitation concept first introduced by the AHA and adapted by different agencies for resuscitation training and education. Previously, the specific actions differed slightly between OHCA and IHCA, as well as between adults and children. The 2025 AHA guidelines have now summarized it into a single concept for OHCA and IHCA, as well as for children and adults. (4,6)

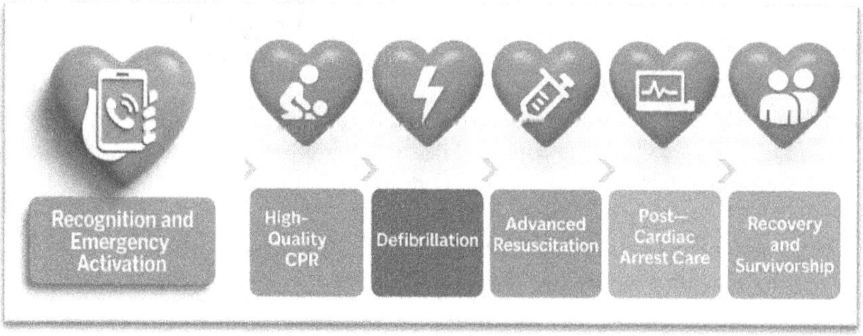

Figure 53.2: Chain of Survival

Adapted from the AHA Chain of Survival 2025, redesigned to highlight the first step as most critical step for LMICs.

In children, respiratory failure is the most common cause of cardiac arrest. Early recognition of a sick child and emergency activation are crucial initial components of the chain of survival. Recognition of a sick child (before cardiac arrest) and emergency treatment at a respiratory distress or failure level to prevent progression to cardiac arrest is a critical and challenging component in India and other LMICs.

Importance of the Chain of Survival

- If any link is missing, the chances of survival drop sharply.
- If every link is strong, outcomes improve, even with basic interventions.
- It provides a stepwise path to follow when seconds feel like storms.
- You may forget what's in your textbook, but in a crisis, if you remember this chain, you know how to save a life.

If you know how to perform CPR, the people around you are safer. But if you also want to be safe, teach it to those around you. Your family members, friends and colleagues. Each person you empower becomes a potential guardian of life in that golden minute when every second counts. As a doctor in training, you should not only master CPR skills, but you should also be able to teach this to others. Sanjeevani Vidya begins with a pair of ordinary hands doing something extraordinary, pressing down on a chest, giving life another chance to beat.

References

1. Del Rios M, Bartos JA, Panchal AR, Atkins DL, Cabañas JG, Cao D, et al. Part 1: Executive Summary: 2025 American Heart Association Guidelines for Cardiopulmonary Resuscitation and Emergency Cardiovascular Care. Circulation. 2025 Oct 21;152 (16_suppl_2):S284-S312.
2. Tiwari L, Jindal A, Gupta V, Taneja LN, Garg R, Edara LR, Chakra Rao SSC. Concept proposal for IRCF national CPR Registry and update on resuscitation guidelines for infants and children. Journal of Pediatric Critical Care. 2022;9(2):48-54.
3. Panchal AR, Bartos JA, Cabañas JG, et al. 2020 American Heart Association Guidelines for Cardiopulmonary Resuscitation and Emergency Cardiovascular Care. Circulation. 2020;142(16_suppl_2):S366–468.
4. Bray JE, Smyth MA, Perkins GD, Cash RE, Chung SP, Considine J, et al. Basic Life Support: 2025 International Liaison Committee on Resuscitation Consensus on Science With Treatment Recommendations. Circulation. 2025 Oct 21;152(16_suppl_1):S34-S71.
5. Soar J, Maconochie I, Wyckoff MH, et al. 2021 International Consensus on Cardiopulmonary Resuscitation and Emergency Cardiovascular Care Science With Treatment Recommendations. Resuscitation. 2021;167:287–303.
6. Nolan JP, Sandroni C, Böttiger BW, et al. European Resuscitation Council Guidelines 2021: Adult advanced life support. Resuscitation. 2021;161:115–51.

Chapter 54: CPR - Psychomotor Domain

Introduction:

In this chapter, we will explore the evidence-based sequence of actions along with specific skills related to CPR. This is the essential algorithm that every healthcare provider must memorise, practice, and execute under pressure with precision and speed. (1-3) You must master each skill before you can execute the complete sequence of life-saving actions. Remember **Recognize-Resuscitate-Review-Refer** sequence.

Recognize

Step 1: Scene-Safety

- Scan the scene to ensure it is safe for both the rescuer and the victim.. Quickly scan for traffic, fire, gas leaks, wires, violence, etc. Do not become another victim.
- Look for circumstantial evidence of poisoning, snakebite, trauma, asphyxia, etc.
- If immediately available, rescuers may use personal protective equipment (PPE) for resuscitation. (3)

Step 2: Assess Responsiveness

- Approach the victim and firmly tap on both shoulders.
- Shout: "Are you okay?"
- If the victim is an infant, tap the sole of the baby's foot or flick the heel.
- If there is no response, time is critical. Even a 5-second delay can cost a life.

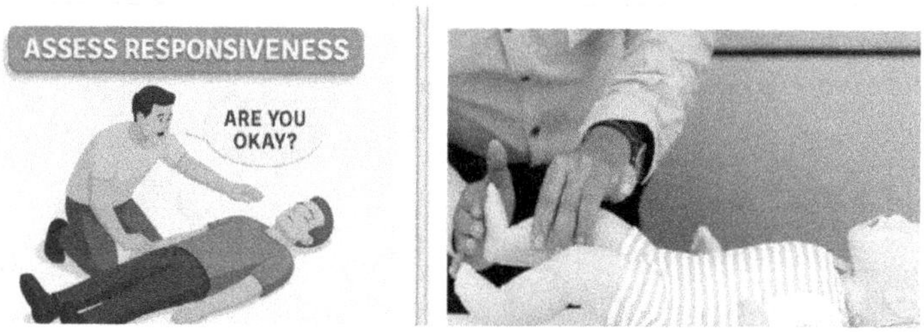

Figure 54.2: Response Assessment in Adults or Children and Infants

Recovery Position

Positioning an injured or ill person is a first-aid intervention to maintain an open airway, prevent aspiration, avoid aggravating suspected spine or pelvic injury, and optimize comfort and breathing. The "recovery" (side-lying) position has long been used for decreased responsiveness with normal breathing.

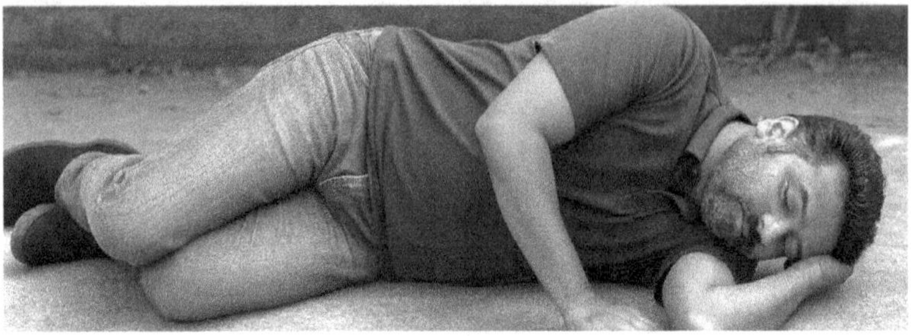

Figure 54.3: Recovery Position

- Place the person in the recovery position if they are non-traumatic, normally breathing, and have decreased alertness.
- If CPR or ventilation is required, position the patient supine.
- Activate EMS for serious illness/injury and stay with the person if safe.
- If the area is unsafe, move to a safer place if you can do so safely.
- With suspected neck, back, hip, or pelvic injury and normally breathing, maintain the victim in a safe position till transport is arranged.
- Allow the awake patient to assume a comfortable position.
- Protect from hypo and hyperthermia.

Evaluate–Identify–Intervene

Time is the currency of Life. The greatest threat emergencies is not ignorance but delay in care deliv Lives are lost if we:

- Fail to 'evaluate' correctly
- Delay in 'identifying' the pathophysiological sta
- Missed the window to 'intervene'

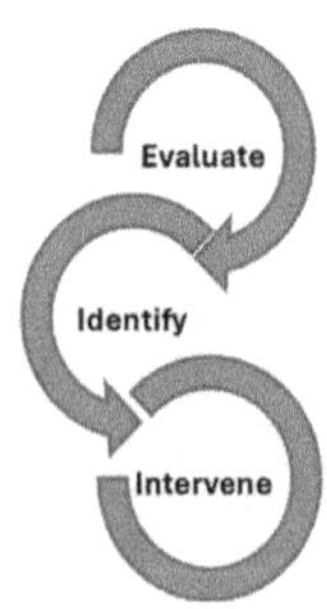

Figure 54.4: Evaluate, Identify and Intervene Approach

You need to get familiar with and master the powerful approach:
Evaluate → Identify → Intervene: and do it fast, correctly, and calmly at each level. You will be trained through case simulations, time-bound drills, and real-life

stories to integrate these instincts into your day-to-day approach.

Step 3: Call for Help and Activate Emergency Medical Services

Activation of the emergency response system is a contextual action. The purpose of activation is to provide immediate on-site support, whenever possible, while administering CPR without delay (within 10 seconds of identifying cardiac arrest).

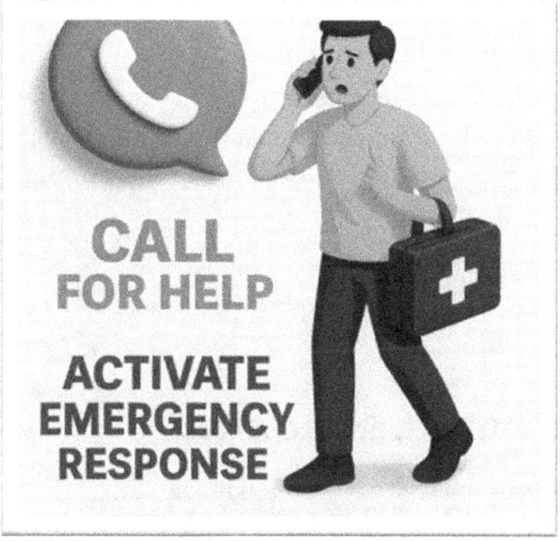

Figure 54.5: Call for Help

Services such as dispatcher-assisted CPR that match the timeline needed to support cardiac arrest victims in out-of-hospital cardiac arrest (OHCA) settings do not exist in India. However, ambulance services for transport to the hospital can be called by dialling 102, 108 or 112 in different states. A practical approach for activation of EMS in case of cardiac arrest in India and similar settings is suggested below. The most important action is to start chest compression within 10 seconds of identifying cardiac arrest.

- If the victim is unresponsive with no signs of life, immediately shout for assistance: "Help! I need an AED and rescuers now!"
- For in-hospital cardiac arrest (IHCA), health care providers should shout for help from nearby healthcare providers while starting onsite CPR (within 10 seconds). The second rescuer should activate the code blue or rapid response teams available in the hospital and a 3rd rescuer should assist the first rescuer in providing CPR.
- If such a uniform dialling or announcement system does not exist in the hospital, delegate the second rescuer the responsibility of getting an AED/manual defibrillator and a crash cart from the nearest ICU / ward or ER and continue CPR with the help of the other (3rd) rescuers onsite, while further help arrives.

- If in a community (OHCA setting), shout for help and quickly assemble a team of two or more lay-rescuers. Ask the second lay-rescuer to activate the ambulance system and obtain the quickest available medical transport service without delaying or stopping CPR for the victim.
- If you are alone, call for help using a mobile device on speaker mode while starting CPR or immediately after the first cycle (2 minutes) of CPR.
- In specific settings, such as airports, malls, office complexes, and certain residential colonies where public access AEDs and first-aid/emergency response kits are available, first lay rescuers should start CPR and instruct the second lay rescuer to retrieve the AED immediately.
- A 3rd lay rescuer should be recruited if available, who should assist the 1st rescuer in providing CPR. The 2nd rescuer should rejoin as soon as possible.
- If you are alone, prioritize chest compressions and ventilation for infants and children over obtaining an AED, so administer 2 minutes of CPR first, then activate emergency response.
- Use your mobile device on speakerphone if possible, and don't leave the victim unless absolutely necessary.

Step 4: Recognize Cardiac Arrest

Consider that the person is in cardiac arrest if he/she is

- Unresponsive.
- Not breathing normally.
- Showing no signs of life.

Signs of life include movements, purposeful activities, normal breathing, response to touch or voice commands and signs of circulation. (3-5)

Role of Pulse Check in Recognising Cardiac Arrest: Accurate assessment of pulse can be difficult, potentially delaying CPR. Lay rescuers should not check a pulse to confirm cardiac arrest. Healthcare providers may check the carotid pulse in adults, the carotid or femoral pulse in children and the brachial pulse in infants, but not for >10 seconds. If unsure, start CPR. (3-5)

Skill Set for Recognition

To recognise cardiac arrest, you need to learn skills of checking responsiveness, breathing, pulse, and other signs of life in adults, children, and infants.

Skill: Check for Responsiveness

Approach the victim and firmly tap on bot unresponsive, it is critical, shout for help.

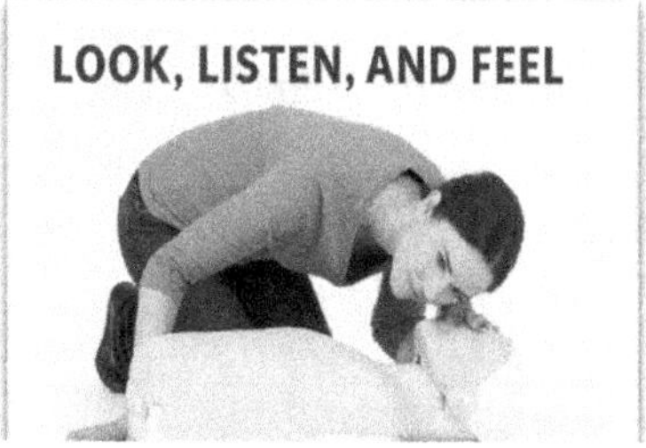

Skill: Check for Breathing

- **Look** for chest rise. The angle of your face should be such that the victim's chest rise is visible to you.
- **Listen** for breathing sounds positioning your ear just above the victim's airway.
- **Feel** the air flow (coming out from the airway) on your cheek. Don't confuse gasping with normal breathing. Gasping = cardiac arrest.

Skill: How to Check for Pulse

Carotid Pulse: Place your two or three fingers on the windpipe (trachea) of the victim. Now, gently move your fingers into the space between the windpipe and the neck muscles. Here you can feel the carotid pulse. It is difficult to find it in infants

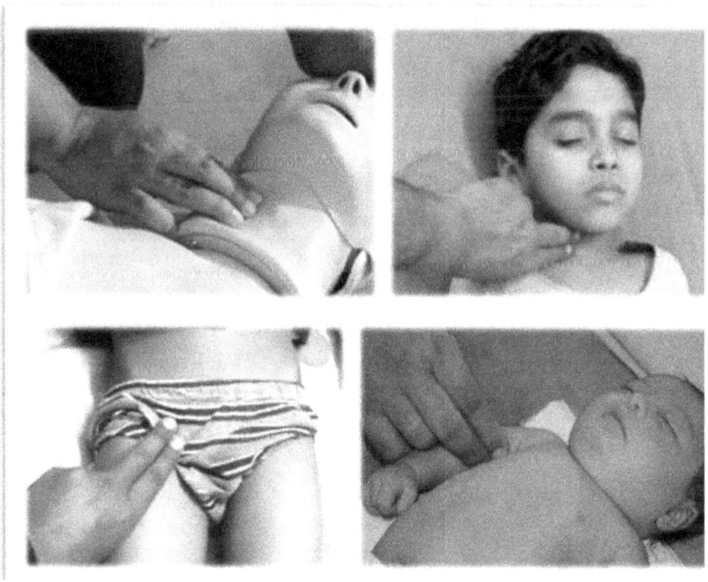

Figure 54.7: Pulse Check Carotid in Adults, Children, Femoral and Brachial

Femoral Pulse: The femoral pulse is easy to palpate in children. To palpate femoral pulse, put two fingers on the upper thigh, midway between the symphysis pubis and hip bone (iliac crest) and just below the crease where the thigh meets the abdomen.

Brachial Pulse: It is easily palpable in infants. Slide two fingers inside the upper arm and palpate the pulse. If you cannot find a pulse within 5-10 seconds, consider it as no pulse.

Skill: Identify Signs of Life

Signs of life include movements, purposeful activities, normal breathing, response to touch or voice commands and signs of circulation. Occasional gasping or agonal breathing is not normal.

Resuscitate

In the absence of signs of life, assume cardiac arrest. Better to start CPR and be wrong than to wait and lose precious time and a life. Depending on the presence of normal breathing and pulse, you should determine your next course of action.

Step 5: Decide next- CPR, Ventilation or Monitoring

Table 54.1: Decision algorithm for next action in CPR

Situation	Action
No breathing and no pulse	• Start CPR: Cycles of chest compression and breathing. • Adults CPR: 30 Compression: 2 breaths for 5 cycles or 2 minutes then review and decide again. • Child and infant CPR: 15 Compressions: 2 ventilation (breaths) for 10 cycles or 2 minutes then review and decide again. • Use AED as soon as available.
No breathing but pulse present	• Give rescue breaths only; No chest compressions. • Adults CPR: 10 breaths/min or each breath after 6 seconds. • Child and infant CPR: 20-30 breaths/ min or each breath after 2-3 seconds. • Review and check breathing and pulse after every 2 minutes.
Normal breathing and pulse present	• Monitor in recovery position; no CPR needed. • Review and check breathing and pulse after every 2 minutes.

For child and infant CPR, some resuscitation councils recommend C:V ratio of 30:2 if only one rescuer is there and 15:2 if more than one rescuers are available. For uniformity and better implementation in India, IAP ALS BLS Group recommends a C:V ratio of 15:2 for infants and children, irrespective of the number of rescuers; however, if rescuers are not trained in infant and child CPR, they should use a 30:2 ratio as used in adults.

Skill Set for Resuscitation

To resuscitate a victim in cardiac arrest, you need certain skills that include giving high-quality chest compressions, opening the airway and delivering effective breaths in adults, children and infants. (3,4)

Skill: Giving High-Quality Chest Compressions

- Place the victim on a firm and flat surface, but do not delay CPR.
- Position: Place the heel of the hand in the centre of the chest corresponding with the lower half of the breastbone (sternum). Place your other hand firmly on top of it and interlock your fingers.
- Consider placing the dominant hand on the sternum.

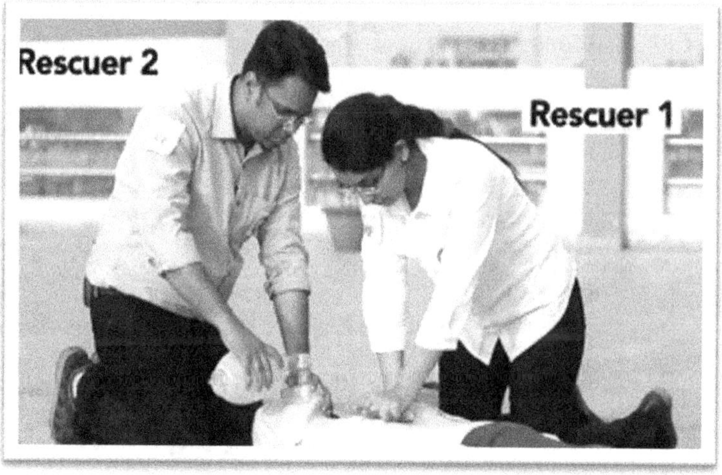

Figure 54.8: Two Rescuer CPR Chest Compression and Ventilation

- Position the patient's torso approximately at the rescuer's knee level to deliver chest compressions effectively. If the victim is on the ground, rescuers should kneel on their knees beside the victim.
- Start chest compression within 10 seconds.
- Depth (push hard): At least 5 cm (but not >6 cm) in adults; 5 cm in children and 4 cm in infants. These numbers correspond to 1/3 of the anteroposterior diameter in different age groups.
- Rate (push fast): 100-120 chest compressions/minute.

- Complete chest recoil.
- Minimise interruptions to as brief as possible and not more than 10 seconds.
- Deliver effective breath for 1 second, giving a visible chest rise.
- Avoid hyperventilation (too fast rate or too much volume).

Child CPR: For a small child, one hand may be sufficient; however, using two hands, with the other hand firmly placed on top, is also acceptable as needed to deliver sufficient force for effective chest compressions.

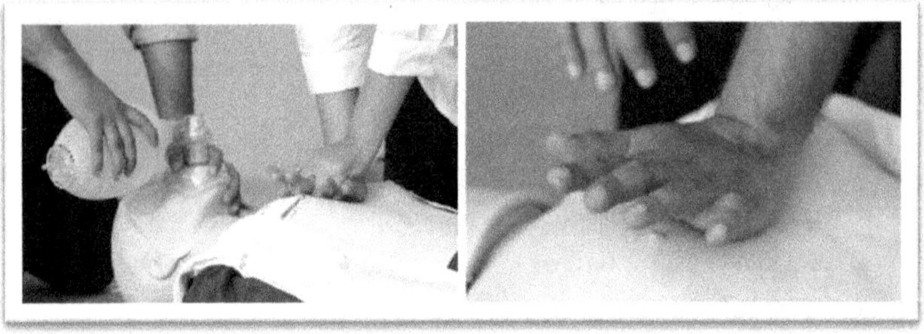

Figure 54.9: Two Hands and One Hand Chest Compression Technique

Infant CPR: One-hand (as above) or two-thumb encircling technique, as shown in the figure below, depending upon the size of the patient and rescuer. The two-finger technique recommended earlier has not been found effective and is not recommended in the 2025 guidelines. (4)

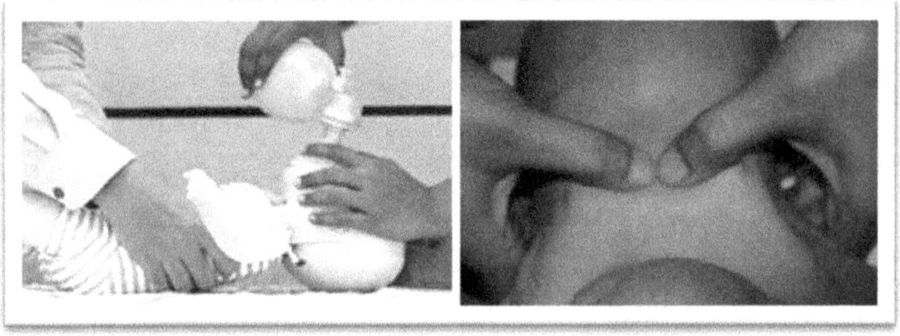

Figure 54.10: Two-Thumb Encircling Hands Technique in Infants

Skill: Continuing CPR

Cycles of chest compressions and ventilation should continue at a ratio of 30:2 for adults and 15:2 for children and infants until the victim revives or an advanced airway is established. To prevent fatigue, rescuers should alternate their roles every 2 minutes, meaning after each five cycles in adults and each 10 cycles in infants and children. The switch should not interrupt compressions for more than 10 seconds. Once an advanced airway (like an endotracheal tube or a laryngeal mask airway) is in place, provide uninterrupted chest compressions (100-120 per minute), with age-appropriate breaths, i.e. 10 breaths per minute in adults (one breath each after 6 sec) and 20-30 per min in infants and children (1 breath after every 2-3 sec), switching roles of rescuers every 2 minutes. (4,5)

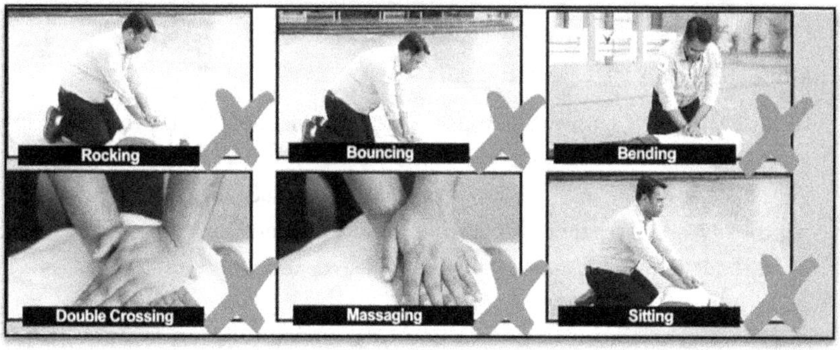

Figure 54.11: Avoid Giving Chest Compressions in These Positions

Skill: Opening the Airway

Use one of the following techniques:

Head-Tilt and Chin-Lift Technique

- Place one hand on the forehead and slightly tilt the head towards the back.
- Lift the chin upward, keeping the fingertips of your other hand under the bony part of the chin.
- This action keeps the airway open by moving the tongue away from the posterior part of the throat.

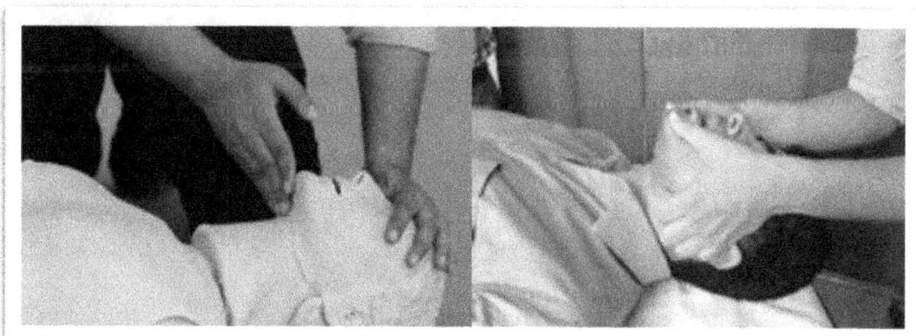

Figure 54.12: Airway Opening Techniques a. Head Tilt Chin Lift b. Jaw Thrust

Jaw-Thrust (If suspected neck or spine injury)

- Position yourself at the head end of the patient.
- Place the heels of both hands on either side of the lower jaw of the patient, fingers resting under the angles of the mandible.
- Apply upward and forward pressure to lift the jaw, without moving the neck.

- Keep the victim's mouth slightly open to allow air to enter.
- Lay rescuers should not use rigid cervical devices for spinal motion restriction for adult head and neck trauma victims. It may be harmful to use if they are not trained for it. (4)

Skill: Delivering Effective Breaths

Use a bag and mask, ensuring a proper seal around the mouth using the E-C clamp technique of bag and mask ventilation for effective breath delivery. When delivering ventilation using a bag-mask device to an adult, one rescuer should use two hands to open the airway and secure a proper seal around the mouth and nose, while a second rescuer should effectively squeeze the bag to deliver effective breaths. (4)

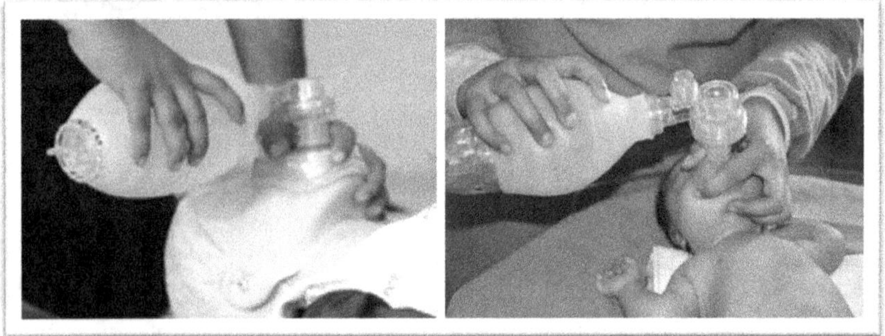

Figure 54.13: E-C Clamp Technique (Adults & Infants)

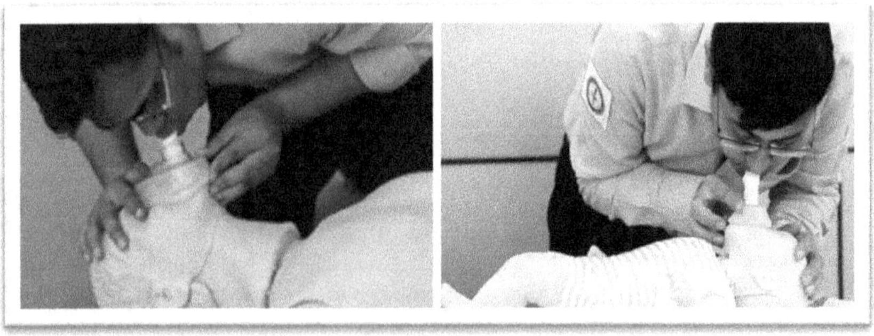

Figure 54.14: Mouth to Mask Ventilation in Adults and Infants

If a bag and mask are unavailable, provide mouth-to-mouth breathing using a barrier device such as a pocket mask or use a piece of cloth (handkerchief, corner of shirt or dupatta) as a barrier in an OHCA setting. When giving mouth-to-mouth breaths to adults, pinch their nose for effective delivery of breath. In small children and infants, you may encircle both the mouth and the nose, depending upon the size of the victim. Provide mouth-to-nose breaths if ventilating through the mouth is not possible.

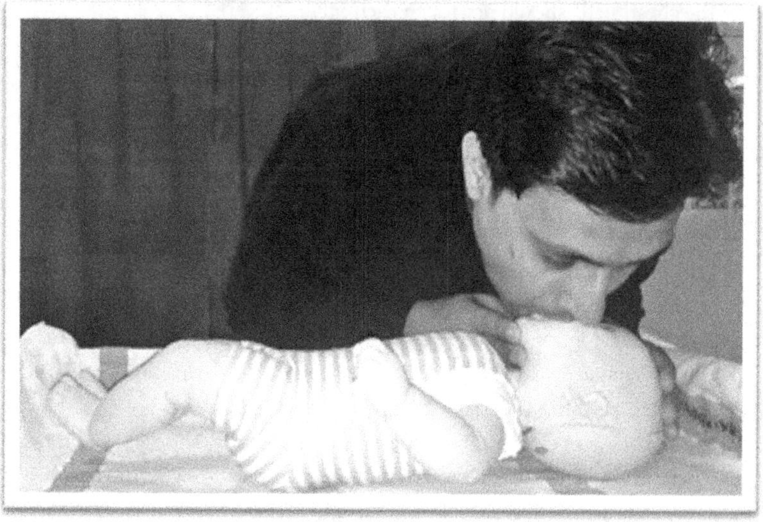

Figure 54.15: Mouth to Mouth-and-Nose Ventilation for Infants

For a patient with a tracheostomy in place, effective ventilation may not be performed via the nose or mouth. In such cases, mask-to-stoma or mouth-to-stoma breath may be given. (4)

- Deliver each breath over one second.
- Achieve a visible chest rise with each ventilation.
- Avoid over-ventilation (risk of gastric inflation and reduced venous return)

A breath that lifts the chest = a breath that matters.

Step 6: Use the AED or defibrillator

As you know, cardiac arrhythmias (VF and pVT) are common causes of cardiac arrest, particularly in adults. These rhythms can often be corrected only by an electric shock delivered through an AED or defibrillator. Immediately on arrival of an AED or defibrillator, use it to identify whether the rhythm is shockable (VF/VT) or non-shockable (asystole/pulseless electrical activity) and deliver a shock if it is indicated. AED automatically identifies the shockable rhythm and gives you voice prompt to deliver shock. Manual defibrillator will display the EEG on its monitor and you need to identify the shockable rhythm and take a decision to deliver shock. The interruption in chest compressions due to shock delivery should be kept as brief as possible, and not more than 10 seconds. (7)

Skill: Using an AED or a Manual Defibrillator in Adults

- Power on the AED and follow prompts.
- Attach the first pad to the right upper side and the second to the left lateral side

of the chest. Pads should not touch each other.

- If a shock is advised, 'clear' the area (do not touch the victim) and press the shock button on the AED. It will deliver the shock, and you will see a sudden, brief contraction or 'twitch' of the patient's chest. Resume CPR immediately after shock delivery without checking for pulse.
- AED will automatically analyse the rhythm every 2 minutes.
- If no shock is advised by the AED, continue chest compressions for 2 min and then check pulse to determine your next step.
- A manual defibrillator does not give voice prompts or action prompts. If you are using a manual defibrillator, switch it on and attach pads or paddles to the chest at the same sites as for AED pads. It will start displaying the ECG rhythm. Identify the rhythm. Asystole and pulseless electrical activity are non-shockable rhythms, so do not deliver shock; continue CPR. Identify shockable rhythms (VF and VT) and deliver 120-200 joules (unsynchronized) for VF and pulseless VT. Using a manual defibrillator is a medical procedure that requires hands-on training and certification for its use.
- The diameter of the paddle or pad electrode for use in adult patients is >8 cm.
- When placing pads on a female victim, adjust the position of the bra; you may not need to remove it. (4)

Skill: Using an AED or a Manual Defibrillator in Infants

- Use a manual defibrillator or a pediatric attenuated AED. If it is not available, use an adult AED.
- Use pediatric pads. If pediatric pads are not available, use adult pads. Attach one pad to the right upper side and another to the left lateral side of the chest. Pads should not touch each other. In infants, pads can be attached in front of the chest and on the back, keeping the heart between two pads.

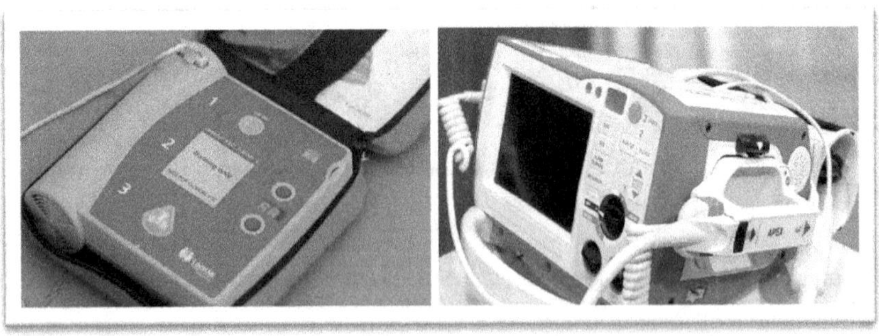

Figure 54.16: AED and Manual Defibrillator

- A manual defibrillator does not give voice prompts or action prompts. If a defibrillator is available, use it as discussed above. Identify shockable rhythms (VF and VT) and deliver 2 joules/kg (unsynchronized) for VF and pulseless VT or do synchronized cardioversion with 0.5-1 joules/kg if it is ventricular tachycardia (VT) with pulse. You may not understand it at this point, but you will during the hands-on session, and that's okay!

The next time you visit an airport or a mall, familiarise yourself with the location of the installed AED. Most airports, malls, railway stations, and public places have AEDs accessible to the public.

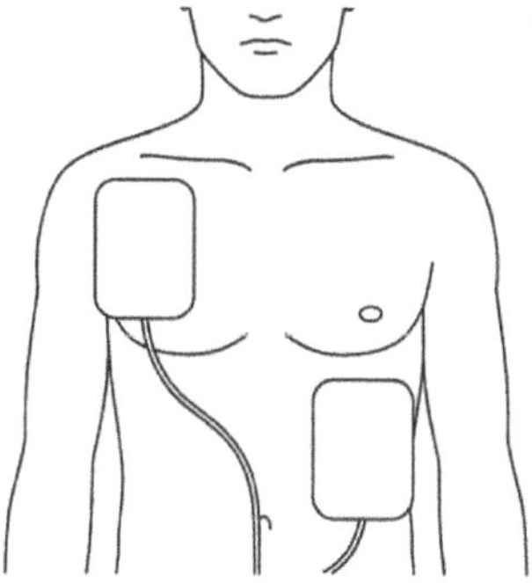

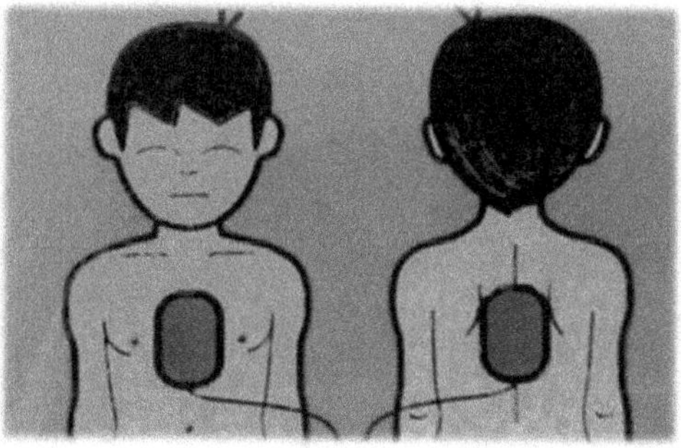

Figure 54.17: A. Position of AED Pads in Adults; B. Anterioposterior in Infants

Review

Step 7: Continue CPR and Reassess Every 2 Minutes

- Continue these 2-minute CPR cycles and reassess for pulse before the next cycle.
- If the victim begins breathing or moving, or if the pulse is detectable, this is referred to as return of spontaneous circulation (ROSC). You should stop CPR once ROSC is achieved.
- If the pulse returns but breathing is absent, stop chest compressions but continue to provide ventilation (breaths) at 10 breaths/min in adults and 20-30 breaths/min in children and infants.
- If no ROSC: continue cycles of CPR + AED analysis.
- Continue CPR, awaiting ambulance and during transport to the hospital.

Refer

Depending upon the setting, hand over care to the advanced life support team as soon as they arrive or the victim reaches to hospital.

Key Differences Between Adult/Adolescent, Child and Infant CPR

Table 54.2: Comparison of Adult/Adolescent, Child and Infant CPR

Feature	Adults and Adolescents	Children	Infants
Cause of Arrest	Cardiac (arrhythmia)	Respiratory (hypoxia, shock)	
Compression: Ventilation	30:2	15:2 (Single or two rescuers). Use 30:2 if not trained in pediatric CPR	
Treatment Emphasis	Early defibrillation	Early ventilation	
CPR depth **1/3 of chest depth**	5–6 cm	~ 5 cm	4 cm
Pulse check	Carotid	Carotid/ femoral	Brachial
Compression technique	Two hands	One or two hands	One hand or 2 thumbs encircle
Only Breaths or breaths with advanced airway	Every 6 sec (10/min)	Every 2-3 sec (20-30/min)	Every 2-3 sec (20-30/min)

References

1. Taneja LN, Tiwari L. BLS for Professionals, 3rd Edition: IAP National Publication House, New Delhi 2018.
2. Tiwari L. Cardiopulmonary Arrest. National Guideline of Indian Academy of Pediatrics 2024-03 | online-resource
3. Kleinman ME, Buick JE, Huber N, Idris AH, Levy M, Morgan SG, et al. Part 7: adult basic life support: 2025 American Heart Association Guidelines for Cardiopulmonary Resuscitation and Emergency Cardiovascular Care. Circulation. 2025;152(suppl 2):S448–S478.
4. Joyner BL, Dewan M, Bavare A, et al. Part 6: pediatric basic life support: 2025 American Heart Association and American Academy of Pediatrics Guidelines for Cardiopulmonary Resuscitation and Emergency Cardiovascular Care. Circulation. 2025;152(suppl 2):S424–S447.
5. Kleinman ME, Brennan EE, Goldberger ZD, et al. Part 5: Adult Basic Life Support and CPR Quality. Circulation.2015;132(18_suppl_2):S414–35.
6. Meaney PA, Bobrow BJ, Mancini ME, et al. Cardiopulmonary resuscitation quality: Improving cardiac resuscitation outcomes both inside and outside the hospital. Circulation. 2013;128(4):417–35.
7. Olasveengen TM, Mancini ME, Perkins GD, et al. Adult basic life support: 2020 International Consensus. Resuscitation. 2020;156:A35–79.

Chapter 55: CPR - Affective Domain

Introduction

Learning CPR is not only about knowing the science (cognitive) or performing the skill steps (psychomotor), it is also about how to deliver it when needed, following all the elements of team dynamics. It encompasses the attitudes, values, and emotions that influence your behaviour in real-life emergencies. This is the affective domain of CPR. In the affective domain, you develop the sense of responsibility, confidence, and compassion needed to step forward when someone's life depends on you. (1)

Table 55.1: Summary of steps and skills needed for BLS/CPR

Steps	Skill needed
Recognize Step 1: Ensure Scene Safety Step 2: Assess Responsiveness Step 3: Call for Help and Activate EMS Step 4: Recognize Cardiac Arrest	Assessment of scene safety Recognize Cardiac Arrest Check responsiveness (adults/infants) Check breathing Check pulses (carotid/femoral/brachial) Identify signs of life Activation of emergency response
Resuscitate Step 5: Decide and perform the next action- CPR, Breaths (ventilation) or Monitoring Step 6: Use AED or defibrillator as it arrives	High quality chest compression Adult CPR Child CPR Infant CPR Opening Airway Head-tilt chin-lift Jaw-thrust Delivering Effective Breaths Bag-mask ventilation E-C Clamp technique Pocket mask ventilation Mouth to mouth ventilation Using an AED and a manual defibrillator in adults and infants
Review Step 7: Continue CPR and Reassess Every 2 Minutes	Identify return of spontaneous circulation (ROSC)
Refer	Structured referral using SBAR

It means overcoming hesitation, fear of failure, or the bystander effect, and instead choosing to act with courage. The affective domain ensures that CPR is not only a technical act of pressing on a chest, but a human skill of saving a life with dignity, courage, and compassion. We will briefly discuss the steps of providing CPR, team dynamics and the importance of debriefing in this chapter. (1) You need to master certain skills to perform each step under the overarching concept of the Recognise-Resuscitate-Review-Refer.

Early Warning Signs and Activation of Code Blue

In most hospital settings, "Code Blue" or calling a rapid response team (RRT) is the universal call for cardiac or respiratory arrest. The Code Blue protocol ensures that a trained, equipped team reaches the patient within seconds, initiating coordinated resuscitation. (3) Before the heart stops, the body often whispers warnings. Recognize early warning signs and call for help to save lives.

Table 55.2: Early warning signs and required actions

Common Pre-Arrest Signs	Action to Take Immediately
Sudden drop in oxygen saturation	Escalate to Rapid Response Team
Altered mental status	Oxygen, glucose, monitor vitals
Bradycardia/tachycardia	Continuous monitoring
Hypotension	Fluid challenge, call for help
Seizure or collapse	Airway support, prepare for CPR

The Crash Cart: Every clinical area should have a fully stocked crash cart. Being familiar with the crash cart can save critical time during an arrest. Regularly check the crash cart for the following contents-

- Bag-mask device, oxygen.
- Defibrillator/AED.
- Emergency drugs (adrenaline, atropine, amiodarone).
- Airway adjuncts (oropharyngeal airway, endotracheal tubes, laryngoscopes).
- Suction apparatus.
- Intravenous access equipment.

Team Dynamics in Resuscitation

Even perfect hands need coordination.

Behind every successful CPR, there are invisible yet essential elements of the code blue team dynamics. Resuscitation is rarely a one-person job. It's a team sport played in chaos, stress, and time pressure. How a team performs, communicates, synchronises, and adapts can significantly influence the outcome as much as the technical skills involved. (2,4) A resuscitation team should function like a well-rehearsed orchestra in which

- Everyone knows their role,
- Everyone listens and
- Everyone adjusts when needed.

Key team members and their roles are summarized in table 55.3. Many times, the availability of all these members is not possible in a busy hospital and team members have to double up their roles.

Table 55.3: Roles and responsibilities of CPR team members

Role	Responsibility
Team Leader	Makes decisions, directs resuscitation
Compressor	Provides chest compressions
Airway Manager	Maintains airway, gives breaths
Defibrillator Operator	Attaches pads, delivers shocks
Medication Nurse	Draws up and gives drugs
Recorder	Documents all events and time stamps

Elements of Effective Team Dynamics

In a well-drilled Code Blue scenario, every second and every person counts. The following are key elements of good team dynamics. When you are part of a team, ensure effective team dynamics for better outcomes. (1)

1. Clear role assignment and understanding it.
2. Clear messages on what to do and what has been done.
3. Closed-loop communication: say the task, confirm when done.
4. Knowing the limitations of the self and individual team members.
5. Constructive intervention.
6. Maintain mutual respect and calmness.
7. Knowledge sharing.
8. Re-evaluation and summarising the code.

In chaos, clarity saves lives.

Prepare with Simulation-Based CPR Training

Many hospitals now conduct mock codes using simulations.

- A mannequin or a real-time virtual tool simulates an arrest
- Real staff respond as they would in a real situation
- Performance is monitored and reviewed by a trained facilitator for accuracy, speed, and teamwork

How it helps

- Practice resuscitation without real risk.
- Improve role clarity and progress.
- Identify system flaws (e.g., equipment availability, response time).
- Build confidence among interns, nurses, and doctors.

You'll forget what you memorized under pressure. But you won't forget what your hands have rehearsed. It is muscle memory.

Debriefing After a CPR Code

After every resuscitation attempt, whether successful or not, a structured debriefing is essential. Debriefing provides the team with an opportunity to review what went well and identify areas for improvement. It is not about blame, but about learning and improving together. Discussion should cover technical aspects (compression quality, airway management, timing of defibrillation), teamwork dynamics (role clarity, communication, leadership), and the emotional experience of team members. A short, focused session of 10-15 minutes (hot debriefing) helps improve future performance, strengthens team cohesion, and provides psychological support to those who may feel distressed. A more detailed cold debriefing is required after an interval. Debriefing transforms each CPR code into a learning opportunity for better care and resilience. (3-5)

Best Practices for Debriefing

- Use a structured framework like "Plus–Delta" (What went well? What could we do differently?).
- Ensure a safe and non-punitive atmosphere where everyone feels heard.
- Assign an experienced facilitator or clinical educator when possible.
- Document key takeaways and follow-up actions.

Why It Matters

Debriefing:

- Reinforces correct techniques and team behavior.
- Prevents repetition of avoidable errors.
- Enhances mutual trust and team bonding.
- Reduces stress, guilt, or burnout among healthcare providers.

Transforms every CPR code into a learning moment—a bridge between doing and becoming better.

ILCOR Ten Steps for Improving CPR Quality and Outcomes

The International Liaison Committee on Resuscitation (ILCOR) has outlined a Ten-

Step Framework to help hospitals improve care for patients experiencing in-hospital cardiac arrest (IHCA). This framework emphasises that saving lives is not only about performing CPR but creating a comprehensive preparedness, execution, and follow-up system using 10 steps in 4 domains as discussed in the table below. (6)

Table 55.4: ILCOR Ten Steps for Improving CPR Quality and Outcomes

Domain	Key Focus Area (Step)	Explanation
Plan and Prepare	1. Governance and Infrastructure	Establish hospital-wide resuscitation governance, policies, and leadership accountability.
	2. Audit and Data Feedback	Implement systems to collect, review, and share data on IHCAs to drive performance improvement.
	3. Training and Competency	Provide regular, hands-on training and assessment for all staff involved in resuscitation.
Prevent	4. Goals of Care and Treatment Limitations	Ensure early discussions and documentation of resuscitation preferences with patients/families.
	5. Identification and Response to Deterioration	Use early warning scores and Rapid Response Teams to prevent cardiac arrest events.
Perform	6. Effective Resuscitation Response	Maintain timely, coordinated team response systems (e.g., code blue) with role clarity.
	7. High-Quality Resuscitation	Adhere to evidence-based CPR practices and monitor quality metrics (depth, rate, etc.).
	8. Post-Arrest Care and Prognostication	Provide structured post-ROSC care, prognostication, and transition to appropriate rehabilitation.
Principles & Culture	9. Person-Centered Care and Family Support	Involve patients/families respectfully, offer counselling and bereavement support.
	10. Staff Support and System Resilience	Promote team debriefing, psychological support, and well-being programs for care providers.

☕ Coffee Moment

It was a pediatric code. The room was crowded. A junior doctor did the compressions, her arms trembling. The nurse counted loudly, the intern ventilated steadily, and the team leader stood clear, calm, sharp, and encouraging. The boy survived. After it was over, they sat in the doctor's lounge. Nobody spoke for a while. Then the nurse whispered, "I've never felt more like a team than I did today."

Sometimes, the best morale-booster is a voice that says: "We've got this. Together."

References

1. BLS for Professionals: IAP Manual of Basic Life Support for Health Care Providers 3rd Edition: IAP National Publication House, New Delhi 2018.
2. Cheng A, Hunt EA, Donoghue A, et al. Examining pediatric resuscitation education using simulation and scripted debriefing. Pediatrics. 2013;132(2):e490–500.
3. Kleinman ME, Buick JE, Huber N, Idris AH, Levy M, Morgan SG, et al. Part 7: adult basic life support: 2025 American Heart Association Guidelines for Cardiopulmonary Resuscitation and Emergency Cardiovascular Care. Circulation. 2025;152(suppl 2):S448–S478.
4. Couper K, Perkins GD. Debriefing after resuscitation. Curr Opin Crit Care. 2013;19(3):188–94.
5. Edelson DP, Litzinger B, Arora V, et al. Improving in-hospital cardiac arrest process and outcomes with performance debriefing. Arch Intern Med. 2008;168(10):1063–9.
6. Nallamothu BK, Greif R, Anderson T, et al. International Liaison Committee on Resuscitation. Ten Steps Toward Improving In-Hospital Cardiac Arrest Quality of Care and Outcomes. Circ Cardiovasc Qual Outcomes. 2023 Nov;16(11):e010491.

Chapter 56: Choking and Airway Obstruction

Introduction

When the breath stops, the clock starts..

Recognizing Choking: When Air Cannot Pass

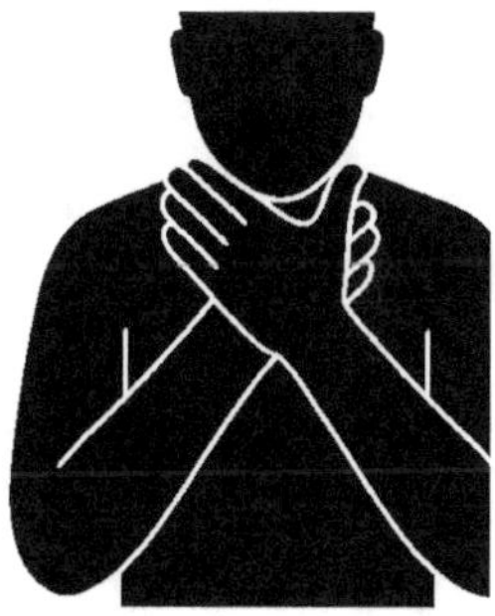

Choking occurs when the airway (windpipe) is blocked due to a foreign object, and air cannot reach the lungs. The victim is unable to speak, breathe, or cough properly. They display the universal choking sign (clutching the throat). Without quick help, the patient turns blue and/or loses consciousness, becomes unresponsive and may develop cardiac arrest. Infants may show respiratory distress or noisy breathing in mild choking and may quickly become unresponsive in severe choking. It is common in children while playing with small toys or eating nuts and grapes, and in adults while eating. Immediate action is life-saving. (1)

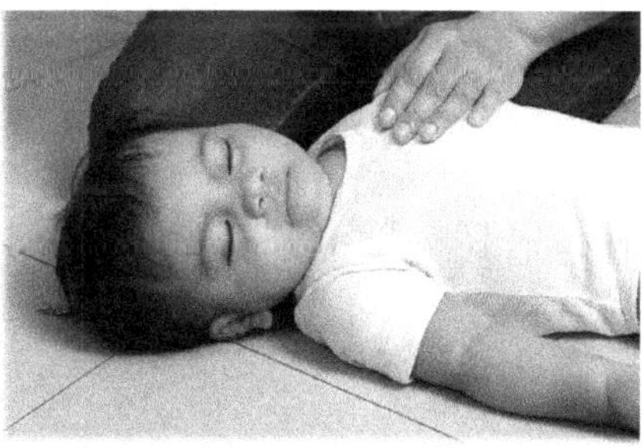

There are two types of choking; mild and severe.

Table 56.1: Mild and severe foreign body airway obstruction

[illegible]	[illegible]
[illegible]	[illegible]
Severe Obstructi	Silent or ineffective cough, clutching the neck (universal choking sign), cyanosis, inability to speak, breathe, or cry

Silent choking suggests severe obstruction where immediate action is needed to save the victim. In people with a pulse, oxygen saturation can drop to dangerously low levels after only 90 seconds of apnoea. Mild obstruction may progress to severe obstruction at any time. If severe obstruction is not treated immediately, the person becomes unresponsive, requiring CPR as well as removal of the foreign body. (2)

Adult and Child (>1 year): Responsive Victim

Ask: "Are you choking?"

- If the person nods yes, encourage coughing if it is effective. In case of mild FBAO, keep them under observation and arrange for definitive care. They may clear the airway by coughing or may develop signs of severe FBAO.
- If unable to cough or speak, act quickly.
- Activate the emergency medical response system for severe FBAO.

Severe FBAO

For adults with severe FBAO, perform repeated cycles of five back blows (slaps) followed by five abdominal thrusts until the foreign body comes out or the person becomes unresponsive. Case reports have described fatal injuries from abdominal thrusts, including aortic dissection and gastric rupture, so back blows followed by abdominal thrusts are now recommended rather than only abdominal thrust for adults with severe FBAO. Back blows are aligned with recommendations for infant victims, where 5 back blows followed by five chest thrusts are recommended. (2,3)

- Stand behind the victim.
- Deliver five back blows (slaps) between the shoulder blades.
- If the foreign body does not come out, perform Heimlich's manoeuvre for abdominal thrust. Wrap your arms around the torso of the victim from their back. Make a fist with your one hand, directing the thumb side of your fist towards the victim.
- Place it just above the navel and grasp it firmly with the other hand.
- Deliver five quick, upward thrusts. (4)
- Repeat cycles of five back blows and five abdominal thrusts until the foreign body comes out or the victim becomes unresponsive. (follow the algorithm for an unresponsive choking victim).

In pregnant or obese patients: Perform chest thrusts rather than abdominal thrusts.

Adult: Unresponsive Choking Victim

1. Lower gently to the ground.
2. Call for help and start CPR.

- Do not check for pulse initially.
- After every set of 30 compressions, open the airway and look in the mouth for a foreign body.
- If the object is visible → remove it carefully (no blind sweeps).
- Deliver two breaths (ventilation).
- Continue cycles of 30:2 CPR until the foreign body comes out or help arrives.

Infants: Responsive Choking Victim

Choking in infants often occurs during feeding on liquids or due to small objects, such as toys, nuts, grapes, or balloons. In case of mild FBAO, keep infants under observation and arrange for definitive management. They may clear the airway by coughing or may develop signs of severe FBAO, as in children and adults. (1,3)

Step-by-step management

- Sit down and lay the infant on your forearm with its face down. Support the head carefully.
- Deliver five back blows (slaps) between the shoulder blades.
- Turn the infant (face-up) and give five chest thrusts (like one hand infant compressions).

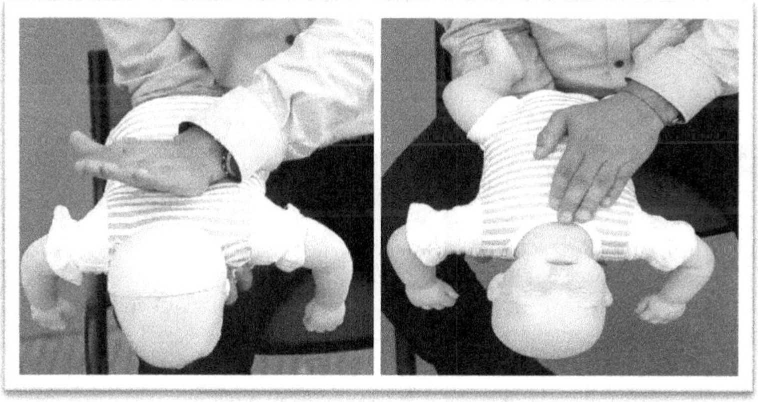

Figure 56.3: Five Back-Blows and Five Chest Thrust in an Infant

- Repeat the sequence of five back blows and chest thrusts until the foreign body comes out or the infant becomes unresponsive.
- Never perform abdominal thrusts on infants. There is a high risk of injury to the liver and stomach. (5)

Infant or Child: Unresponsive Choking Victim

- Begin CPR immediately

- Start with chest compressions without checking for pulse.
- Open the airway and check for visible objects.
- Remove the foreign body if seen.
- Deliver two gentle breaths.
- Repeat cycles of 15:2 (30:2 if you are not trained for infant CPR).

What Not to Do

- Do not give water or try to "wash down" the object.
- Do not perform blind finger sweeps.
- Do not delay CPR if the victim becomes unresponsive.
- Do not shake the child or turn them upside down violently. (6)

☕ Coffee Moment

A resident doctor in the pediatric OPD noticed a mother panicking with a blue-faced toddler. The child had been playing with coins, and she suspected one had been swallowed. The young doctor didn't waste time. He picked the child up, gave five back blows followed by chest thrusts, and with a sharp gasp, the child coughed out a tiny 1-rupee coin. The mother cried. The doctor exhaled deeply. A small life restored. Sometimes, the smallest tools become instruments of miracles.

References

1. BLS for Professionals: IAP Manual of Basic Life Support for Health Care Providers 3rd Edition: IAP National Publication House, New Delhi 2018.
2. Kleinman ME, Buick JE, Huber N, et al. Part 7: adult basic life support: 2025 American Heart Association Guidelines for Cardiopulmonary Resuscitation and Emergency Cardiovascular Care. Circulation. 2025;152(suppl 2):S448–S478.
3. Joyner BL, Dewan M, Bavare A, de et al. Part 6: pediatric basic life support: 2025 American Heart Association and American Academy of Pediatrics Guidelines for Cardiopulmonary Resuscitation and Emergency Cardiovascular Care. Circulation. 2025;152(suppl 2):S424–S447.
4. Heimlich HJ. A life-saving maneuver to prevent food-choking. JAMA. 1975;234(4):398–401.
5. Maconochie IK, Aickin R, Hazinski MF, et al. Pediatric Basic Life Support and Pediatric Advanced Life Support: 2020 Guidelines. Circulation. 2020;142(16_suppl_2):S469–523.
6. National Health Service (UK). Choking – First aid. NHS; 2023.

Chapter 57: CPR in Special Circumstances

Introduction

Emergencies don't always follow algorithms. Here are some special situations where you need to take additional or slightly different steps while performing CPR.

CPR in Drowning

Drowning victims experience hypoxic cardiac arrest from water in the airway. Managing the airway and reversing hypoxia is critical. (1) When respiratory arrest is addressed by breaths that interrupt the drowning process, the death rate is lower (44%) than in those cases that progress to cardiac arrest and receive CPR (93%). (2)

Key Actions

- Rescuers must consider personal safety, equipment availability, and distance to shore when determining whether to perform in-water breaths. (2)
- Prioritize ventilation before beginning chest compressions. However, if you are not trained or unable to provide breaths, go ahead with chest compressions.
- Trained rescuers should provide breaths using the most readily available methods (mouth-to-mouth, pocket mask, or bag-mask ventilation).
- Clear the airway of debris or water, remove wet clothing, and warm the victim.
- Trained drowning rescuers may initiate in-water or on-the-boat CPR if the expected time to reach on shore is more than five minutes.
- CPR with breaths should be initiated before applying an AED. (2)
- Although shockable rhythms are uncommon in drowning victims, use an AED once available to analyse and deliver a shock if indicated. (1,3)

CPR in Hypothermia

Accidental hypothermia causes progressive depression of cardiac conduction, myocardial contractility, and respiratory drive. Severe hypothermia may result in bradyarrhythmias, ventricular fibrillation, or asystole. In hypothermic cardiac arrest, survival with good neurological outcome is possible even after prolonged resuscitation, particularly when rewarming is integrated with high-quality CPR. (1,2)

Key Actions

- Suspect cardiac arrest early and initiate standard high-quality CPR.
- Rewarming should occur concurrently with resuscitation, using both passive and active methods that are appropriate to the available resources.

- Handle the victim gently, as rough movement may precipitate ventricular fibrillation due to myocardial irritability.
- Use an AED or defibrillator if a shockable rhythm is present, although the hypothermic heart may be less responsive.
- If VF or pulseless VT persists, avoid repeated excessive defibrillation attempts, and continue CPR while rewarming progresses.
- Extracorporeal life support (ECMO/ECLS) should be considered when available, as it allows controlled rewarming and circulatory support.
- $ETCO_2$ to unreliable to predict outcomes in hypothermic cardiac arrest.
- Do not terminate resuscitation solely because of hypothermia. Prognostic tools (such as HOPE or ICE scores) may assist in decision-making. (1,2)

Key Principle

In hypothermic cardiac arrest, effective CPR combined with active rewarming should be continued whenever feasible, as hypothermia itself may be reversible and compatible with survival.

CPR in Hyperthermia

Life-threatening hyperthermia (core temperature ≥40°C) leads to cellular injury, circulatory collapse, and malignant arrhythmias. Cardiac arrest in hyperthermia is primarily driven by extreme temperature–related physiological failure. Rapid temperature reduction, initiated concurrently with standard resuscitation, is essential for survival. (1)

Key Actions

- Initiate standard high-quality CPR immediately if cardiac arrest occurs.
- Begin active cooling at the same time as CPR and advanced life support, as hyperthermia is a reversible cause of arrest.
- Ice-water immersion is the preferred cooling method when feasible, as it provides the fastest and most effective temperature reduction.
- If ice-water immersion is unavailable, tepid-water immersion or tarp-assisted ice-water cooling may be used as alternatives.
- Cool rapidly, aiming for a temperature reduction of at least 0.15°C per minute.
- Discontinue active cooling when core temperature reaches approximately 38.6°C, to avoid overshoot hypothermia.
- Use standard defibrillation and medications according to cardiac arrest algorithms; no modifications are recommended solely due to hyperthermia.
- Dantrolene is not indicated for hyperthermia due to heat stroke or environmental causes (use is limited to malignant hyperthermia). (1,2)

Key Principle

In hyperthermic cardiac arrest, CPR and rapid active cooling must proceed simultaneously; delaying cooling reduces the chance of successful resuscitation.

CPR in Trauma

Traumatic cardiac arrest results primarily from reversible causes such as severe hemorrhage, hypoxia, tension pneumothorax, cardiac tamponade, or traumatic brain injury,. rather than primary cardiac pathology. Survival depends on rapid identification and correction of these causes, alongside high-quality CPR. (1)

Key Actions

- Initiate high-quality CPR immediately when cardiac arrest is identified, while simultaneously addressing reversible traumatic causes.
- Control catastrophic hemorrhage without delay, using direct pressure, tourniquets, pelvic binders, or hemostatic measures as appropriate.
- Ensure effective airway management and oxygenation, as hypoxia is a common precipitant of traumatic arrest.
- Relieve tension pneumothorax promptly if suspected, using needle decompression or chest tube insertion.
- Assess for and treat cardiac tamponade in penetrating chest trauma, with emergent pericardiocentesis or thoracotomy if expertise and resources permit.
- Use defibrillation only if a shockable rhythm is present, recognizing that traumatic cardiac arrest most often presents with non-shockable rhythms.
- Minimize interruptions to CPR, but prioritize life-saving trauma interventions that directly address the cause of arrest.
- Early transport to a trauma-capable facility is essential; prolonged resuscitation without correction of underlying injuries is unlikely to be successful. (1,2,4)

Key Principle

In traumatic cardiac arrest, CPR alone is insufficient; survival depends on rapid correction of reversible causes, especially hemorrhage and hypoxia.

CPR in Pregnancy

Cardiac arrest during pregnancy is rare but potentially survivable for both mother and fetus when managed promptly and appropriately. Physiological changes of pregnancy, including aortocaval compression by the gravid uterus, increased oxygen consumption, and reduced functional residual capacity, significantly affect resuscitation. High-quality CPR with early uterine displacement and timely perimortem delivery are critical to maternal and fetal outcomes. (2)

Key Actions

- Initiate standard high-quality CPR immediately when cardiac arrest is identified; pregnancy alone does not alter compression rate or depth.
- Relieve aortocaval compression as soon as CPR begins by manual left uterine displacement. Manual displacement is preferred over lateral tilt, as it allows effective chest compressions.

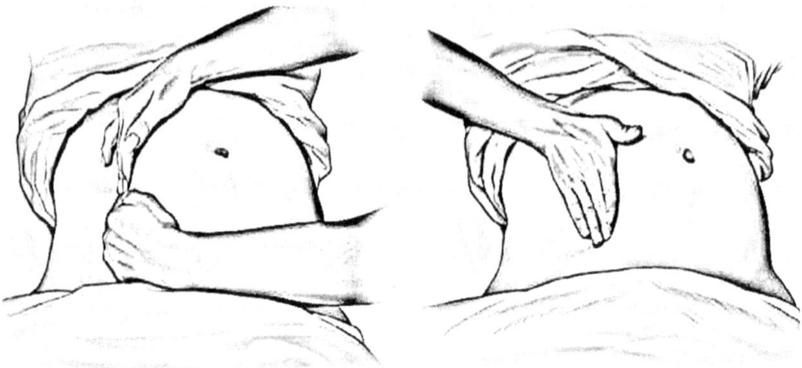

Figure 57.1: Manual Left Lateral Displacement of Uterus

- Prioritize early airway management and oxygenation, as pregnant patients desaturate rapidly due to reduced pulmonary reserve.
- Use defibrillation without delay when indicated; standard energy doses are recommended and are safe in pregnancy.
- Identify and treat reversible causes of maternal cardiac arrest, with special attention to obstetric causes (e.g., hemorrhage, preeclampsia/eclampsia, amniotic fluid embolism).
- Prepare for perimortem cesarean delivery (resuscitative hysterotomy) if return of spontaneous circulation is not achieved within 5 minutes of arrest in a patient with a uterus at or above the umbilicus (approximately ≥20–24 weeks gestation).
- Perimortem cesarean delivery is performed to improve maternal resuscitation, with potential fetal survival as a secondary benefit.
- Continue maternal resuscitation throughout delivery, and ensure neonatal resuscitation support is available. (1,2)

Key Principle

In maternal cardiac arrest, relieving aortocaval compression and restoring maternal circulation take precedence; timely perimortem cesarean delivery can be life-saving for the mother and may also improve fetal survival.

CPR during Respiratory Pandemics

Your safety is your patient's top priority. A sick rescuer can't save lives. (1,5)

Key Actions

- Safety First: Always wear appropriate PPE, mask (N95 or higher), eye protection, gloves, and gown.
- Prefer bag-mask ventilation with a HEPA filter.
- Avoid mouth-to-mouth breathing.
- Limit the number of rescuers.
- Prioritize intubation by an experienced provider using closed-circuit oxygenation.

CPR in Snakebite Victims

Cardiac arrest following snakebite commonly results from secondary causes, like neurotoxic paralysis leading to respiratory failure and hypoxia, rather than primary cardiac pathology. Less frequent causes include severe shock, massive bleeding, or anaphylaxis. Early ventilatory support and timely CPR can be lifesaving. (6)

Key Actions

- Ensure rescuer safety and call for urgent transport to a healthcare facility with antivenom and ventilatory support.
- Recognize early respiratory failure, especially in neurotoxic envenomation (ptosis, slurred speech, shallow or absent breathing).
- Provide breathing or bag-mask ventilation promptly if breathing is inadequate; do not wait for cardiac arrest to support ventilation.
- If the victim becomes unresponsive with absent or abnormal breathing, initiate standard high-quality CPR without delay.
- Chest compressions, defibrillation, and medications follow standard CPR protocols; no modification in compression technique or energy doses is required.
- Do not delay CPR to reapply splints, pressure bandages, or limb immobilization; maintain immobilization only if it does not interfere with resuscitation.
- In hospital settings, remain alert for anaphylaxis, including antivenom-related reactions, and manage per standard resuscitation and anaphylaxis protocols. (6,7)

Key Principle

In snakebite-related arrest, CPR is standard, but early and effective ventilation is crucial, as respiratory paralysis and hypoxia are the most common reversible causes.

Electric Shock and Lightning Strike

Arrhythmias are a common cause of cardiac arrest in this situation. (1,3)

Key Actions

- Ensure the scene is safe before approaching.
- Begin CPR immediately if the victim seems unresponsive or pulseless.
- Internal burns and arrhythmias are common; defibrillation is key.
- Victims may experience brief asystole with full recovery if promptly resuscitated.
- Lightning can stop a heart, but not your hands.

Prone CPR

In ICUs, when a patient is very sick and being ventilated in the prone position, it may be difficult to immediately turn them supine. If an adult patient being nursed in a prone position develops cardiac arrest, turn the patient supine before initiating chest compressions. If the patient cannot be safely turned supine, rescuers may consider performing CPR in the prone position with the following adjustments. (8)

Key Actions

- Deliver compressions between the vertebral levels T7 and T10.
- Position your hands over the thoracic spine and apply gentle downward pressure.
- Compression rate and compression-to-ventilation ratio same as standard CPR.
- As soon as possible, resume supine position and continue standard CPR.
- CPR in the prone position is less effective, but it is better than no CPR.

Family Presence During CPR

Family presence during cardiopulmonary resuscitation (FPDR) refers to the practice of allowing family members to be present during active resuscitation efforts. Evidence suggests that, when appropriately supported, family presence does not interfere with the quality of resuscitation and may improve family understanding, psychological outcomes, and trust in the healthcare team. (9)

Key Actions

- Offer family members the option to be present during CPR when resources and trained staff are available to support them.
- Assign a dedicated team member (nurse, social worker, or physician) to explain ongoing actions, provide emotional support, and escort them if needed.
- Maintain patient dignity, safety, and resuscitation quality as the highest priorities.
- Do not allow family presence if it compromises team performance, patient

safety, or poses a risk to staff.

- Respect cultural values, patient preferences, and institutional policies when making decisions about family presence.
- Document the offer and family response, as well as any reasons for discontinuation if family presence is stopped. (9)

Key Principle

When supported by trained staff, family presence during CPR is safe, ethical, and may reduce long-term psychological distress without compromising resuscitation outcomes.

When to Stop CPR (Termination of Resuscitation)

Decisions to terminate cardiopulmonary resuscitation are among the most challenging aspects of emergency care. Termination should be based on clinical judgment, response to resuscitation, underlying cause, and available resources, rather than elapsed time alone. (1)

Key Actions

- Continue CPR while reversible causes (hypoxia, hypovolemia, tension pneumothorax, tamponade, toxins, thrombosis, hypothermia) are addressed.
- Follow the validated termination-of-resuscitation (TOR) rules of your institute, where applicable, including organ donation programs.
- Special circumstances (hypothermia, pregnancy, lightning, drug overdose) may justify prolonged resuscitation.
- Communicate clearly and compassionately with family members when termination is considered or declared.
- Document the decision making process, including clinical findings, treatments provided, and team consensus.

Key Principle

CPR should be stopped when continued resuscitation is medically futile, all reasonable interventions have been attempted, and ongoing efforts no longer offer a meaningful chance of survival.

When NOT to Start CPR

CPR should be started in case of a cardiac arrest by default. However, there are certain predefined conditions and orders for not starting CPR, such as

- Unsafe environment for rescuers.
- Presence of valid DNR orders.

- Definite signs of irreversible death (decapitation, rigour mortis, decomposition).

☕ Coffee Moment

An intern returning from night duty saw a crowd gathered. A man had collapsed near a tea stall, and the people watching stood frozen. The intern stepped forward and checked the pulse—there was none. Activated emergency response. Compressions began. Minutes later, the AED arrived. A shock was delivered. A groan followed. A pulse regained. When the ambulance arrived, she stepped aside. Her hands trembled with fatigue. The tea stall owner handed her a hot cup, and her eyes glistened.

"You saved him," he whispered.

At times, your clinical training extends into the world. At times, the road becomes your ward.

References

1. Soar J, Böttiger BW, Carli P, et al. European Resuscitation Council Guidelines 2021: Special circumstances. Resuscitation. 2021;161:152–219.
2. Cao D, Arens AM, Chow SL, et al. Part 10: Adult and Pediatric Special Circumstances of Resuscitation: 2025 American Heart Association Guidelines for Cardiopulmonary Resuscitation and Emergency Cardiovascular Care. Circulation. 2025 Oct 21;152(16_suppl_2):S578-S672.
3. Perkins GD, Graesner JT, Semeraro F, et al. European Resuscitation Council Guidelines 2021: Epidemiology and outcomes. Resuscitation. 2021;161:61–79.
4. Jeejeebhoy FM, Zelop CM, Lipman S, et al. Cardiac arrest in pregnancy: A scientific statement from the AHA. Circulation. 2015;132(18):1747–73.
5. Tiwari L, Taneja LN, Gupta S, et al. IAP ALS Update on Resuscitation Guidelines During COVID-19 Pandemic. Indian Journal of Pediatrics. 2021;88:469-475.
6. World Health Organization. *Guidelines for the management of snakebites.* 2nd ed. Geneva: WHO; 2016.
7. Avau B, Borra V, Vandekerckhove P, De Buck E. The Treatment of Snake Bites in a First Aid Setting: A Systematic Review. PLoS Negl Trop Dis. 2016 Oct 17;10(10):e0005079.
8. Kleinman ME, Buick JE, Huber N, Idris AH, Levy M, Morgan SG, et al. Part 7: adult basic life support: 2025 American Heart Association Guidelines for Cardiopulmonary Resuscitation and Emergency Cardiovascular Care. Circulation. 2025;152(suppl 2):S448–S478.
9. Elmer J, Atkins DL, Daya MR, et al. Part 3: Ethics: 2025 American Heart Association Guidelines for Cardiopulmonary Resuscitation and Emergency Cardiovascular Care. Circulation. 2025 Oct 21;152(16_suppl_2):S323-S352.

Chapter 58: CPR Awareness and Community Readiness

Introduction

A nation that knows CPR becomes a nation that saves itself. Every minute without CPR after a cardiac arrest reduces survival chances by 7–10%. In India alone, 7-10 lakhs of out-of-hospital sudden cardiac arrest occur each year, many witnessed, but untreated, because bystanders don't know what to do. Imagine the difference if:

- Every schoolchild knew compressions.
- Every office had an AED.
- Every home had a CPR-trained member.
- Every bystander turns into a lay rescuer.

Empowering the community plays a crucial role in survival. (1-3)

CPR Certification: For Students and HCWs

You are not truly trained in CPR until you have

- Practiced compressions on a mannequin.
- Ventilated with a bag mask.
- Followed a complete CPR sequence with team dynamics under the supervision of a trained facilitator in examination conditions.

Must-Have Certifications

CPR (BLS) Awareness Training: For all citizens, including school children.

CPR/BLS/BCLS Provider Course: This course is designed for all MBBS students, nursing students, and healthcare workers in India. Medical colleges and hospitals typically offer it in collaboration with organizations such as the Indian Academy of Pediatrics (IAP) and the Indian Resuscitation Council Federation (IRCF) to ensure the quality and adherence to benchmark standards. (1,3-5)

Table 58.1: Summary of skills learned during a CPR certification course

Skill	What You Practice
Adult, child, and infant CPR	Step-by-step compressions and rescue breaths.
Use of AED	Pad placement, safety checks, shock delivery.
Choking relief	Back blows, abdominal thrusts, chest thrusts.
Team dynamics	Role assignment, communication, CPR as a team.
Post-arrest care basics	ROSC steps, oxygenation, documentation.

Scan QR Code at the end of this chapter to access your online CPR certification module. Complete the video-based module and assessment to receive your certificate in your inbox.

CPR Instructor Training (optional) – for those who wish to teach others.

Creating CPR-Ready Institutions

Whether it's your hospital, college, or society, becoming CPR-ready involves:

- CPR training for all staff and students.
- Visible display of AEDs and CPR posters.
- Periodic mock codes.
- CPR instructor teams and student ambassadors.
- Linkage with local emergency services.
- Make your hospital a place where resuscitation is not a formality, but a culture!
- CPR for School Children and Families.

Kids Save Lives

Start early; children aged 12 years and older can learn CPR and perform effective compressions. However, CPR training should be started early as children from the age of 4-7 years can make an emergency call. They can also follow AED instructions and can play a significant role in the chain of survival if appropriately trained. (6)

- Use engaging modules, including cartoons, songs, and role-playing exercises.
- Empower teachers and parents as first responders.
- Conduct CPR camps in schools, villages, malls, and offices with at least annual repetition.
- The "CPR4Schools" and "Kids Save Lives" initiatives are already creating a new generation of lifesavers. Join the movement. (2, 7)

🎥 Video-Based CPR Learning Modules

"Knowing what to do is the first step. Practising it with your hands is when it becomes life-saving." Now, it's time to bring everything to life through visual learning and hands-on experience. This structured training will provide you with the skills, confidence, and rhythm of real-world CPR. (4)

This module aims to help you recognise, understand, and internalise the core elements of high-quality resuscitation.

The Science Behind CPR

Understand cardiac arrest and the importance of timely chest compressions and ventilation.

Recent Updates in CPR Guidelines

Stay aligned with evidence-based protocols, including compression depth, rate, and CPR sequences.

How to Use an AED

Learn the proper and safe use of AEDs before encountering them in real life.

Team Dynamics in Resuscitation

Activating the emergency response system, forming a team, assigning roles, ensuring effective communication, and providing timely feedback all save lives. Effective CPR is a team effort, and further improvement can be achieved through debriefing.

Hands-On CPR Training Sessions

Objective

By the end of this module, you should be able to initiate and lead high-quality CPR for an adult cardiac arrest victim, either as a single rescuer or as part of a team. These sessions provide authentic learning, engaging your hands, voice, eyes, and heart in harmony. You'll rotate through skill stations and participate in guided practice with immediate feedback.

Scene Safety Assessment: Rescuers must prioritize their own safety to save lives.

Recognition of Cardiac Arrest: Practice swiftly and accurately, checking for responsiveness, breathing, and pulse.

Breathing with a Barrier Device or Bag-and-Mask Ventilation: Learn to deliver breaths safely with a pocket mask. Practice effective breathing with the Ambu bag, mastering the 'E and C' technique for achieving a proper seal and ventilation.

Single Rescuer CPR: Master compressions and breaths at a 30:2 rhythm on a mannequin.

Two-Rescuer CPR and use of AED: Administer compressions, breaths, and defibrillation in a coordinated manner within a real resuscitation team.

Practice-While-Watching (PWW) Video Stations: Synchronize your actions as you watch video demonstrations of chest compression and ventilation. This serves as a powerful tool for building muscle memory.

Simulation Session on Complete CPR Sequence: Collaborate as a team to make quick decisions and execute smoothly.

Tip: Perfection will come with time. Focus on rhythm, coordination, and presence.

Scan this QR Code to Begin Your CPR Certification Journey

Figure 58.1: QR Code for IAP CPR Awareness Program for Citizens

☕ Coffee Moment

The Teenager Who Saved His Father

At a railway station in Bhopal, a man collapsed. Not breathing, no signs of life. His heart had stopped. His 16-year-old son, who attended a CPR training session just a month ago at his school, recognized cardiac arrest. He started compressions and shouted for help. A nurse from the crowd joined. Another lay rescuer brought an AED from a nearby public access AED kiosk at the railway station. The man survived. When asked how he knew what to do, the boy simply said: "We had this CPR session at school. I remembered the song we used – *CPR do… CPR do.. cardiac arrest mein CPR do...*"

CPR is not just a medical skill. It's a ripple that saves lives.

A Lifesaving Legacy

You are now entering a world where your hands can heal and your mind can guide. CPR is the first skill that connects that potential. You can learn CPR while also training laypersons, family, and friends in it.

Please don't wait for your internship to learn it.

Don't stop at yourself; train others.

Don't hesitate when the moment comes.

Because the life you save may be that of your loved one, also.

References

1. Tiwari L, Jindal A, Gupta V, Taneja LN, Garg R, Edara LR, Chakra Rao SSC. Concept proposal for IRCF national CPR Registry and update on resuscitation guidelines for infants and children. Journal of Pediatric Critical Care. 2022;9(2):48-54.
2. Tiwari L, et al. More than 302 million people reached and over 2,200,000

trained in cardiopulmonary resuscitation worldwide: The 2021 ILCOR World Restart a Heart initiative. Resuscitation Plus. 2023;14:100375. doi:10.1016/j.resplu.2023.100375

3. Bhoi S, Thakur N, Aggarwal P, et al. Impact of CPR training on the knowledge and attitude of school children in India. Indian J Crit Care Med. 2014;18(8):516–22.
4. Taneja L, Tiwari L. BLS for Professionals: IAP Manual of Basic Life Support for Health Care Providers 3rd Edition: IAP National Publication House, New Delhi 2018.
5. Berdowski J, Berg RA, Tijssen JG, Koster RW. Global incidences of out-of-hospital cardiac arrest and survival rates. Resuscitation. 2010;81(11):1479–87.
6. Del Rios M, Bartos JA, Panchal AR, Atkins DL, Cabañas JG, Cao D, et al. Part 1: executive summary: 2025 American Heart Association Guidelines for Cardiopulmonary Resuscitation and Emergency Cardiovascular Care. Circulation. 2025;152(suppl):S284–S312.
7. Perkins GD, Handley AJ, Koster RW, et al. European Resuscitation Council Guidelines 2015: Resuscitation education and implementation. Resuscitation. 2015;95:288–301.

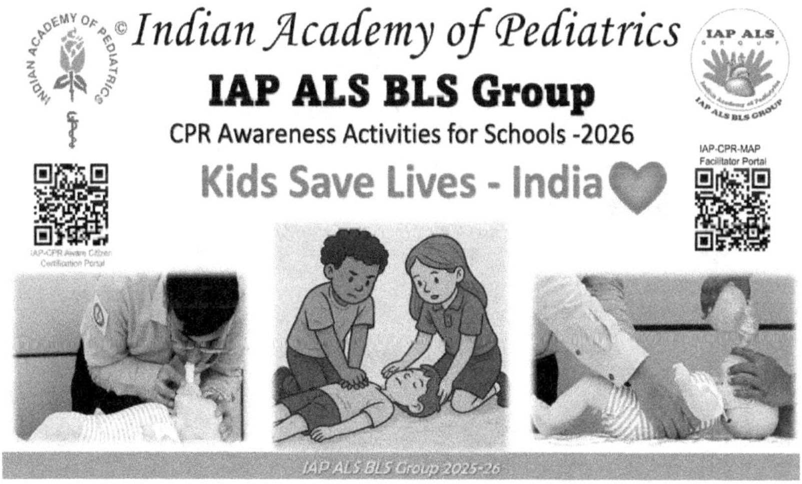

Figure 58.2: Kids Save Lives Initiative on CPR Awareness in India

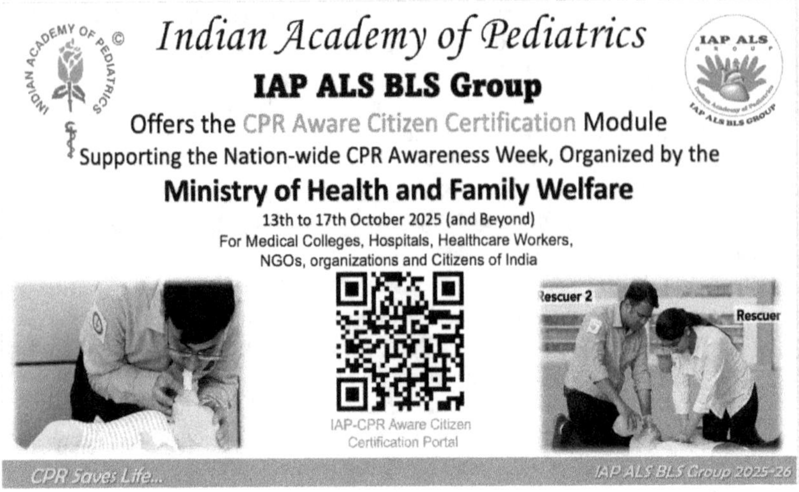
Indian Academy of Pediatrics
IAP ALS BLS Group
Offers the CPR Aware Citizen Certification Module
Supporting the Nation-wide CPR Awareness Week, Organized by the
Ministry of Health and Family Welfare
13th to 17th October 2025 (and Beyond)
For Medical Colleges, Hospitals, Healthcare Workers,
NGOs, organizations and Citizens of India
IAP-CPR Aware Citizen
Certification Portal
Rescuer 2
Rescuer
CPR Saves Life...
IAP ALS BLS Group 2025-26

Figure 58.3: CPR Awareness Initiative for Healthcare Workers

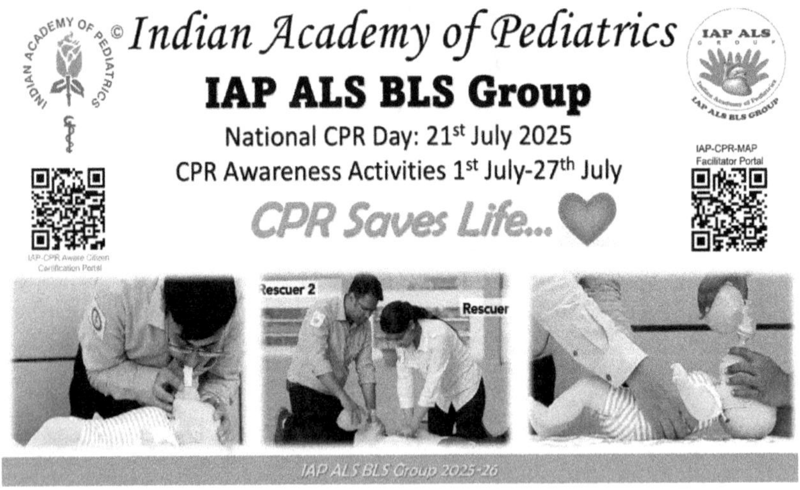

Figure 58.4: CPR Awareness Day of the Indian Academy of Pediatrics

Rescue

Rescue is about the first hands that reach out when someone collapses, gasps, or cries out.
These moments are unfiltered: raw, urgent, often chaotic. They don't wait for degrees or specialist training. They demand composure, clarity, and courage.

As a medical student, you will face them sooner than you expect: in hostels, rural postings, hospital corridors, or even on a roadside. The skills here are not advanced therapies, but fundamental life-saving actions: pressing a wound, rolling a patient onto their side, mixing ORS correctly, or administering aspirin at the right moment.

What makes these simple steps profound is their timing. When done early and correctly, they tilt destiny, turning potential death into survival.

This section will guide you through the most critical emergencies, not to overwhelm you, but to prepare.

Think of it as your first shield and your first bridge. Mastering these skills means that wherever you are, you carry the power to make a difference.

S No.	Rescue: At a Glance
1.	**Chapter 59** - First Aid: Which Emergencies Matter Most India's burden of preventable deaths: why CPR, bleeding control, drowning rescue, burns, and poisoning matter most.
2.	**Chapter 60** - First Aid in Medical Emergencies: WHO's structured ABCDE approach Recognize, Resuscitate, Review, Refer.
3.	**Chapter 61** - Heart Attack Aspirin, early recognition, and the golden 10 minutes.
4.	**Chapter 62** - Stroke FAST recognition, why "time is brain," and safe transfer.
5.	**Chapter 63** - Anaphylaxis When allergies turn fatal: epinephrine as the life-saving drug.
6.	**Chapter 64** - Presyncope, Syncope, and Shock From simple fainting to circulatory collapse: what to do.
7.	**Chapter 65** - Decreased Consciousness The recovery position: why sometimes the safest help is restraint.
8.	**Chapter 66** - Hypoglycemia Sugar as medicine: quick fixes that prevent brain damage.
9.	**Chapter 67** - Snakebite and Stings Do it R.I.G.H.T. in snakebite and first things first in scorpion, jellyfish, bees and wasp stings.
10.	**Chapter 68** - Common Poisonings From pesticides to kerosene: what to do and what not to do. Handle opioid overdose.
11.	**Chapter 69** - The First Look That Saves a Child The Pediatric Assessment Triangle: a gaze that guides action.
12.	**Chapter 70** - Childhood Diarrhoea and Pneumonia ORS, zinc, antibiotics: simple packets that save millions.
13.	**Chapter 71** - Status Asthmaticus & Acute Respiratory Distress When wheeze becomes silence: recognizing the red flags.
14.	**Chapter 72** - Seizures and Status Epilepticus First things first: protecting airway, preventing harm and controlling seizures.

Chapter 59: First Aid- Which Emergencies Matter Most

Introduction

Welcome to your journey as a medical student. Medicine involves more than textbooks, stethoscopes, or wards. It is about quick, delicate and life-changing moments. Someone collapses. A child struggles to breathe. A worker arrives in the ER covered in fumes. In these moments, seconds matter. For India, with its large population, diverse geography, and unique health issues, identifying the most critical emergencies and skills that save lives quickly is the first step towards becoming a doctor who makes a difference.

This chapter introduces the evidence, reviewing data from the WHO, ICMR, NCRB, ILCOR and other sources. It explores the causes of preventable death and disabilities and highlights key first-aid recommendations with updated best possible evidence and skills to learn.

First aid: First aid is the immediate assistance provided to a person suffering from an acute illness or injury by a trained or untrained individual, using available resources, until professional medical care is accessible or condition no longer requires urgent intervention. Its scope depends on the rescuer's knowledge, skill, available equipment, and the safety of the environment. (1)

The Ground Reality: What the Numbers Say

Out-of-hospital cardiac arrest (OHCA): The global incidence is approximately 55 per 100,000 person-years. There is no reliable data from India in the absence of cardiac arrest registries, but assuming a similar incidence, an estimated number of OHCAs in India is 785,000 annually, about 2,150 per day. (2)

Road traffic accidents (RTAs): 1,68,491 people died in road traffic accidents in India in the year 2022 (460 per day). Timely bleeding control, airway support, and safe transport are key interventions to save lives in RTAs. (3,4)

Cardiovascular and cerebrovascular emergencies: Heart attacks and strokes are time-critical emergencies and leading causes of death in India. (5,6) Aspirin for suspected heart attacks and early recognition of stroke can significantly change the outcome.

Snakebite: India alone accounts for approximately 58,000 deaths annually from snakebites. Most of these deaths occur in rural areas and during the monsoon season. Many are preventable through proper first aid and prompt referral.

Drowning: WHO calls drowning an "urgent and overlooked" issue; India's monsoon rivers, wells, and ponds become traps for children and young adults. Here, early rescue, ventilation and CPR are life-saving.

Burns: Domestic and industrial burns are common in India, causing deaths, lifelong disability and stigma. Cooling a burn with running water for ≥20 minutes is a simple first aid measure to improve outcomes if provided immediately. (1)

Poisonings, especially pesticides: Organophosphate poisoning is commonly reported in India. Early detection, removal from exposure, and airway management are crucial life-saving steps until antidotes are given.

Childhood diarrhoea and pneumonia: Despite progress, diarrhoeal disease remains a leading cause of under-5 mortality. WHO/UNICEF emphasize ORS and zinc as simple, scalable first-line interventions.

These numbers are more than statistics. They are faces you will encounter in your future wards and emergency rooms. These are the reasons why your first-aid training is essential and not optional.

How to Prioritise Emergencies

Not all emergencies are the same. Consider two questions: Which conditions cause the most preventable death or disability in India, and where does first aid have the greatest impact quickly? Evidence suggests that emergencies, which are common, can be rapidly fatal without intervention, and are highly responsive to simple, teachable steps, are the most critical. (7,8)

Priority list: major trauma/bleeding (RTIs), cardiac arrest and chest pain (suspected MI), stroke, drowning, burns, snakebite, poisoning (especially organophosphates), heat illness, anaphylaxis, hypoglycaemia, and under-5 diarrhoea/dehydration.

Mastering a small set of essential, versatile skills for these scenarios will have the greatest impact on the skill development of a new medical student.

Skills That Move the Needle of Life

Basic Life Support (BLS) for Cardiac Arrest

Learning to perform effective chest compressions and rescue breaths is the most critical skill you must acquire. Immediate CPR can double or even triple survival in out-of-hospital cardiac arrest.

Bleeding Control in RTA

Severe bleeding can be fatal within minutes. Evidence indicates that direct pressure, pressure dressings, and (when indicated and trained) tourniquet application are among the most effective life-saving first-aid measures.

First Aid Updates 2025

The International Liaison Committee on Resuscitation (ILCOR) has recently published its general and specific recommendations for first aid. These recommendations and good practice statements (GPS) are integrated throughout the chapters, but we have also summarized them in the table below to bring to your attention important changes, in case you have previously read them or taught during your orientation sessions. You may find the topics and recommendations random at first glance, but they will make sense when you go through the chapters related to relevant topics. (1,9)

Table 59.1: Updated general recommendations during first aid

Topic	Updated recommendations or good practice statements
Use of Pulse Oximetry in FA	First aid providers using oximeters should be proficient and aware of limitations (e.g., cold extremities, poor perfusion, nail polish). Pulse oximetry should *not* replace physical assessment.
Providing Supplemental Oxygen in FA	First aid providers should be trained to administer supplemental oxygen in different conditions with hypoxia or with the risk of hypoxia. They should be able to titrate O_2 in COPD to avoid high-flow O_2 and maintain SpO_2 88–92%. Without withholding it in life-threatening hypoxia (SpO_2 <88%).
Recovery Position for FA	Use recovery position for persons with decreased responsiveness (non-traumatic) with monitoring for breathing and airway obstruction. If there is uncertainty of signs of life, immediate assessment should be done in supine position.

First Aid in Medical Emergencies

Table 59.2: Updated recommendations for first aid in medical emergencies

Topic	Updated recommendations or good practice statements
Recognition of Anaphylaxis	Recognition improves only with repeated training; untrained persons should not be expected to reliably recognize anaphylaxis.
Second Dose of Epinephrine in anaphylaxis	A second epinephrine dose may be given by autoinjector if symptoms persist after the first dose.
Foreign-Body Airway Obstruction	Use back blows followed by abdominal thrusts (>1 year) or chest thrusts (<1 year). Extract visible item from mouth. No blind finger sweep.
Bronchodilators	Trained providers may assist individuals with asthma

	to use prescribed inhalers during breathing difficulty.
Early Aspirin for Chest Pain	Early administration of aspirin (chewed or swallowed) is suggested in adults with non-traumatic chest pain
Glucose Administration in hypoglycemia	Use oral (swallowed) glucose for conscious individuals. If not available, use oral + buccal glucose gel. Sublingual glucose for uncooperative children.
Dietary Sugar for Hypoglycemia	Use glucose tablets first-line. If unavailable, dietary sugar (small candies, sugar cubes, juice) may be used.
Recognition of Stroke	Use validated stroke scales: FAST, Cincinnati, Melbourne, Los Angeles. Check blood glucose if available.
Recognition of Sepsis	Encourages awareness of early sepsis signs: altered mentation, tachycardia, fever, rapid breathing.
Postpartum Hemorrhage- Manual Uterine Massage	Laypersons may provide uterine massage in low-resource settings if trained and when no professional care available.
Postpartum Hemorrhage Lay Interventions	Community responders should be trained for early intervention and referral.
Naloxone in Opioid Emergency	If available, trained rescuers should administer naloxone during suspected opioid related cardiac arrest while continuing CPR.
Counter-Pressure for Syncope	Lay providers may teach physical counter-pressure maneuvers (leg crossing, arm tensing) to prevent vasovagal syncope.
Unintentional Injury from CPR	Minor rib or chest injuries should not deter bystanders from performing CPR.

First Aid in Trauma Emergencies

Table 59.3: Updated recommendations for first aid in trauma emergencies

Topic	Updated recommendations or good practice statements
Spinal Motion Restriction	Use manual spinal stabilization instead of full immobilization where resources limited. Maintain neutral alignment and minimize unnecessary movement.
Cryotherapy for Epistaxis	Topical cooling or compression may reduce bleeding.
Bleeding Control – Manual Pressure	Strong recommendation: direct manual pressure is first-line for external bleeding.
Use of tourniquets	Use tourniquets only if direct pressure fails. Commercial devices preferred over improvised
Hemostatic	When available, use hemostatic dressings as adjuncts to

Dressings	direct pressure.
Burn Cooling	Cool burns with running water for ≥20 min as soon as possible; avoid ice.
Dental Avulsion	Reimplant tooth immediately if possible; or store in milk, saline, or saliva.
Compression Wrap	Elastic compression wrap may be used for closed joint injuries.
Preservation of Amputated Part	Wrap part in moist sterile gauze, seal in bag, place on ic, avoid direct freezing.

First Aid in Environmental Emergencies

Table 59.4: First aid in environmental emergencies (2025)

Topic	Updated recommendations or good practice statements
Exertion-Related Dehydration	Encourage oral rehydration with water or electrolyte solution at first sign of dehydration.
Tick Removal	Remove tick with fine-tipped tweezers grasping close to skin, pulling upward steadily.
Treatment of Jellyfish Stings	Rinse with vinegar (acetic acid 4–6%) where effective species known. Avoid freshwater or alcohol rinsing. Use tweezers to remove tentacles.

Why this matters

Your actions in the first minutes can determine survival. You might be the only trained person present when someone collapses; in rural postings, referral can take hours. As the first intern in the ER, your basic skills can buy time and save lives. Master these skills now.

References

1. Djärv T, Douma MJ, Carlson JN, Singletary EM, Berry DC, Bradley RN, et al. First aid: 2025 International Liaison Committee on Resuscitation Consensus on Science With Treatment Recommendations. Circulation. 2025;152(suppl 1):S250–S282.
2. Yan S, Gan Y, Jiang N, Wang R, Chen Y, Luo Z, et al. The global survival rate among adult out-of-hospital cardiac arrest patients who received cardiopulmonary resuscitation: a systematic review and meta-analysis. Crit Care. 2020;24(1):61.
3. Ministry of Road Transport and Highways. Road Accidents in India 2022 [Internet]. New Delhi: MoRTH; 2023 Oct 30 [cited 2025 Sep 1]. Available from: https://morth.nic.in/sites/default/files/RA_2022_30_Oct.pdf
4. Ministry of Road Transport & Highways. Good Samaritan Guidelines—Notification 21 Jan 2016 & SOP; Supreme Court order 30 Mar 2016 [Internet]. [cited 2025 Sep 1]. Available from: https://morth.gov.in/

5. India State-Level Disease Burden Initiative Collaborators. India: Health of the Nation's States—The India State-Level Disease Burden Initiative [Internet]. New Delhi: ICMR, PHFI, IHME; 2017 [cited 2025 Sep 1]. Available from: https://www.icmr.gov.in/reports
6. Prabhakaran D, et al. The burgeoning cardiovascular disease epidemic in Indians. Lancet Reg Health–Southeast Asia. 2023;7:100097.
7. American Heart Association; American Red Cross. 2024 Guidelines for First Aid—Focused updates summary [Internet]. 2024 Nov 14 [cited 2025 Sep 1]. Available from: https://professional.heart.org/en/science-news/2024-aha-and-american-red-cross-guidelines-for-first-aid.
8. Singletary EM, Zideman DA, De Buck E, et al. 2020 International Consensus on First Aid Science with Treatment Recommendations. Circulation. 2020;142(16 Suppl 2):S284–S303.
9. Hewett Brumberg EK, Douma MJ, Alibertis K, Charlton NP, Goldman MP, Harper-Kirksey K, et al. 2024 American Heart Association and American Red Cross Guidelines for First Aid. Circulation. 2024;150:e519–e579.

Chapter 60: First Aid in Medical Emergency

Introduction

Emergencies do not wait for a specialist's availability. Very often, the first responder is a layperson, nurse, medical student, intern or community health worker. Knowing what to do in the first crucial minutes can make the difference between life and death. The World Health Organization (WHO) has developed a structured, evidence-based algorithm for medical emergencies. This chapter introduces the approach and helps you build a visual memory of the sequence, so that actions are instinctive when time is short.

First Aid Algorithm

It is a simple, systematic, and step-by-step flow that is adaptable to different settings, ranging from rural clinics to tertiary care hospitals. It follows the **Recognise-Resuscitate-Review-Refer** flow with the ABCDE approach in recognition as well as resuscitation.

1. Recognize – Spot the Emergency Early

Quick recognition: It saves critical time.

- **Scene safety:** It is important for both, rescuer and the patient.
- **Look for clues:** Empty pill bottles, vomitus, signs of trauma, insect bite or envenomation and behaviour of the crowd.
- **Check responsiveness:** Call out by name or say 'hello,' and tap their shoulders.

ABCDE assessment

- **Airway:** Is it clear, maintainable with simple measures like position, suctioning or oral/nasal airway or not maintainable by simple measures and needs advanced airway measures such as intubation or insertion of a laryngeal mask airway (LMA)? Is the patient speaking or choking?
- **Breathing:** Is there chest movement? What is the rate, depth, work of breathing, any abnormal sound and SpO_2?
- **Circulation:** Pulse rate, pulse volume, perfusion/capillary filling time, skin colour and temperature and blood pressure.
- **Disability:** Level of consciousness (AVPU: Alert, Verbal, Pain response, Unresponsive), size and reaction of pupils and blood sugar.
- **Exposure:** Look for signs of bleeding, injuries, rashes, bites, or burns.

Example: A hostel cook collapses suddenly. You note sweating, chest pain, and altered responsiveness → Recognized as a possible cardiorespiratory failure due to acute coronary syndrome.

2. Resuscitate – Immediately Stabilize Life-Threats

Once recognized, act fast. Treat first what kills first.

- **Airway:** Clear obstructions and secretions. Place the person in a recovery position if unconscious but breathing.
- **Breathing:** Administer oxygen using different devices, assist ventilation, and give bronchodilators for asthma.
- **Circulation:** Control bleeding, apply pressure dressings, start IV fluid resuscitation and vasoactive drugs for shock, and provide CPR if indicated.
- **Disability:** Position, correct low sugar, treat seizures.
- **Exposure:** Stop bleeding, correct ambient temperature.

Principle: These interventions provide a survival window until definitive care becomes available.

3. Review – Reassess and Monitor

- First aid is not a one-time task to be forgotten. Constant monitoring and reassessment are crucial as the clinical condition evolves over time.
- Recheck ABCDE after every intervention.
- Record vital clinical signs (heart rate, pulse, BP, respiratory rate, SpO_2, consciousness) at regular intervals and additionally as needed.
- Document specific actions, timing, and the patient's response.
- Anticipate complications: airway care, worsening shock, and cardiac arrest.

Tip: Always think two steps ahead. If giving oxygen, ask: What if they stop breathing?

4. Refer – Ensure Definitive Care

- First aid is the bridge, not the destination.
- Call for ambulance/transport early.
- Use SBAR handover (Situation, Background, Assessment, Recommendation).
- Please send along notes on interventions and vital signs.
- If feasible, have trained staff accompany the patient.

Principle: A good referral is part of first aid, as it prevents the repetition of errors and builds trust.

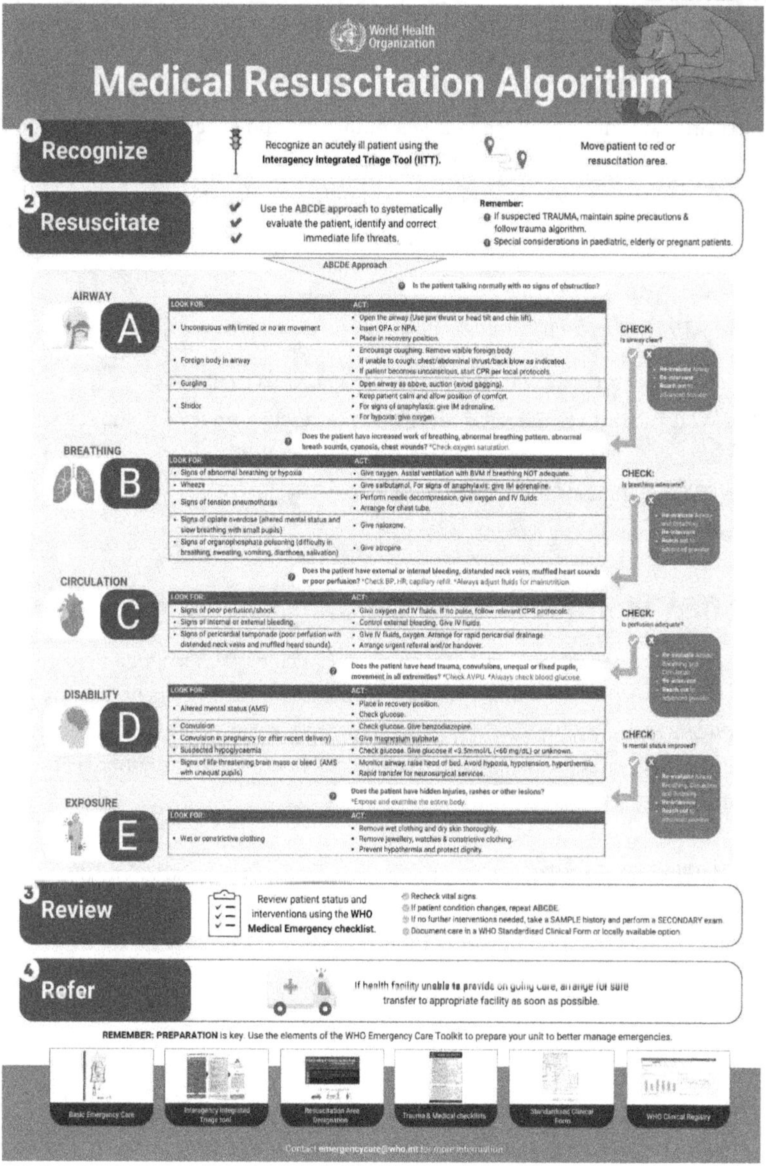

Figure 60.1: WHO Medical Resuscitation Algorithm
(used with written permission from WHO)

Case Snapshot

A 45-year-old man collapses in the hospital corridor. You witness it and quickly scan the area to ensure it is safe. You recognize that he is unresponsive, his breathing is shallow, and his pulse is palpable.

You resuscitate the patient and take quick sequential actions- call for help, put him in recovery position, start oxygen and monitor. Prepared to deliver chest compressions and use an AED if needed. You review and check the airway, breathing and circulation, monitor pulse and oxygen saturation, and check the random blood sugar level, which is 40 mg/dL (low). You arrange to give a 10% dextrose bolus and arrange a quick transfer. He is stabilized and referred to the emergency department with proper handover. The structured approach ensures no critical step is missed, even under stress.

Learning Points

- Emergencies need a structured approach; panic leads to mistakes.
- The WHO algorithm integrates recognition, resuscitation, review, and referral as a flow.
- The ABCDE framework is central to this approach.
- Safe transfer and clear handover are part of first-aid.

☕Coffee Moment

Imagine being the one who spots danger early, the person who recognized a choking child in the cafeteria or a fainting classmate in the lab. In that moment, you are not 'just a student'; you are the first doctor in someone's chain of survival. That is the power of first aid, ordinary hands with minimal resources doing extraordinary things that save lives.

References

1. World Health Organization. WHO First Aid Guidelines. Geneva: WHO; 2016.
2. World Health Organization. Basic Emergency Care: Approach to the Acutely Ill and Injured. Geneva: WHO; 2018.
3. Zideman DA, Singletary EM, De Buck ED, et al. European Resuscitation Council Guidelines for First Aid: 2021 Update. Resuscitation. 2021;161:270–290.
4. International Liaison Committee on Resuscitation (ILCOR). First Aid Task Force Recommendations. Circulation. 2015;132(16 Suppl 1):S287–S303.

Chapter 61: Heart Attack

It's 7 a.m. in your hostel when the security guard bursts in, clutching his chest. He is sweating, pale, and gasping, "*Dard... seene mein dard* (Pain...chest pain)." Some bystanders urge him to lie down and breathe deeply, while others run to get water. You recognize this could be a heart attack. There's no time to waste—the next 10 minutes could decide his life.

Introduction

Acute Coronary Syndrome (ACS) and Myocardial Infarction (MI) are commonly known as "Heart Attack". It occurs when blood flow to the heart is blocked, typically by a clot in a coronary artery (the arteries that supply blood to the heart muscles). In India, heart attacks are likely to happen about a decade earlier than in Western populations, often affecting men in their 40s and 50s. Recently, it has been noted to increasingly affect women also. Early recognition and immediate first aid, including aspirin administration and rapid transport to a cardiac facility, can save a life. [1,2)

Recognize Warning Signs

- Central chest pain (pressure, tightness, heaviness, burning), often radiating to the arm, jaw, or back and lasting over 10 minutes.
- Cold sweats, nausea, and vomiting.
- Shortness of breath, dizziness, and fainting.
- May present atypically in women, the elderly, or diabetics as fatigue and breathlessness without pain. (2-4)

Critical Skill

Aspirin for a Suspected Heart Attack and CPR if cardiac arrest

Why it matters: During the first minutes of a suspected heart attack, platelet activation causes coronary thrombosis. Chewing aspirin quickly offers a rapid antiplatelet effect and is among the most impactful first-dose interventions recommended in first aid guidelines. (1,3,4)

First Aid Steps

- **Activate EMS/ Ambulance (102/108/112) early**. Keep the patient sitting upright or semi-reclined for comfort. Reassure calmly to reduce anxiety and cardiac workload.
- **Give aspirin if there is no allergy and no contraindication:** 160–325 mg of non-enteric-coated ("chewable") aspirin, chewed and swallowed. If only enteric-coated tablets are available, crush or chew them to speed absorption. Water sips

are allowed. (1,3,4)

- **Administer medications early**: Administer Nitroglycerine (for known heart condition) and provide supplemental oxygen if available.
- **Monitor ABCs and Start CPR if needed**: Be prepared for sudden cardiac arrest. Start CPR if the person becomes unresponsive and is not breathing normally; use an AED as soon as available.
- **Hand over** to EMS with the time of symptom onset and the dose of aspirin already given.

Do *not* give aspirin if

- Known aspirin allergy or history of severe asthma triggered by NSAIDs.
- Active bleeding or known bleeding disorder.
- Signs of stroke; aspirin is not the first aid for acute stroke.
- Suspected aortic dissection (sudden "tearing" chest/back pain, unequal pulses).

What NOT to Do

- Substituting painkillers (ibuprofen, diclofenac, paracetamol) for aspirin—these do not provide the needed antiplatelet effect.
- Delaying EMS while hunting for tablets. Call first, then give aspirin.
- Enteric-coated tablets should be swallowed whole—chew for a faster effect.

Outcome

Early aspirin administration and swift transport for reperfusion therapy (thrombolysis or angioplasty) significantly reduce mortality and complications. Delays are often due to misinterpretation of symptoms, lack of awareness, and transportation issues. First aid can bridge this critical gap. (1,2,4)

Learning Points

- Time is life: every minute counts in heart attacks.
- The first-aid trifecta is recognise early → call 112 → give chewable aspirin (160–325 mg), while preparing for CPR/AED if the patient deteriorates.
- If chest pain, suspect MI unless proven otherwise.
- Aspirin is the single most important first aid drug.
- Ensure rapid hospital transfer; first aid is not definitive care.

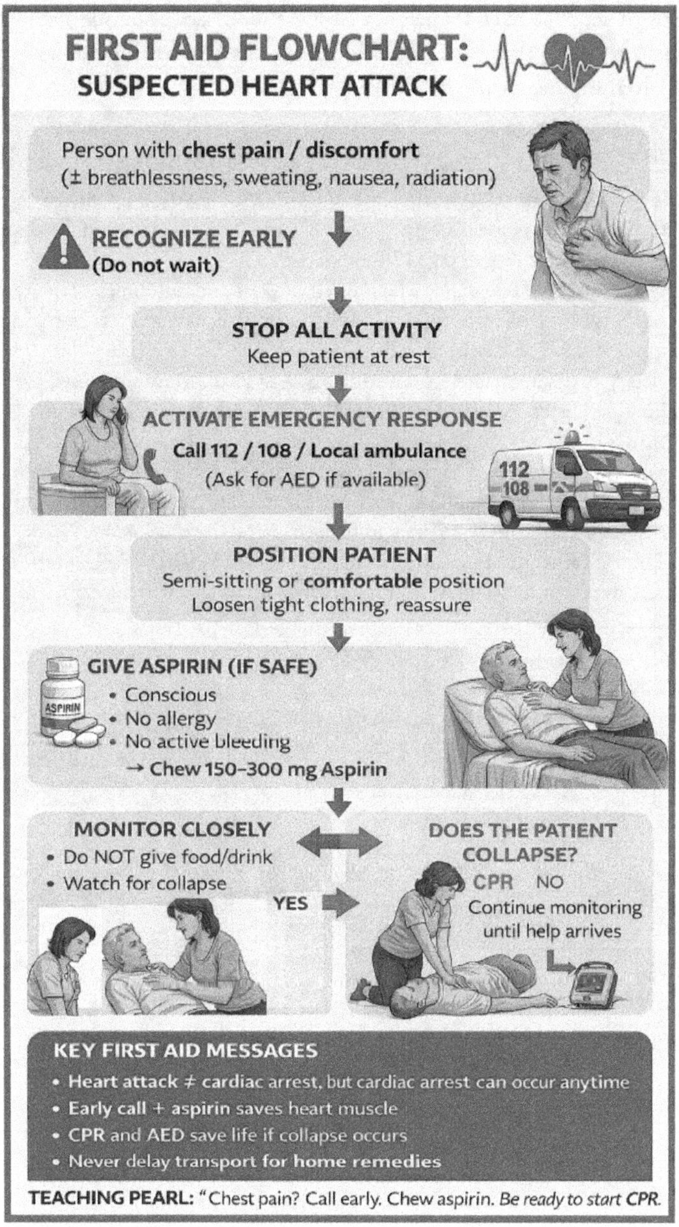

Figure 61.1: First Aid Flowchart for Heart Attack

Coffee Moment

Later, the student replayed the guard's frightened eyes in the OPD canteen. "All I did was give aspirin and keep him calm until the ambulance came," she thought. Her professor smiled: "Exactly. Sometimes saving a life is about buying time until the cath lab takes over." The coffee felt like the beat of a heart that had almost stopped but was given another chance.

References

1. Antman EM, Hand M, Armstrong PW, et al. 2007 focused update of the ACC/AHA 2004 guidelines for the management of ST-elevation myocardial infarction. Circulation. 2008;117(2):296–329.
2. Xavier D, Pais P, Devereaux PJ, et al. Treatment and outcomes of acute coronary syndromes in India (CREATE): a prospective analysis of registry data. Lancet. 2008;371(9622):1435–42.
3. Singletary EM, Zideman DA, De Buck ED, et al. 2020 International Consensus on First Aid Science With Treatment Recommendations. Circulation. 2020;142(16_suppl_1):S284–S334.
4. Hewett Brumberg EK, Douma MJ, Alibertis K, Charlton NP, Goldman MP, Harper-Kirksey K, et al. 2024 American Heart Association and American Red Cross Guidelines for First Aid. Circulation. 2024;150:e519–e579.
5. O'Gara PT, Kushner FG, Ascheim DD, et al. 2013 ACCF/AHA guideline for the management of ST-elevation myocardial infarction. Circulation. 2013;127(4):e362–425.

Chapter 62: Stroke

During a morning lecture, a 62-year-old retired teacher sitting in the front row suddenly drops his pen, struggles to speak, and his face appears lopsided. Some students think he is just dizzy, but you recall the "FAST" warning signs of stroke. The clock is ticking; every minute without treatment means brain cells are dying.

Introduction

Stroke is a sudden neurological deficit caused by interruption of blood supply to the brain (ischemic or hemorrhagic). It is one of the leading causes of death and disability, with delayed recognition and transportation being major barriers to survival. The role of the first aid provider is not treatment but rapid recognition, reassurance, and urgent transfer to a hospital with stroke facilities. (1,2)

Recognizing FAST for Stroke

Why it matters: Stroke is a race against time; brain cells die every minute. Use FAST to identify it quickly and take action.

F - Face: Ask the person to smile and check for drooping or asymmetry.
A - Arms: Ask to raise both arms and see if one drifts down or cannot be lifted.
S - Speech: Listen for slurred speech, wrong words, or inability to speak.
T - Time: Record the time symptoms started or the last time the person was well and call 112 immediately. Do not wait for symptom improvement.

Additional clues include sudden weakness or numbness, changes in vision, imbalance, and a severe headache. (2,3)

First Aid Steps

1. Call emergency help immediately: Stroke is a "time is brain" emergency. The typical patient loses 1.9 million neurons each minute if the stroke is untreated. (4) Arrange immediate transfer to the nearest hospital with a CT scan and a stroke unit.

2. Position & Reassure: Lay patient with head elevated around 30°, ensure airway is open; loosen tight clothing and reassure to reduce anxiety.

3. Oxygen (if available): Provide oxygen if the patient is breathless or hypoxic.

4. Nil per oral: Do not give food, water, or medicines by mouth (risk of aspiration).

5. Monitor vitals and glucose level: If unresponsive and no breathing/pulse → start CPR. Hypoglycemia can mimic a stroke.

6. Record onset time: Note the exact time symptoms started; this is critical for thrombolysis (the tPA window is up to 4.5 hours in ischemic stroke).

What NOT to Do

- Do not give aspirin or any medication unless advised by a doctor. Some strokes are hemorrhagic, and aspirin may worsen bleeding.
- Do not ignore "minor" symptoms; It may be transient ischemic attacks (TIA).
- Do not delay transfer by seeking home remedies.

Outcome

If recognized and treated within the "golden window," many stroke patients benefit from thrombolysis or mechanical thrombectomy. Delay leads to irreversible brain injury and disability. First aiders can significantly influence outcomes by reducing pre-hospital delays, which remain a major challenge in India. (1,5,6)

Learning Points

- Use FAST to recognize stroke quickly.
- Do not give anything orally; protect the airway and immediate transport.
- Record the time of onset; this guides hospital treatment.

☕ Coffee Moment

Later, in the college canteen, the student absentmindedly stirred her tea. She couldn't shake the image of the teacher's crooked smile and slurred words. Her senior whispered, "Remember: when you see a stroke, you don't panic, you act. One call, one quick decision, and you save a lifetime of speech, movement, and dignity." The tea tasted stronger, heavy with the weight of minutes that matter more than hours.

References

1. Johnson W, Onuma O, Owolabi M, Sachdev S. Stroke: a global response is needed. Bull World Health Organ. 2016 Sep 1;94(9):634-634A.
2. Powers WJ, Rabinstein AA, Ackerson T, et al. Guidelines for the Early Management of Patients With Acute Ischemic Stroke: 2019;50(12):e344-e418.
3. Singletary EM, Zideman DA, De Buck ED, et al. 2020 International Consensus on First Aid Science With Treatment Recommendations. Circulation. 2020;142(16_suppl_1):S284–S334.
4. Saver JL. Time is brain--quantified. Stroke. 2006 Jan;37(1):263-6.
5. Hewett Brumberg EK, Douma MJ, Alibertis K, Charlton NP, Goldman MP, Harper-Kirksey K, et al. 2024 American Heart Association and American Red Cross Guidelines for First Aid. Circulation. 2024;150:e519–e579.
6. Pandian JD, Gall SL, Kate MP, et al. Prevention of stroke: a global perspective. Lancet. 2018;392(10154):1269–78.

Chapter 63: Anaphylaxis

During a hostel dinner, a 19-year-old student develops itching, swelling around the eyes, and difficulty breathing after eating peanuts. Within minutes, she collapses, gasping for air. Friends panic; some suggest water, while others want to rub balm on her chest. You check her bag and find an epinephrine auto-injector. Your action in the next 60 seconds will determine whether she survives.

Introduction

Anaphylaxis is a severe, life-threatening allergic reaction triggered by exposure to allergens, including foods (such as peanuts, seafood, milk, and eggs), insect stings, latex, or certain medications. It is a medical emergency due to airway obstruction, bronchospasm, and circulatory collapse. In India, food-related anaphylaxis is increasingly recognized, but awareness and access to epinephrine remain limited. Prompt recognition and administration of epinephrine are crucial for survival. (1,2)

Recognition

- **Skin/mucosal signs:** Hives, itching, flushing, swelling (angioedema of lips, eyes, tongue).
- **Respiratory signs:** Wheeze, stridor, hoarseness, shortness of breath.
- **Circulatory signs:** Dizziness, syncope, weak pulse, hypotension, shock.
- **GI signs:** Nausea, vomiting, abdominal cramps.
- **Clue:** Rapid onset (minutes to hours) after allergen exposure leading to airway, breathing, or circulatory compromise. It is anaphylaxis. (2-6)

First Aid Steps

1. Call for help immediately: Begin CPR if unresponsive, not breathing or has no pulse. Activate emergency services. Lay the patient supine with their legs raised (or in a sitting position if severe breathlessness is present); avoid standing or walking.

2. IM Epinephrine: Give IM epinephrine in the mid-outer thigh (through clothing if needed). Do not give SC or in the buttocks. Do not dilute epinephrine (available as a 1:1000 or 1 mg/mL) further for IM injection in anaphylaxis. An autoinjector can be self-administered. (5)

- Adults/adolescents: 0.5 mg IM (0.5 mL).
- Children: 0.01 mg/kg (0.01 mL/kg) IM, max 0.5 mg per dose.
- Quick estimate- 0.1 mL for infants, 0.3 mL for children and 0.5 mL for adolescents and adults.
- Auto-injectors: 0.3 mg for ≥30 kg, 0.15 mg for 10–30 kg. (1,3)
- Repeat every 5–10 minutes if airway, breathing, or circulation problems persist

or recur.

- If β-blocker exposure is suspected, IV glucagon is a reasonable option. (4)
- Administer rapid isotonic fluids in cases of shock.
- If the patient develops cardiac arrest, a standard IM epinephrine dose may not suffice; proceed with ALS/PALS dosing/route. (4,5)

3. Supportive care: Provide oxygen if available; administer a short-acting beta agonist (salbutamol) inhaler for wheezing; give IV fluids for shock when trained; antihistamines and steroids are also used later, but are not first-line treatments and must not delay epinephrine.

4. Hospital transfer: All patients require observation for at least 4–6 hours due to the risk of biphasic reaction (recurrence after initial recovery). (2) Refractory cases need treatment escalation even upto ECMO support. (4)

What NOT to Do

- Do not delay epinephrine while searching for IV access or giving antihistamines.
- Do not make the patient stand or walk suddenly (risk of collapse).
- Do not assume one injection is enough; recurrence is possible.

Outcome

Timely administration of epinephrine helps most patients recover fully. Delays in recognizing symptoms or relying on alternative remedies like water or home treatments often lead to preventable deaths. Raising awareness among students, teachers, and communities is crucial, especially for those with known food or insect sting allergies.

Learning Points

- Anaphylaxis means acting quickly. Epinephrine is life-saving.
- Recognize early signs: skin, airway, breathing, or circulatory compromise.
- Suspect early → position → IM epinephrine to the thigh → repeat if needed → support ABC and transfer. This sequence saves lives.
- Food allergies such as peanuts, seafood, and milk are common triggers in India.
- All patients require monitoring due to the risk of biphasic reactions.

☕ Coffee Moment

Later, in the hospital canteen, the student who administered epinephrine sipped her tea with trembling hands. "I thought she was choking on food. I didn't know it could

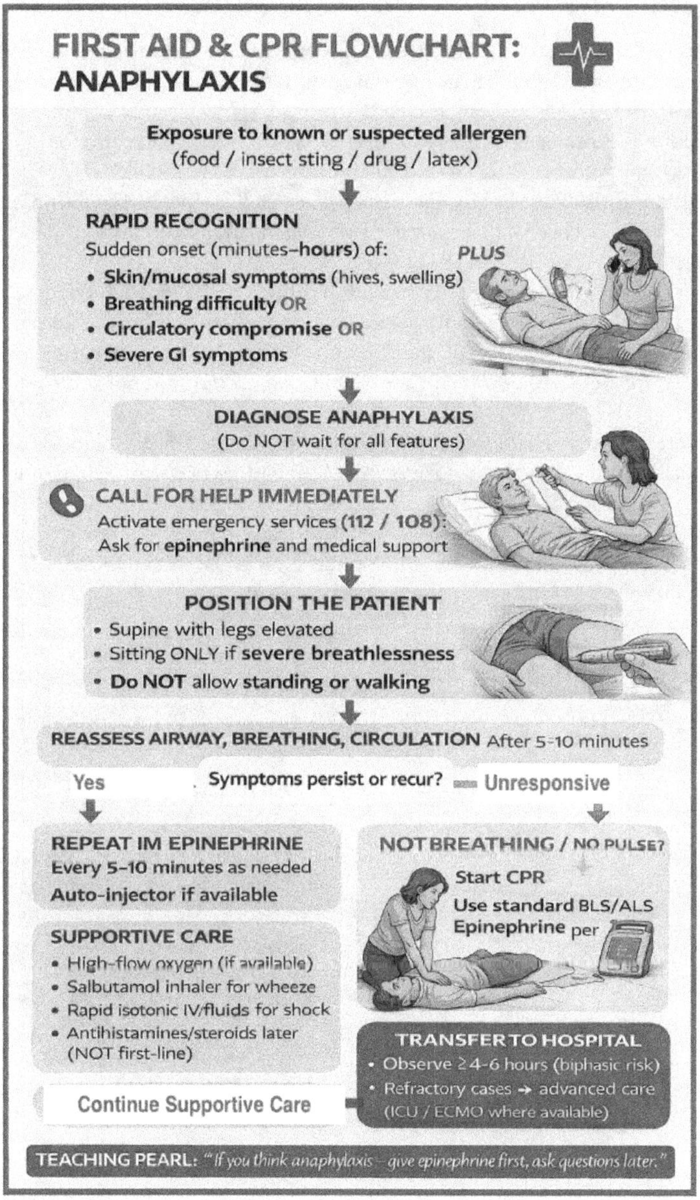

Figure 63.1: First Aid in Anaphylaxis

be so sudden," she whispered. Her senior replied gently, That's anaphylaxis. It doesn't give you time to think, only to act if you are prepared. And you acted. The tea felt better, a quiet reminder that courage in crisis is sometimes measured in seconds.

References

1. Simons FE, Ardusso LR, Bilo MB, et al. World Allergy Organization guidelines for the assessment and management of anaphylaxis. World Allergy Organ J. 2011;4(2):13–37.
2. Cardona V, Ansotegui IJ, Ebisawa M, et al. World Allergy Organization anaphylaxis guidance 2020. World Allergy Organ J. 2020;13(10):100472.
3. Singletary EM, Zideman DA, De Buck ED, et al. 2020 International Consensus on First Aid Science With Treatment Recommendations. Circulation. 2020;142(16_suppl_1):S284–S334.
4. Cao D, Arens AM, Chow SL, Easter SR, Hoffman RS, Lagina AT III, et al. Part 10: adult and pediatric special circumstances of resuscitation: 2025 American Heart Association Guidelines for Cardiopulmonary Resuscitation and Emergency Cardiovascular Care. Circulation. 2025;152(suppl 2):S578–S672.
5. Hewett Brumberg EK, Douma MJ, Alibertis K, Charlton NP, Goldman MP, Harper-Kirksey K, et al. 2024 American Heart Association and American Red Cross Guidelines for First Aid. Circulation. 2024;150:e519–e579.
6. Tiwari L. Anaphylaxis: IAP textbook of pediatric and neonatal emergencies. 1st Edition. Jaypee Brothers Medical Publishers New Delhi/ London. 2020 ISBN 978-93-5270-982-3: 121-127.

Chapter 64: Presyncope, Syncope, and Shock

During morning rounds, a 19-year-old MBBS student experiences dizziness, excessive sweating, and briefly collapses while standing in the crowded ward. Friends panic, shouting for water. You notice her pale face and weak pulse. She regains consciousness within seconds but looks frightened. Everyone is confused. Was the 'blacking out' something more serious?

Introduction

Syncope is a sudden, temporary loss of consciousness caused by reduced blood flow to the brain, often preceded by presyncope (dizziness, blurred vision, sweating, nausea). While many cases are harmless (vasovagal faint), syncope can also indicate serious issues like arrhythmias, dehydration, or shock. In India, fainting in crowded or hot environments is common, but shock resulting from trauma, bleeding, or infection is a leading cause of preventable deaths. Recognizing and responding appropriately can save lives. (1)

Recognition

- **Presyncope:** Lightheadedness, sweating, nausea, tunnel-vision.
- **Syncope:** Brief loss of consciousness with spontaneous recovery.
- **Shock:** Rapid, weak pulse, clammy skin, low blood pressure, altered sensorium or persistent unresponsiveness.

Key difference: Syncope recovers quickly, while shock persists and worsens without intervention. (2)

First Aid Steps

- **Immediate positioning**: Lay the person flat on their back, elevate legs about 30 cm (Trendelenburg-like position) to improve blood flow to the brain, and loosen tight clothing.
- **Airway & Breathing**: Ensure the airway is open. If unresponsive and not breathing, start CPR.
- **Identify and treat triggers:** Vasovagal is often due to standing for long time, pain, fear, heat. Hypoglycemia is common in diabetes. Shock is commonly due to trauma, bleeding, severe infection, or dehydration.
- **Specific measures:** Syncope usually resolves in minutes. Reassure, offer oral fluids once awake. (3,4) Shock requires specific actions - control bleeding with direct pressure and dressings, keep the victim warm with a blanket, avoid giving food or drink if unconscious or surgery is anticipated, and urgent transfer.

- **Monitoring & Transfer:** Even after recovery, unexplained syncope, recurrent fainting, or shock warrants hospital assessment to find the underlying cause. (1,3)

What NOT to Do

- Do not make the patient sit upright or stand immediately after fainting.
- Do not splash water or slap repeatedly—focus on maintaining proper positioning and ensuring the airway is clear.
- Do not delay transfer in case of suspected shock.

Outcome

Most fainting episodes resolve with simple positioning and reassurance. Shock is a red flag that requires rapid intervention and hospital management (IV fluids, blood transfusion, antibiotics, surgery depending on cause). Delays can be fatal.

Learning Points

- Differentiate between benign fainting and serious shock.
- Position the patient flat and elevate their legs, then check the airway.
- In shock, stop the bleeding, keep warm, and transfer to the hospital immediately.
- Never ignore recurrent or unexplained syncope; seek medical evaluation.

☕ Coffee Moment

Later, the fainted student laughed shyly while sipping lime water in the hostel mess. "I felt everything closing in, like I was drifting away," she said. Her friends teased, "Funny how a simple act, lying you down and raising your legs, brought you back." The tea on the table tasted different that day. A quiet reminder that life sometimes hangs by posture, patience, and presence of mind.

References

1. Shen WK, Sheldon RS, Benditt DG, et al. 2017 ACC/AHA/HRS guideline for the evaluation and management of patients with syncope. Circulation. 2017;136(5):e60–122.
2. Singletary EM, Zideman DA, De Buck ED, et al. 2020 International Consensus on First Aid Science With Treatment Recommendations. Circulation. 2020;142(16_suppl_1):S284–S334.
3. Hewett Brumberg EK, Douma MJ, Alibertis K, Charlton NP, Goldman MP, Harper-Kirksey K, et al. 2024 American Heart Association and American Red Cross Guidelines for First Aid. Circulation. 2024;150:e519–e579.
4. Vincent JL, De Backer D. Circulatory shock. N Engl J Med. 2013;369(18):1726–34.

Chapter 65: Decreased Consciousness

A 50-year-old man suddenly slumps in his chair in the outpatient waiting area. He is breathing but unresponsive. Attendants shout for water and try to force it into his mouth. You rush in, realizing that if he aspirates, he may die. Within seconds, you must secure his airway and place him in the correct position.

Introduction

Decreased consciousness can result from metabolic, neurological, or systemic causes—such as hypoglycemia, seizures, stroke, infections, intoxication, or postictal states. Unlike trauma-related coma, these are non-traumatic but equally serious conditions. The first aid provider's priority is to secure the airway, ensure breathing, and maintain circulation while preventing aspiration or injury. Simply placing a patient in the recovery position can help prevent complications and provide time until definitive care is available. (1,2)

Recognition

- The victim is unresponsive to voice or pain.
- Breathing may be normal, shallow, or noisy (such as snoring or gurgling).
- Pulse is present, but the patient is not interacting.
- No signs of external trauma.
- **Key distinction:** Patient is alive but unable to protect their airway. (2,3)

First Aid Steps

1. Rapid Assessment (ABC): Check responsiveness by tapping and calling loudly. Assess airway, breathing (chest rise, 10 seconds), and circulation (pulse).

2. Place in Recovery Position: If breathing and pulse are present but unconscious: Gently roll the patient onto their side. Keep the lower arm extended, and flex the upper knee to stabilize. Tilt their head slightly back, keep their mouth open and face downward to allow secretions to drain. This prevents aspiration of saliva or vomitus.

3. Airway Care: Remove dentures or loose foreign bodies if visible. Do not attempt forceful clearance unless the obstruction is obvious.

4. Oxygen: Provide oxygen by mask if breathing is inadequate but present.

5. Monitor Vitals for Any Deterioration: If breathing stops → start CPR. If seizures occur → protect from injury, do not insert objects into the mouth.

6. Urgent transport for altered consciousness cases for hospital evaluation (glucose, stroke, intoxication, infection). Carry the patient in the lateral position. (2-4)

What NOT to Do

- Do not give oral fluids or food—there is a risk of aspiration.
- Do not shake the patient violently or slap them.
- Do not leave the patient supine and unattended.

Outcome

Proper positioning and airway protection often prevent aspiration pneumonia and hypoxic injury. Delay or improper handling (e.g., force-feeding liquids) can cause avoidable complications and death. Definitive treatment depends on the cause—IV dextrose for hypoglycemia, antiepileptics for seizures, antibiotics for meningitis, or advanced stroke care.

Learning Points

- The recovery position saves lives in unconscious but breathing patients.
- Protect the airway, monitor breathing, and transfer quickly.
- Never feed or force liquids into an unconscious patient.
- Altered consciousness is always a medical emergency.

☕ Coffee Moment

That evening, while sipping coffee in the canteen, the student recalled how everyone instinctively tried to pour water into the man's mouth. "We think helping means giving something," he reflected. His mentor replied, "Sometimes helping means withholding, a safe position, an open airway, and patience until the experts take over."

References

1. Nolan JP, Sandroni C, Bottiger BW, et al. European Resuscitation Council and European Society of Intensive Care Medicine Guidelines 2021: Post-resuscitation care. Resuscitation. 2021;161:220–69.
2. Singletary EM, Zideman DA, De Buck ED, et al. 2020 International Consensus on First Aid Science With Treatment Recommendations. Circulation. 2020;142(16_suppl_1):S284–S334.
3. Hewett Brumberg EK, Douma MJ, Alibertis K, Charlton NP, Goldman MP, Harper-Kirksey K, et al. 2024 American Heart Association and American Red Cross Guidelines for First Aid. Circulation. 2024;150:e519–e579.
4. Adams JG, Walls RM. Rosen's Emergency Medicine: Concepts and Clinical Practice. 9th ed. Philadelphia: Elsevier; 2018.
5. Wijdicks EFM. The diagnosis of stupor and coma. 4th ed. New York: Oxford University Press; 2014.

Chapter 66: Hypoglycemia

You are posted in the emergency OPD when a middle-aged diabetic man is rushed in by his colleagues. He had skipped lunch and, during a meeting, suddenly began sweating, trembling, and speaking incoherently before collapsing. He is barely conscious; his friends are trying to force water into his mouth. You have only minutes to prevent brain damage.

Introduction

Hypoglycemia is defined as blood glucose below 70 mg/dL. It may lead to seizures, coma, or death if not treated. It most commonly occurs in patients with diabetes using insulin or oral hypoglycemics, but it can also happen in children with infections, prolonged fasting, or metabolic disorders. Lack of awareness often results in harmful first aid practices such as force-feeding liquids to unconscious patients, which risks aspiration. Timely recognition and simple interventions can be life-saving. (1)

Recognition

Early (autonomic) symptoms include sweating, tremors, palpitations, hunger, irritability, and anxiety. Late (neuroglycopenic) symptoms are confusion, slurred speech, seizures, altered behaviour, drowsiness, and coma. Any diabetic with abnormal behaviour or loss of consciousness must be assumed hypoglycemic until proven otherwise. (2)

First Aid Steps

- **Check responsiveness, breathing, and pulse**: If the patient is unresponsive, not breathing, and has no pulse, initiate CPR.
- **If the patient is alert and can swallow:**
  Administer 15–20 g of fast-acting carbohydrate such as sugar solution, (3–4 level teaspoons of sugar dissolved in water).
  150–200 mL of fruit juice or regular (non-diet) soda.
  Glucose tablets: usually 4 tablets × 4 g (about 16 g).
  Glucose gel: 1 tube, approximately 15 g, rubbed on gums or inside cheeks if the patient can manage secretions.
- **If semi-conscious but able to cooperate**: Use buccal glucose or rub honey/glucose gel inside the cheek. Do not give large volumes orally.
- **If unconscious or unresponsive but breathing normally:** Do not attempt to feed orally, place in recovery position, and arrange rapid transfer to hospital for IV dextrose (25–50 mL of 50% dextrose) or IM/SC glucagon if available.
- **Recheck every 15 minutes:** If symptoms persist, repeat the oral glucose and test blood sugar. Once recovered, provide a carbohydrate-rich snack (such as

bread, fruit, or biscuits) to help prevent recurrence. (3-5)

What NOT to Do

- Do not force food or fluids into an unconscious patient (risk of aspiration).
- Do not delay transport if IV/IM therapy is needed.
- Do not assume recovery is permanent; rebound hypoglycemia may occur.

Outcome

With prompt first aid, hypoglycemia usually reverses without complications. Delay may cause seizures, irreversible brain injury, or death. Educating diabetic patients and their families about early warning signs and keeping glucose sources readily available can help prevent recurrence. (3–5)

Learning Points

- Hypoglycemia is a common and reversible emergency in diabetics.
- Oral glucose is safe only if the patient is conscious and can swallow.
- Never feed an unconscious patient; IV dextrose or glucagon is necessary.
- Education and preparedness (carrying glucose, snacks) are the best prevention.

☕ Coffee Moment

After the patient stabilized with IV dextrose, the student sat in the hospital canteen with her tea. "It looked so dramatic, sweating, shaking, then collapsing," she reflected, and all it took was sugar. Her mentor added, "That's hypoglycemia; big danger, simple remedy. If you remember it once, you'll never forget."

References

1. Nakhleh A, Shehadeh N. Hypoglycemia in diabetes: An update on pathophysiology, treatment, and prevention. World J Diabetes. 2021 Dec 15;12(12):2036-2049.
2. Singletary EM, Zideman DA, De Buck ED, et al. 2020 International Consensus on First Aid Science With Treatment Recommendations. Circulation. 2020;142(16_suppl_1):S284–S334.
3. ILCOR First Aid Task Force: Hypoglycaemia—methods and recommendations [Internet]. 2025 Mar 28. Available from: https://ilcor.org/
4. Kalra S, Mukherjee JJ, Venkataraman S, et al. Hypoglycemia: The neglected complication. Indian J Endocrinol Metab. 2013;17(5):819–34.
5. Hewett Brumberg EK, Douma MJ, Alibertis K, et al. 2024 American Heart Association and American Red Cross Guidelines for First Aid. Circulation. 2024;150:e519–e579.

Chapter 67: Snakebite and Stings

During your rural posting, a 15-year-old boy is rushed in by his parents after being bitten near the ankle while working in the paddy fields. The village crowd insists on tying a tight rope above the bite and cutting the wound to "suck out the poison." The boy is sweating and frightened. He looks at you and pleads, "Will I die?"

Introduction

Snakebite is a major health concern in India, causing many deaths, especially in rural areas. India has the highest snakebite deaths due to limited care access, reliance on traditional remedies, and antivenom delays. (1) First aid helps reduce complications and improve survival chances until proper treatment can be administered.

Snakebite

How to Identify

History and local symptoms like pain, swelling, bleeding, or fang marks.

Systemic features like ptosis, difficulty swallowing, respiratory distress (neurotoxic), bleeding gums, hematuria, shock (hemotoxic) and muscle pain, dark urine (myotoxic). Non-venomous bites have local pain/swelling without systemic toxicity.

First Aid Steps

Do it R.I.G.H.T

R – Reassure the patient

Most snakes are non-venomous. Even in cases of venomous bites, timely treatment can save lives. Calm the victim; panic increases heart rate and spreads venom faster.

I – Immobilize the limb

Splint the bitten limb, as in a fracture. The use of pressure immobilization bandaging can be potentially harmful. Keep it at the heart level. Immobilization slows systemic absorption.

GH – Get to the Hospital immediately

Shift the patient quickly but gently to the nearest medical facility. Only anti-snake venom (ASV) can neutralize venom. Do not waste time on traditional remedies. Ensure supportive care (airway, breathing, circulation, ventilatory support).

T – Tell the truth about harmful practices

Tell correctly about bite timing, swelling progression, and snake species if identified. Educate the community: no cutting, sucking, tying tourniquets, applying herbs, or giving alcohol.

What NOT to Do (Common Misconceptions)

- Do not apply a tight tourniquet (causes gangrene).
- Do not cut, suck, or apply herbal paste to the wound.
- Do not attempt to catch or kill the snake.
- Do not give alcohol or stimulants.

Outcome

With correct immobilization, reassurance, and rapid hospital transfer, most patients survive even serious bites. Delays, improper first aid, and harmful practices significantly increase morbidity and mortality. (5)

Learning Points

- Snakebite is a time-critical emergency; survival depends on immobilization and rapid hospital care.
- ASV is a definitive treatment.
- Avoid harmful practices (such as cutting, sucking, and tourniquet use) that are still prevalent in rural India.

Scorpion Sting

Scorpion stings inject neurotoxic venom through a curved telson at the tail's tip. Most cause local pain and swelling; a few species (e.g., Mesobuthus tamulus, the Indian red scorpion) can produce a life-threatening autonomic storm. Venom stimulates massive neurotransmitter release (acetylcholine and catecholamines), leading to hypertension, tachycardia, pulmonary edema, and cardiac failure. Children are more vulnerable due to their smaller body mass. (6)

Treatment Recommendations

- Ensure scene safety and reassure the patient to minimise the spread of venom, which increases with agitation.
- Clean the wound with soap and water; avoid incision, suction, or tourniquet.
- Apply lidocaine (if the skin is intact) or a cool compress with ice to reduce local pain and swelling.
- Over-the-counter acetaminophen and NSAID agents to alleviate local pain.
- Immobilize the affected limb below heart level to slow lymphatic spread.

- Monitor for systemic signs such as excessive salivation, sweating, vomiting, tachycardia, or breathlessness.
- If any systemic features develop, activate EMS immediately. Treatment includes IV fluids, prazosin, and specific antivenom, where available.
- Keep the person calm and continuously observe them during transport.

Jellyfish Sting

Jellyfish envenomation occurs when nematocysts (stinging cells) discharge venom into the skin, producing pain, redness, and sometimes systemic reactions such as muscle cramps or collapse. Different species release different toxins. Box-jellyfish (Chironex fleckeri) stings can be fatal; most coastal Indian species cause local injury. Freshwater or urine rinsing can trigger the discharge of more nematocysts. Only certain solutions inactivate stingers.

Treatment Recommendations

- Move the victim out of the water; reassure and restrict movement to slow the spread of venom.
- Remove any remaining tentacles by gently lifting or pulling them using gloves or tweezers, avoiding direct manual contact.
- Rinse the affected area with seawater (not freshwater) to remove the tentacle if mechanical removal is not possible.
- Apply vinegar (4–6 % acetic acid) for at least 30 seconds to inactivate undischarged nematocysts of Australian box jellyfish species.
- Immerse or apply hot water (≥ 45 °C) to the affected area for 20 minutes to relieve pain.
- Topical lidocaine (10%-15% or 4%–5%) inhibits nematocyst discharge or decreases pain from stings by the tentacles of multiple jellyfish species.
- Provide standard wound care. If systemic symptoms (chest pain, breathing difficulty, collapse) occur, activate EMS and treat according to the anaphylaxis protocol. (6)

Wasp and Bee Sting

Hymenoptera stings (wasps, bees, hornets) inject venom, causing localized pain, redness, and swelling. Occasionally, they can trigger systemic allergic or anaphylactic reactions. Bee stingers remain attached to the venom sac and continue to inject toxin, whereas wasps can sting repeatedly. Local reactions are typically due to histamine release; severe reactions involve IgE-mediated anaphylaxis, which can lead to airway and cardiovascular compromise. (6)

Treatment Recommendations

- Remove the stinger promptly by scraping sideways with a firm object (card, nail); do not squeeze.
- If a person experiences anaphylaxis due to a sting, they should self-administer an epinephrine autoinjector if available.
- If signs of anaphylaxis (wheezing, swelling of lips or tongue, dizziness) are present, administer IM epinephrine and activate EMS immediately. (6)
- Wash the area with soap and water and apply a cold compress for 10 minutes on and 10 minutes off to reduce pain and swelling.
- Elevate the affected limb and apply topical ice or cold packs.
- Use over-the-counter analgesic agents for pain, antihistamines or topical steroids for local itching.
- Multiple stings, particularly in children, require medical observation for systemic toxicity.
- Stings to the eye require immediate medical attention.

☕ Coffee Moment

Later that night at the rural health centre, the medical student said, "All I did was keep his leg still and reassure." Her mentor smiled: "Sometimes the simplest act of doing what matters makes the difference between life and death. The coffee felt grounding—like a quiet reminder of their profound responsibility.

References

1. World Health Organization. Snakebite envenoming: a strategy for prevention and control. Geneva: WHO; 2019.
2. Warrell DA. Snake bite. Lancet. 2010;375(9708):77–88.
3. Kasturiratne A, Wickremasinghe AR, de Silva N, et al. The global burden of snakebite: a literature analysis and modelling based on regional estimates of envenoming and deaths. PLoS Med. 2008;5(11):e218.
4. Kumar M, Tiwari L. Snake bite–a review. J Pediatr Crit Care. 2018;5(6):34–41. doi:10.21304/2018.0506.00442
5. Suraweera W, Selvaraj S, Jagadeeshan M, et al. Trends in snakebite deaths in India from 2000 to 2019. *eLife*. 2020;9:e54076.
6. Hewett Brumberg EK, Douma MJ, Alibertis K, Charlton NP, Goldman MP, Harper-Kirksey K, et al. 2024 American Heart Association and American Red Cross Guidelines for First Aid. Circulation. 2024;150:e519–e579.

Chapter 68: Common Poisonings

During your rural posting, a farmer is brought to the health sub-centre after ingesting pesticide during a family dispute. He is sweating, drooling, and struggling to catch his breath. Family members beg you to give him milk and salt water to vomit out the poison. You recall your first aid training: the wrong step here could kill him.

Introduction

Poisoning is a leading cause of illness and death in India, especially in rural areas. Common causes include organophosphate insecticides, kerosene ingestion in children, plant toxins (castor beans, oleander), alcohol intoxication, and household cleaners. Most fatalities result not from a lack of antidotes but from delayed treatment, harmful traditional practices, and aspiration during forced vomiting. The role of the first aid provider is to stabilize the patient, prevent further absorption, and ensure prompt transfer to the hospital. (1,2). For quick telephonic assistance, one can contact the National Poison Centre, AIIMS Delhi, at the Toll-Free Number.-1800116117. Tel No.-011-26589391, 011-26593677.
E-mail: npicaiims2010@gmail.com.

Recognition (Common Signs)

- **Organophosphates (pesticides):** Excessive salivation, sweating, pinpoint pupils, muscle twitching, breathing difficulty ("SLUDGE" syndrome: Salivation, Lacrimation, Urination, Defecation, GI upset, Emesis).
- **Opioid Poisoning:** Coma, pinpoint pupils, and respiratory depression (triad). Other features - bradycardia, hypotension, hypothermia, decreased bowel sounds, pulmonary edema, cyanosis, and cardiac arrest due to hypoxia.
- **Kerosene/volatile hydrocarbons:** Cough, choking, breathlessness, chemical pneumonia.
- **Plant toxins:** Nausea, vomiting, irregular heartbeat (cardiac arrhythmias).
- **Alcohol intoxicationn:** Slurred speech, incoordination, vomiting, coma.
- **Household cleaners (acids, alkalis, bleach):** Mouth burns, drooling, difficulty swallowing, abdominal pain. (2,3)

First Aid Steps

Ensure rescuer safety

Wear gloves/mask if available. Avoid exposure to fumes or vomit. (4)

Airway, Breathing, Circulation (ABC)

Assess responsiveness, pulse, and breathing. If absent → start CPR. Use a barrier device for rescue breaths if needed; avoid unprotected mouth-to-mouth.

Do NOT induce vomiting in specific poisonings

Especially risky with kerosene or corrosive substances (danger of aspiration and additional injury). If ingested, avoid neutralizing with opposite chemicals (e.g., acid vs alkali).

Supportive measures

If conscious and able to swallow, give sips of clean water or milk for corrosives to dilute, but only if no airway compromise. Keep the patient in the recovery position if unconscious but breathing.

Hospital transfer

Crucial for additional treatment and antidotes such as atropine and pralidoxime in organophosphorus poisoning, antiarrhythmics in oleander poisoning, ventilatory support for kerosene-related lung injury, and gastric lavage or activated charcoal in various other cases. Carry the container or label of the ingested substance for identification. (2,4) Your priority is decontamination, supporting ABC, and rapid transport. Early, thorough decontamination reduces absorbed dose and protects healthcare workers and bystanders.

Critical Skills and Specific Treatment

Organophosphate exposures

Decontamination: Remove the patient from the exposure area by moving them to fresh air. In cases of liquid or skin contact, carefully remove contaminated clothing (cut it off rather than pulling it over the head), place the clothing in double plastic bags, and wash the affected skin and hair thoroughly with plenty of water (preferably with soap) for at least 10–15 minutes. Be sure to prevent contamination of yourself and the surroundings by directing runoff away from others. For eye contact, rinse with clean water or saline for 15 minutes. If inhaled, ensure the patient moves to fresh air and loosen restrictive clothing. (4,5)

Opioid poisoning

Prompt airway management and assisted ventilation. Inj naloxone (antidote) intravenously (0.1 mg/kg, max 2 mg), repeated every 2–3 minutes until spontaneous breathing resumes. Continuous infusion may be required. Oxygen, intravenous fluids, and monitoring for recurrence of respiratory depression. In suspected heroin or fentanyl overdose, early naloxone administration can be lifesaving and should not be delayed for laboratory confirmation. Prioritize airway/ventilation and CPR; administer naloxone without delaying CPR. (4, 6)

What NOT to Do

- Do not give salt water, mustard water, or raw eggs.
- Do not attempt home remedies or delay referral.
- Do not force liquids into an unconscious patient.

Outcome

Survival depends on the rapid recognition, airway support, and timely administration of antidotes. Harmful interventions at the community level, such as forceful vomiting and delay in referral, remain a major cause of preventable deaths.

Emergency Room Management

1. Airway & Breathing: Oxygen, suctioning secretions, intubation and ventilation for respiratory failure.

2. Decontamination: Skin wash, gastric lavage with activated charcoal, as ingestion was recent.

3. Antidotes: Excess secretions, pinpoint pupils, wheeze, and bradycardia suggest cholinergic toxicity. Atropine and Pralidoxime are antidotes

Atropine - 1.8–3 mg IV, repeated every 5–10 min, till secretions controlled and heart rate was >80 (Children: 0.05 mg/kg IV). Maintenance infusion is often required.

Pralidoxime (2-PAM): 30 mg/kg (1–2 g) IV over 30 min, repeat in 12 hrs or continuous infusion (children: 20–50 mg/kg IV).

4. Supportive Care: IV fluids for hypotension, seizure control, and bronchodilators.

5. Monitoring: Continuous ECG, SpO_2 for stabilisation and identify Intermediate Syndrome (respiratory muscle weakness at 24–96 hrs) and Delayed Neuropathy (weeks later). (1,3)

Learning Points

- Do not induce vomiting; seek immediate medical attention so that gastric lavage can be performed for certain poisonings.
- Prioritize airway, breathing, and safe transport to the hospital.
- Carry the sample and its container, along with the label, for diagnosis.
- Awareness is essential: most poisonings can be prevented through safe storage and community education.

☕ Coffee Moment

Later, at the health centre canteen, the student stared into his chai, recalling the farmer's glassy eyes. Everyone thought induced vomiting would save him. The senior replied, First aid is not about doing more, but doing the right thing. Sometimes, restraint is the real intervention. The tea felt heavy, flavoured with the quiet responsibility of holding back harmful hands.

References

1. Eddleston M, Buckley NA, Eyer P, Dawson AH. Management of acute organophosphorus pesticide poisoning. Lancet. 2008;371(9612):597–607.
2. Singletary EM, Zideman DA, De Buck ED, et al. 2020 International Consensus on First Aid Science With Treatment Recommendations. Circulation. 2020;142(16_suppl_1):S284–S334.
3. Srivastava A, Peshin SS. An epidemiological study of poisoning cases reported to the National Poisons Information Centre, All India Institute of Medical Sciences, New Delhi. Hum Exp Toxicol. 2005;24(6):279–85.
4. Hewett Brumberg EK, Douma MJ, Alibertis K, Charlton NP, Goldman MP, Harper-Kirksey K, et al. 2024 American Heart Association and American Red Cross Guidelines for First Aid. Circulation. 2024;150:e519–e579.
5. World Health Organization. Clinical management of acute pesticide intoxication: prevention of suicidal behaviours [Internet]. Geneva: WHO; 2008 [cited 2025 Sep 1]. Available from: https://apps.who.int/iris/handle/10665/44020
6. Cao D, Arens AM, Chow SL, Easter SR, Hoffman RS, Lagina AT III, et al. Part 10: adult and pediatric special circumstances of resuscitation: 2025 American Heart Association Guidelines for Cardiopulmonary Resuscitation and Emergency Cardiovascular Care. Circulation. 2025;152(suppl 2):S578–S672.

Chapter 69: The First Look That Saves a Child

Introduction

Sometimes, all it takes is a trained eye, a calm heart, and a moment of mindful observation to change the course of a life.

When a child arrives at the emergency room breathless, pale, in their caregiver's arms, what is the first thing a doctor does?

Do we rush for tests, wait for vitals or begin treatment based on a possible diagnosis?

The art and science of evaluating a critically ill child begins with a vigilant gaze and a structured method. It is known as the Pediatric Assessment Triangle, followed by primary assessment, secondary assessment, and, if necessary, diagnostic testing. After each evaluation stage, we identify the problem in the pathophysiological state and intervene to prevent its progression. This cycle is known as the **Evaluate–Identify–Intervene (EII)** cycle. You will learn about making pathophysiological diagnoses and implementing life-saving interventions during your pediatric postings in the MBBS program.

This chapter explores the journey of clinical reasoning, the process that can help you save lives confidently.

1. The Pediatric Assessment Triangle (PAT)

The PAT is your first impression, a quick visual and auditory scan that takes only a few seconds. No equipment is needed. Only your eyes, ears, and awareness. PAT includes three vital aspects.

Appearance: Is the child alert, crying, responsive, and interacting or listless, floppy, and vacant?

Work of Breathing: Are they breathing comfortably or with effort? Look for flaring nostrils, grunting, and chest retractions.

Circulation to the Skin: Is the skin pink and warm or pale, mottled, blue? Any signs of poor perfusion?

Why it matters: PAT doesn't provide a diagnosis. It offers insight into the severity of the child's condition and which system - respiratory, circulatory, or neurological - may be affected. It helps prioritize your next steps quickly.

Like a mother's glance that instantly knows something is wrong, PAT is your intuitive, trained response.

2. The Primary Assessment: A–B–C–D–E

Once you **identify** through PAT that the child is unwell, you must act quickly with life-saving interventions such as providing oxygen, connecting to monitors for further assessment, and alerting your team, including nursing officers, interns, and resident doctors, for possible assistance. In case the child is unresponsive with no signs of life, assume that child is in cardiac arrest, and you must immediately activate code blue and start CPR. (1)

If CPR is not indicated, we move in close to evaluate further, identify the problem, and quickly intervene to stabilise. This is the primary assessment, focusing on life-threatening problems.

A –Airway: Is the airway open and protected?

B –Breathing: Rate, effort, chest rise, breath sounds and O_2 saturation (SpO2).

C –Circulation: Heart rate, pulse, perfusion, skin temperature, and blood pressure.

D –Disability: Level of consciousness, AVPU scale, pupils.

E –Exposure: Temperature, rashes, trauma, hidden clues.

This step is dynamic; you identify the problem and intervene with corrective actions. This could include opening the airway, administering oxygen, controlling bleeding, inserting intravenous cannulas for fluid resuscitation, etc. This is not just a clinical examination; it is a rescue in real time. (1,2)

3. The Secondary Assessment: Filling in the Story

Once the child is stable or being stabilized, we dive deeper with a focused history and head-to-toe examination. The mnemonic **SAMPLE** helps:

S – Signs & Symptoms

A – Allergies

M – Medications

P – Past medical history

L – Last meal or intake

E – Events leading up to illness or injury

Here, you're building trust, listening to caregivers, and gently uncovering what brought the child to this point. You also examine the child systematically — from head to toe — picking up subtle signs that may hold big clues. “This is where the child is no longer a case, but a story you begin to understand.” (2-5)

Approach to A Sick Child

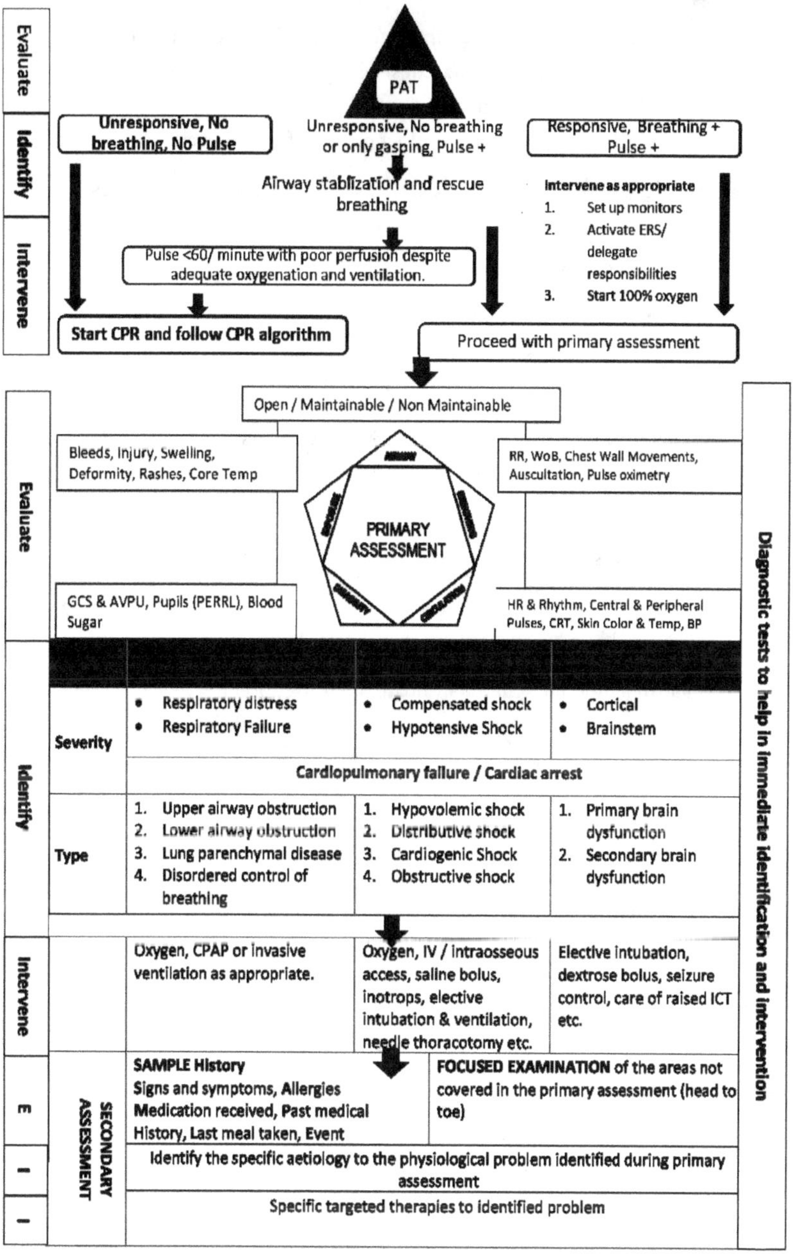

Figure 69.1: Approach to a Sick Child

4. Diagnostic Testing: To Support, Not to Replace

While your evaluation, identification, and intervention are underway, you also decide what tests are needed. Whether it's a chest X-ray, a blood gas, or a CT scan, tests must be chosen purposefully, guided by your clinical suspicion. A test cannot replace a missed airway. A lab report cannot undo a delay in fluid resuscitation.

Thus, diagnostics are partners, not leaders, in your decision-making process.

☕ Coffee Moment

You walk into the emergency room and see a child in distress. You observe the triangle: he is pale, grunting, and limp. You quickly support his airway, call for help, start oxygen, connect monitors, and check the pulse.

Within seconds, you've begun saving a life. Such moments, when all your training comes into action, will keep coming to you. It starts with respecting the process: from PAT, to Primary, to Secondary, and then testing.

"Every child deserves a doctor who sees beyond symptoms, who listens, watches, and acts with wisdom and heart."

As you move ahead in your medical journey, let this sequence be your guide:

Evaluate, identify, intervene, then reevaluate, identify, and intervene again until your patient is stabilized. Master this rhythm — it will stay with you across wards, emergencies, and even in the quiet hours when no one else knows what to do.

It is not just how we assess.
It is how we care.

Reference

1. Taneja LN, Tiwari L. BLS for professionals. Third Edition 2018.
2. Pediatric Advanced Life Support Provider Manual, New 2015 American Heart Guidelines, Pg. 29-67.
3. Hazinski MF. Children are different. In: Hazinski MF, ed. Nursing care of critically ill child. 3rd ed. St Louis, MO: Mosby; 2013:1-18
4. Rogers' Handbook of Pediatric Intensive Care, Fifth Edition 2017, pg. 217-272.
5. WHO. Emergency Triage Assessment and Treatment (ETAT). Geneva: World Health Organisation;2005

Chapter 70: Childhood Diarrhoea and Pneumonia

At a rural health camp, a mother rushes in with her 2-year-old son. He has been passing watery stools since morning and now appears lethargic, with sunken eyes and dry lips. Another mother nearby seeks help for her 4-year-old girl, who is coughing severely, breathing rapidly, and making grunting noises. Both children are in danger unless simple lifesaving measures are taken immediately.

Introduction

Diarrhoea and pneumonia are the two leading causes of under-five mortality globally, particularly in low- and middle-income countries like India. Together, they account for nearly one-third of all preventable childhood deaths. (1,2)

Recognition

Diarrhoea: Frequent loose/watery stools. Signs of dehydration: sunken eyes, dry mouth, lethargy, poor skin turgor, excessive thirst, or inability to drink. Rapid loss of fluids and electrolytes → dehydration, shock, and death.

Pneumonia: Lung infection causing hypoxia, respiratory distress, and sepsis. Child presents with cough and/or fever and fast breathing [>50 breaths/min (2–12 months), >40/min (1–5 years)]. Chest indrawing, grunting, inability to feed, and bluish lips are danger signs.

First Aid Steps

Critical Skill For Diarrhoea

- Rehydration saves lives. Use WHO low-osmolarity ORS: mix the entire sachet in 1 L of water, stir until dissolved, and discard any leftovers after 24 hours.
- If ORS is not available, prepare home solution with 6 level teaspoons of sugar plus ½ level teaspoon of salt in 1 L of water. Switch to ORS as soon as possible. Continue breastfeeding and usual foods with small, frequent sips after each stool.
- Administer approximately 75 mL/kg over 4 hours, then reassess. Additionally, administer 10 mL/kg after each stool to replace ongoing losses.
- Watch for danger signs such as lethargy, persistent vomiting, blood in stool, extreme thirst or inability to drink, sunken eyes, or fever - refer immediately.
- Add zinc for 10–14 days to lower duration and recurrence risk: 10 mg/day for infants under 6 months, 20 mg/day for those 6 months or older.
- Teach to prepare ORS correctly (incorrect concentration can cause harm), to use clean cups/spoons, and to seek care if intake is poor or symptoms worsen.

Critical Skill For Pneumonia

- Keep airway clear, position upright and provide oxygen support.
- Paracetamol for fever and comfort.
- Antibiotic: Amoxicillin 40 mg/kg orally first dose (max single dose: 1 g).
- If unable to take orally (severe disease/danger signs): Ampicillin 50 mg/kg IM/IV plus Gentamicin 7.5 mg/kg IM/IV.
- Alternative: Cotrimoxazole 4 mg/kg (trimethoprim component) orally.
- Refer the child urgently for hospital care if they exhibit any signs of danger.

What NOT to Do

- Do not stop feeding during diarrhoea and do not give anti-diarrhoeal drugs.
- Do not ignore fast breathing or chest indrawing, as it may indicate pneumonia.

Outcome

Most diarrhoeal deaths are preventable with timely ORS, zinc, breastfeeding, and early referral. It has significantly reduced child mortality as the most effective first-line treatment. (4,5) Pneumonia outcomes improve with early recognition and the administration of antibiotics.

Learning Points

- ORS + zinc saves lives in diarrhoea. Danger signs demand urgent referral.
- Pneumonia must be suspected in every child with a cough and fast breathing.

☕ Coffee Moment

Student shared coffee with her mentor: "It felt so simple—sugar, salt, water, and a mother's reassurance. Yet, it saved a life today." The mentor smiled: "Sometimes the smallest packets of care—ORS and oxygen—are the biggest miracles in child health."

References

1. WHO. Pocket Book of Hospital Care for Children. 2nd ed. Geneva: World Health Organization; 2013.
2. UNICEF/WHO. Diarrhoea: Why children are still dying and what can be done. Geneva: WHO; 2009.
3. United Nations Inter-agency Group for Child Mortality Estimation. Levels & Trends in Child Mortality: 2022 Report. New York: UNICEF; 2022.
4. World Health Organization. Diarrhoeal disease—fact sheet [Internet]. 2024 Mar 7 [cited 2025 Sep 1].
5. World Health Organization. Zinc supplementation in the management of diarrhoea (WHO eLENA) [Internet]. 2023 Aug 9 [cited 2025 Sep 1].

Chapter 71: Status Asthmaticus & Respiratory Distress

It is a humid evening on a playground when a 14-year-old boy with a history of asthma suddenly starts wheezing loudly and clutching his chest. His inhaler is empty. Within minutes, he is gasping, unable to speak full sentences, lips turning bluish. Friends rush to you, shouting, "He's choking!" You realize this is not a foreign body or simple asthma attack but a life-threatening status asthmaticus.

Introduction

Status asthmaticus is a severe, sustained asthma attack that does not respond to the usual doses of inhaled bronchodilators. It can rapidly progress to respiratory failure and cardiac arrest. Acute respiratory distress may also occur in other conditions - severe allergic reactions, pneumonia, trauma, or inhalational injuries. Poor access to inhalers, delayed recognition, and reliance on home remedies often worsen outcomes. First aid is crucial to support breathing until hospital care is available. (1)

Recognition

Acute Severe Asthma: Wheezing, cough, chest tightness, difficulty speaking full sentences, use of accessory muscles and flaring nostrils.
Impending respiratory failure (red flags): Severe breathlessness, exhaustion, silent chest (no breath sounds despite effort), cyanosis (bluish lips/nails), altered sensorium, tachycardia or bradycardia.
Key Point: If the patient cannot complete a sentence or is unable to lie down due to breathlessness → consider it an emergency. (2)

First Aid Steps

1. **Call for help immediately**: Prepare for urgent transfer to the hospital.

2. **Positioning**: Make the patient sit upright, leaning slightly forward (like tripod).

3. **Reliever medication (if available)**: Assist the patient in using a short-acting beta-agonist (SABA) inhaler (salbutamol), and use a spacer if possible. If no spacer is available, improvised options, such as a plastic bottle spacer, can help. If a nebuliser is available, administer salbutamol with oxygen flow. (3, 4)

4. **Oxygen (if available)**: Administer high-flow oxygen to maintain SpO_2 >94%.

5. **Monitor airway and circulation**: Be prepared to initiate CPR if the patient becomes unresponsive and pulseless. (3, 4)

6. **Avoid triggers and exertion:** Remove the patient from smoke, dust, or allergens if present, do not allow lying flat; maintain an upright position. Suspect complications

early; ventilate with low RR/VT to avoid air trapping; ECMO if refractory. (3)

What NOT to Do

Do not force the patient to lie down.
Do not delay hospital transfer, waiting for complete relief with inhalers.
Do not give sedatives; they can worsen respiratory depression.

Outcome

With early recognition, inhaler support, and oxygen, patients may stabilize until they can be transferred to the hospital. Delays can lead to respiratory arrest, requiring intubation and ventilatory support. Education on asthma action plans, inhaler technique, and availability of reliever medication are essential for long-term prevention. (4)

Learning Points

Severe asthma attack with inability to speak or "silent chest" = emergency.
Sit upright, support breathing, administer reliever medication if available.
Oxygen and urgent transfer to hospital are vital.
Never underestimate an attack; status asthmaticus kills silently and quickly.

☕ Coffee Moment

After the boy was stabilized in the emergency ward, the student's heart was still pounding while sipping coffee. "I kept thinking, what if the inhaler had worked, what if we had wasted time?" he murmured. His senior replied, "Asthma doesn't give many chances. You did what actually mattered, acted quickly and moved him to care."

References

1. Global Initiative for Asthma (GINA). Global strategy for asthma management and prevention, 2023 update. Available at: https://ginasthma.org
2. Singletary EM, Zideman DA, De Buck ED, et al. 2020 International Consensus on First Aid Science With Treatment Recommendations. Circulation. 2020;142(16_suppl_1):S284–S334.
3. Cao D, Arens AM, Chow SL, et al. Part 10: adult and pediatric special circumstances of resuscitation: 2025 American Heart Association Guidelines for Cardiopulmonary Resuscitation and Emergency Cardiovascular Care. Circulation. 2025;152(suppl 2):S578–S672.
4. Hewett Brumberg EK, Douma MJ, Alibertis K, Charlton NP, Goldman MP, Harper-Kirksey K, et al. 2024 American Heart Association and American Red Cross Guidelines for First Aid. Circulation. 2024;150:e519–e579.

Chapter 72: Seizures and Status Epilepticus

You are organizing a CPR training session for school children. Walking through the school corridor, a 10th-grade student suddenly falls to the ground, stiffens, and begins to jerk violently. His classmates scream; one tries to hold his arms, and another attempts to pour water into his mouth. You recall your training: seconds matter, and the wrong move can be fatal.

Introduction

Seizures are episodes of abnormal electrical activity in the brain, presenting as convulsions, altered awareness, or unusual behaviours. Status epilepticus is a seizure lasting more than 5 minutes or repeated seizures without recovery in between. Seizures are often mismanaged due to myths: attempts to force objects into the mouth, restrain the patient, or apply traditional remedies. Proper first aid can prevent aspiration, trauma, and progression to status epilepticus and death. (1)

Recognition

- **Generalised tonic-clonic seizure**: loss of consciousness, stiffening, jerking movements, frothing, tongue biting.
- **Partial seizures**: twitching, altered awareness, staring spells.
- **Status epilepticus**: continuous seizure >5 min or ≥2 seizures without recovery.
- **Febrile seizures:** convulsions that occur during fever in children aged 6 months to 5 years, lasting less than 15 minutes, and the child recovers quickly. Febrile seizures are usually self-limiting, but can conceal serious infections. (2, 3)
- **Sepsis warning signs:** lethargy, poor feeding, persistent vomiting, stiff neck, cold extremities, rapid breathing, altered consciousness. (3,4)

First Aid Steps

1. Ensure safety: Clear the area of sharp objects and furniture, and cushion the head.
2. Protect the airway: Do not put anything in the mouth, such as spoons, keys, or fingers. Keep the patient in the recovery position as soon as the jerks stop to allow saliva or vomit to drain. (2,3)
3. Do not restrain movements: Restraining can cause injury. (3)
4. Time the seizure: Most seizures last 1–3 minutes. If it exceeds 5 minutes, treat it as status epilepticus-call for emergency help immediately.
5. After seizure (post-ictal phase): The patient may be drowsy, confused, or sleepy. Reassure them and allow rest. Monitor airway, breathing, and pulse.
6. Hospital transfer when needed: first seizure, prolonged (>5 min), recurrent seizures, breathing difficulty, injury, or poisoning suspicion → urgent transfer. (4)

What NOT to Do

- Do not force-feed water, milk, or medicines during a seizure.
- Do not put any objects in the mouth.
- Do not delay referral if red flags are present.

Outcome

Most seizures resolve spontaneously without harm if the airway is protected and the patient is not restrained. Delay in recognizing status epilepticus or improper practices, such as forcing objects or liquids, can lead to hypoxia, trauma, and death. In hospitals, treatment includes IV benzodiazepines, antiepileptic drugs, and supportive care.

Learning Points

- Seizures are typically self-limiting; first aid helps prevent complications.
- Airway safety and side positioning are key interventions.
- Status epilepticus lasting over 5 minutes is a life-threatening emergency.
- Avoid practices based on myths and misconceptions that can cause harm.

☕ Coffee Moment

With a cup of tea, a medical student replayed the scene he witnessed when some villagers brought a seizing child to CHC. The jerks, the fear, the crowd shouting advice. "I did nothing fancy; cushioned his head, rolled him on his side and waited while the specialist medical officer loaded some injections," he thought. Professor smiled: "That's first aid. Sometimes saving a life means knowing what not to do."

References

1. Fisher RS, Acevedo C, Arzimanoglou A, et al. ILAE official report: A practical clinical definition of epilepsy. Epilepsia. 2014;55(4):475–82.
2. Singletary EM, Zideman DA, De Buck ED, et al. 2020 International Consensus on First Aid Science With Treatment Recommendations. Circulation. 2020;142(16_suppl_1):S284–S334.
3. Hewett Brumberg EK, Douma MJ, Alibertis K, et al. 2024 American Heart Association and American Red Cross Guidelines for First Aid. Circulation. 2024;150:e519–e579.
4. WHO. Pocket Book of Hospital Care for Children. 2nd ed. Geneva: WHO; 2013.

Impact

Traumatic Emergencies

Impact is the sudden collision between health and harm; the motorbike skid, the fall from scaffolding, the stray cricket ball, the collapsing roof. It is uninvited, abrupt, and often merciless.

For doctors, it is the moment when chaos demands clarity, and fear demands skill.

In this section, you will step into the frontline of trauma care. You will learn how to stop the bleeding, protect the brain, stabilise the spine, preserve a limb, and safeguard vision or a smile. The goal is not just to know the steps, but also to have the ability to act swiftly in the midst of a storm when every minute matters.

First aid begins with steady hands, a clear head, and the courage to act.

S No.	Impact: At a Glance
1.	**Chapter 73** Trauma Resuscitation and Life-Threatening Bleeding First aid in trauma and uncontrolled haemorrhage: WHO algorithm for trauma resuscitation, direct pressure, tourniquets, wound packing: how minutes decide survival.
2.	**Chapter 74** Head Injuries From concussions on the field to life-threatening brain trauma: spotting red flags and protecting the brain.
3.	**Chapter 75** Spinal Injuries Immobilization and careful handling that prevent paralysis when every movement matters.
4.	**Chapter 76** Musculoskeletal Injuries, Fractures & Dislocations Sprains, fractures, dislocations: learning immobilization and avoiding harmful “traditional” practices.
5.	**Chapter 77** Crush Injuries Hidden dangers after rescue: crush syndrome, toxins, and the importance of fluids and careful release.
6.	**Chapter 78** Eye Injuries Chemical burns, blunt trauma, penetrating injuries: preserving sight when seconds matter.
7.	**Chapter 79** Dental Emergencies Avulsed and fractured teeth: saving smiles with correct first aid and timely referral.

Chapter 73: Trauma Resuscitation and Bleeding Control

Introduction

Trauma is one of the leading causes of preventable deaths, particularly in young adults. Road crashes, falls, burns, and violence claim lives not because care is impossible to save, but because the right care is delayed. The World Health Organization (WHO) provides a structured Trauma Algorithm to guide first responders and clinicians in providing immediate, organized care that stabilizes patients and prepares them for definitive treatment. To help you apply it in practice, we use the same 4Rs framework -Recognize, Resuscitate, Review, Refer with the ABCDE sequence embedded in resuscitation. (1-3)

1. Recognize: Spot and Prepare

Scene Safety: Ensure the environment is safe from fire, traffic, or violence.

Universal Precautions: Use gloves, mask, and eye protection.

Quick Scan: Identify obvious injuries and rapidly assess for life threats.

Begin ABCDE: Immediately start structured assessment of Airway, Breathing, Circulation, Disability, and Exposure. (1,2)

Example: At a roadside accident, you recognize that a patient is bleeding heavily and gasping, which signals the need for immediate life-saving action.

2. Resuscitate: Stabilize Life-Threatening Injuries (ABCDE)

A. Airway with Cervical Spine Protection

Assume every trauma patient has a cervical spine injury until proven otherwise.
Open airway using 'jaw thrust', not head tilt–chin lift.
Suction blood or secretions. Insert an oropharyngeal/nasopharyngeal airway if needed.
Consider an advanced airway management if obstruction persists.

B. Breathing

Expose the chest and look for asymmetry, wounds, or paradoxical movement.
Treat immediate killers:

Tension pneumothorax → needle decompression, chest tube.

Open pneumothorax → occlusive dressing.

Massive hemothorax → chest tube, fluids, urgent surgery referral.

Give high-flow oxygen to all trauma patients.

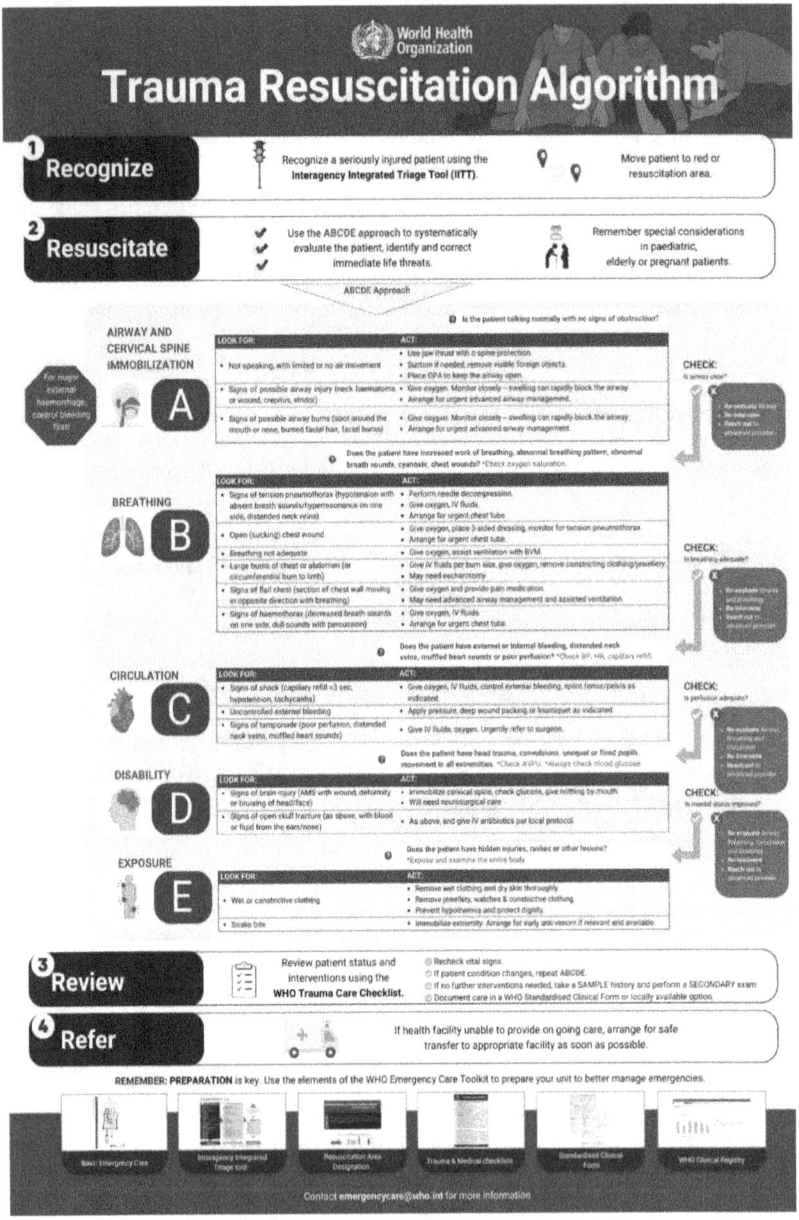

Figure 73.1: Trauma Resuscitation Algorithm

(Used with permission from WHO)

C. Circulation with Haemorrhage Control

Control external bleeding with direct pressure, pressure dressings, or a tourniquet.
Assess pulse, BP, and skin perfusion.
Initiate IV/IO access and administer fluids for shock, preferably warmed crystalloids.
Look for hidden bleeding: chest, abdomen, pelvis, long bones.

D. Disability (Neurological Status)

Rapid check using AVPU (Alert, Voice, Pain, Unresponsive).
Assess pupils for size and reactivity.
Consider reversible causes like hypoglycemia or hypoxia.

E. Exposure and Environment

Fully expose the patient to detect hidden injuries.
Prevent hypothermia by using warm blankets, warmed IV fluids, and maintaining a controlled environment.
Principle: Treat first what kills first. Never move to the next step without addressing immediate threats.

3. Review: Reassess and Monitor

Repeat the ABCDE assessment after every intervention.
Monitor vitals, level of consciousness, and response to treatment.
Document all findings and interventions clearly.
Anticipate deterioration: airway collapse, re-bleeding, or shock.

4. Refer: Definitive Care and Handover

Arrange safe transfer to a trauma-capable facility.
Maintain spinal precautions and bleeding control during transport.
Use structured handover (SBAR: Situation, Background, Assessment, Recommendation).
Provide details of injuries, interventions given, and the patient's response.

Case Snapshot: Motorcycle Crash

A 19-year-old motorcyclist is brought in after colliding with a truck.

Recognize: He is unresponsive with a visible chest injury and bleeding leg wound.

Resuscitate: Airway secured with jaw thrust, cervical spine immobilized; tension pneumothorax decompressed; bleeding leg controlled with tourniquet; fluids started.

Review: Repeat ABCDE, monitor vital signs, and stabilize with oxygen and splinting.

Refer: Transferred urgently with spinal precautions to a tertiary trauma centre.

Outcome: Early recognition and structured resuscitation stabilized the patient, enabling definitive surgery.

Learning Points

Trauma resuscitation follows the 4Rs: Recognize, Resuscitate, Review, Refer.
ABCDE is the backbone of resuscitation.
Cervical spine protection and bleeding control are trauma-specific priorities.
Hypothermia prevention is a key part of trauma care.
Clear communication and structured referral save lives as much as interventions.

☕ Coffee Moment

After a trauma shift, you may recall the blood, the chaos, the adrenaline. But think of the patient who was left alive because you kept your order when the world around you was in disorder. That's the silent pride of trauma care, calm minds saving broken bodies.

Bleeding Control in RTA

You're at a bus stop when a young man falls from a motorbike. Blood spurts from a deep thigh wound, quickly soaking his jeans. Onlookers panic, pressing handkerchiefs weakly on the wound. You remember: uncontrolled bleeding can kill within minutes; this is the moment to act.

Introduction

Severe bleeding is one of the leading preventable causes of trauma deaths. Life-threatening haemorrhage may occur from road accidents, industrial injuries, assaults, or disasters. First aid aims to stop bleeding, maintain circulation, and buy time until surgical care is available. (5-8)

Recognition

Spurting or pooling of blood (especially arterial).
Soaking through clothes rapidly.
Pale, clammy skin, weak rapid pulse.
Confusion, collapse → signs of shock.

First Aid Steps

Critical Skill: Bleeding Control

Why it matters: Severe external bleeding after an RTA can be fatal within minutes.

Your task is to identify the haemorrhage, stop it quickly, and transport the patient to care. (5-8)

Recognize Life-threatening Bleeding: Look for spurting or pooling blood, clothing or dressings rapidly soaked through, partial or complete amputation, or deep wounds in the groin, axilla, neck, or other junctional sites. Expose quickly but preserve privacy and warmth. If safe, activate 112 and enlist lay rescuers. Use gloves or a clean barrier if available. (5-7)

Step 1 - Apply Direct Pressure (the first and most crucial step): Place a clean cloth or gauze directly on the wound and press firmly with both hands. Maintain steady pressure for several minutes without "peeking." If bleeding slows, secure a pressure bandage to free your hands; if blood soaks through, add more layers without removing the initial layer. (8)

Step 2 - Wound Packing for Deep or Junctional Wounds: If the wound is deep and located in the groin, axilla, or neck (areas where tourniquets cannot be applied), pack it tightly with gauze (hemostatic gauze, if available) until the cavity is filled, then apply firm pressure. Packing combined with pressure enhances control when bandaging alone is insufficient. (4,6)

Step 3 - Tourniquet for life-threatening limb bleeding: If heavy limb bleeding continues despite direct pressure or multiple wounds prevent sustained pressure, apply a commercial windlass tourniquet 5–7 cm above the wound (not over a joint). Tighten it until bleeding stops and note the time. Do not remove or periodically loosen it. Improvised tourniquets with a width of≥ 2 inches are reasonable if no commercial device is not available. (8)

Step 4 - Hemostatic Agents (if available): If bleeding persists or pressure is impractical, hemostatic dressings, combined with pressure, improve the time to control bleeding compared to pressure alone. (8)

Step 5 - Position & Support: Lay the patient flat, elevate legs if no fracture suspected. Keep warm with a blanket and monitor responsiveness and breathing.

Step 6 - Urgent Transfer: All cases require surgical evaluation; time is critical.

What NOT to Do

Do not remove soaked dressings or impaled objects; blindly clamp vessels; apply powders.

Do not apply a tourniquet loosely (it may increase bleeding) or use tight circumferential dressings that occlude venous return only.

Do not waste time looking for perfect materials; use what's available.

Outcome

Early bleeding control significantly improves survival. Improvised tourniquets and continuous direct pressure can save lives, especially in prehospital environments. Definitive care involves surgical repair, blood transfusion, and intensive monitoring.

Learning Points

Severe bleeding kills fast; minutes matter.
Direct pressure is the cornerstone of first aid.
Tourniquets save lives when pressure fails.
Always transfer urgently for definitive care.

☕ Coffee Moment

Later, sipping tea in the trauma ward, the student replayed the moment the spurting stopped under her hand. "It felt like the world paused when the bleeding slowed," she thought. Her mentor added softly: "That pause is the life you bought."

References

1. World Health Organization. Trauma Algorithm. Geneva: WHO; 2018.
2. World Health Organization. Basic Emergency Care: Approach to the Acutely Ill and Injured. Geneva: WHO; 2018.
3. American College of Surgeons Committee on Trauma. Advanced Trauma Life Support (ATLS®): Student Course Manual. 10th ed. Chicago: ACS; 2018.
4. Zideman DA, Singletary EM, De Buck ED, et al. European Resuscitation Council Guidelines for First Aid: 2021 Update. Resuscitation. 2021;161:270–290.
5. Kauvar DS, Lefering R, Wade CE. Impact of hemorrhage on trauma outcome: an overview of epidemiology, clinical presentations, and therapeutic considerations. J Trauma. 2006;60(6 Suppl):S3–11.
6. Singletary EM, Zideman DA, De Buck ED, et al. 2020 International Consensus on First Aid Science With Treatment Recommendations. Circulation. 2020;142:S284–334.
7. International Liaison Committee on Resuscitation (ILCOR). Control of severe, life-threatening external bleeding in the out-of-hospital setting: Tourniquets—Systematic review & CoSTR [Internet]. 2020 Jan 4 [cited 2025 Sep 1].
8. Hewett Brumberg EK, Douma MJ, Alibertis K, Charlton NP, Goldman MP, Harper-Kirksey K, et al. 2024 American Heart Association and American Red Cross Guidelines for First Aid. Circulation. 2024;150:e519–e579.

Chapter 74: Head Injuries

During a football game on campus, a 20-year-old player collides with another student and falls to the ground. He gets up, looks dazed, and complains of a headache. Minutes later, he vomits and has difficulty recalling the score. The crowd discusses whether to let him rest on the bench. You realize this could be a concussion instead of "just a bump."

Introduction

Head injuries can range from mild concussions to severe traumatic brain injuries (TBI). In India, common causes include road traffic accidents, falls, and occupational injuries. In this chapter, you will get an orientation to first aid in head injuries, ranging from a concussion to severe brain trauma.

Concussion Injury

A concussion is a mild traumatic brain injury caused by direct or indirect head impact, leading to temporary brain dysfunction. While many recover fully, missed or mismanaged concussions can progress to complications, including second impact syndrome or intracranial bleeding. First aid providers must recognize red flags, prevent further injury, and ensure safe referral. (1,2)

Recognition

Symptoms: headache, dizziness, nausea, confusion, memory loss, blurred vision.

Signs: imbalance, slurred speech, delayed response, irritability.

Red flags (urgent referral): repeated vomiting, seizures, loss of consciousness lasting over 1 minute, unequal pupils, worsening headache, and drowsiness. (3,4)

First Aid Steps

Stop the activity immediately and remove the person from play or work. (2)

Assess responsiveness and ABCs (airway, breathing, circulation).

If unconscious but breathing, place in recovery position; if not breathing, start CPR.

Do not allow a return to play on the same day, even if symptoms improve.

Use a cold compress on the scalp swellings.

Monitor closely for 24 hours. Worsening headache, confusion, or seizures require immediate hospital transfer.

A hospital evaluation is recommended for all cases of head injury. Even mild cases require medical clearance before resuming activity.

What NOT to Do

Never ignore or underestimate a head injury.
Avoid giving sedatives or alcohol (as they mask symptoms).
Do not permit the patient to return to play or drive home alone.

Outcome

With prompt recognition, monitoring and rest, most concussion injuries resolve within 7-14 days. Failing to identify complications can lead to permanent brain damage or death. Structured 'return-to-play' or 'return-to-learn' protocols are crucial for students and athletes.

Learning Points

A concussion is a brain injury, not a simple knock.
Remove from play, monitor carefully, and seek medical evaluation.
Red flags demand immediate transfer.

Severe Head Trauma

A 40-year-old construction worker falls from scaffolding. He briefly regains consciousness, then becomes drowsy. Blood is trickling from his ear, and his breathing is irregular. Bystanders think he's just "stunned" and want to let him relax in a comforting position. You realize this could be a serious head injury with a risk of brain bleeding.

Severe head trauma can lead to brain swelling, bleeding (such as subdural, extradural, and intracerebral haemorrhages), and death if not recognized early. First aid aims to protect the brain by maintaining airway, breathing, and circulation, and preventing further harm. (2,5,6)

Recognition

Altered consciousness (drowsiness, confusion, coma).

Severe or worsening headache.

Vomiting, seizures.

Bleeding or CSF leak from the ear or nose.

Unequal pupils, weakness or paralysis.

Irregular breathing or pulse (signs of raised intracranial pressure). (4,5)

Scene safety & Good Samaritan protections

Why it matters: Before approaching the casualty, scan for hazards such as fast-moving traffic, fuel leaks, fires, unstable vehicles, debris, electricity, chemicals, and potential crowd aggression.

Make the area safer by activating hazard lights, using bystanders as spotters, calling 112, and only entering if it seems reasonably safe. Wear gloves or improvise a barrier; avoid contact with blood or secretions.

Prioritise catastrophic bleeding → airway/breathing → circulation, but avoid moving the patient unnecessarily if a spinal injury is suspected.

Recovery position: Keep the person lying on their back. If they are vomiting or drowsy, place them in the recovery position while ensuring their spine is protected.

Good Samaritan framework: It protects you when giving honest, good-faith help. Good Samaritans are not liable for civil or criminal actions, and they cannot be forced to reveal their identity or detained for lengthy questioning. Hospitals must provide immediate care without demanding upfront payment from good Samaritans. Police statements may be brief and voluntary. These protections are derived from MoRTH guidelines and the 2016 Supreme Court order, allowing for prompt action without fear.

First Aid Steps

1. ABCs first: Ensure airway, use jaw-thrust instead of head-tilt if a cervical injury is suspected. Provide oxygen if available. If the patient is not breathing, start CPR and activate EMS (2)

2. Position: If possible, keep the patient flat with the head slightly elevated to 30°. If vomiting occurs, place the patient in the recovery position with their neck supported. (4,6)

3. Control bleeding: Apply gentle pressure to scalp wounds. If a skull fracture is suspected (bone fragments or open wound), cover with a sterile dressing and avoid applying pressure on protruding bone.

4. Immobilization: Suspect spinal injury and stabilize neck and back.

5. Monitor: Check pulse, breathing, and responsiveness every 2 minutes. Watch for deterioration (drowsiness, unequal pupils).

6. Transport urgently: Early hospital transfer is critical for CT scans and neurosurgical intervention.

What NOT to Do

Do not allow the patient to "sleep it off."
Do not give sedatives or alcohol.
Do not attempt to wash deep wounds or remove bone fragments.

Outcome

Early recognition and urgent neurosurgical care save lives in head injuries. Delay often leads to irreversible brain damage.

Learning Points

Altered consciousness after trauma; assume severe head injury.
Protect the airway and immobilize the spine.
Urgent referral is the key; time lost is brain lost.

☕ Coffee Moment

After transferring the worker, the student sat with a steaming cup of coffee. "It looked like he wanted to sleep, but inside his brain was swelling." His mentor nodded: "In trauma, the calmest faces sometimes hide the stormiest battles. That's why we must never ignore the quiet signs."

References

1. McCrory P, Meeuwisse W, Dvorak J, et al. Consensus statement on concussion in sport—the 5th international conference. Br J Sports Med. 2017;51(11):838–47.
2. Hewett Brumberg EK, Douma MJ, Alibertis K, Charlton NP, Goldman MP, Harper-Kirksey K, et al. 2024 American Heart Association and American Red Cross Guidelines for First Aid. Circulation. 2024;150:e519–e579.
3. Giza CC, Kutcher JS, Ashwal S, et al. Summary of evidence-based guideline update: evaluation and management of concussion. Neurology. 2013;80(24):2250–7.
4. Singletary EM, Zideman DA, De Buck ED, et al. 2020 International Consensus on First Aid Science With Treatment Recommendations. Circulation. 2020;142:S284–334.
5. Dewan MC, Rattani A, Gupta S, et al. Estimating the global incidence of traumatic brain injury. J Neurosurg. 2019;130(4):1080–97.
6. American College of Surgeons. Advanced Trauma Life Support (ATLS) Student Course Manual. 10th ed. Chicago: ACS; 2018.

Chapter 75: Spinal Injuries

On a rainy evening, a 25-year-old biker skids and crashes into a roadside barrier. He is conscious but cannot move his legs. Friends try to lift him by the arms to put him in a car. You rush in, realizing that careless handling could turn a survivable injury into permanent paralysis.

Introduction

Spinal injuries occur in road traffic accidents, falls, diving incidents, and industrial trauma. The biggest risk is secondary spinal cord damage caused by improper movement during rescue. First aid providers must assume spinal injury in all trauma cases with neck or back pain, neurological deficits, or unconsciousness. (1,2)

Recognition

- Severe pain or tenderness in the neck or back.
- Weakness, numbness, or paralysis in the limbs.
- Loss of bladder and bowel control.
- Obvious deformity or abnormal position of the spine.

In unconscious trauma patients, suspect spinal injury until proven otherwise. (2,3)

First Aid Steps

1. Protect the airway and breathing without moving the neck

If the airway needs to be opened, use the jaw-thrust manoeuvre (not the head-tilt manoeuvre). If CPR is needed, maintain neck stabilization. Maintain the person as still as possible and activate the EMS or ambulance. (4)

2. Manual cervical stabilization

Hold the victim's head firmly in a neutral position with both hands. Do not twist, flex, or extend the neck. ILCOR recommend against routine spinal immobilization for patients with penetrating trauma (e.g., gunshot or knife wounds). (4)

3. Immobilization

Use a cervical collar if it is available and you are trained to use it. Immobilize the head with sandbags or rolled towels if the collar is absent. Place on a firm surface (spine board) using the log-roll technique, with at least 3–4 helpers to maintain spine alignment. Current recommendations are against the routine use of rigid cervical collars and long spine boards for spinal immobilization by lay rescuers. (4)

4. Transport

Transfer on a spine board or firm stretcher.

Keep spine straight during movement.

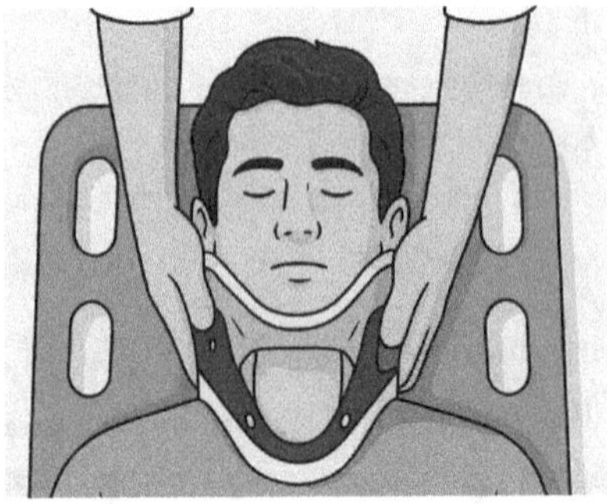

What NOT to Do

Do not lift the patient by arms or legs.
Do not allow the patient to sit or walk "to test movement."
Do not twist the body of the victim while moving onto the stretcher.

Outcome

Proper immobilization prevents secondary cord injury and permanent paralysis. Definitive management requires imaging, neurosurgical review, and intensive care.

Learning Points

- Always suspect spinal injury in trauma.
- Stabilize neck and spine first, even before transport.
- Wrong handling can be as dangerous as the accident itself.

Coffee Moment

At the hospital canteen, the student remembered the stillness of the biker's eyes. "He trusted me when I told them not to move him," he said. His senior replied, "Sometimes saving a spine is about saving patience, convincing others to slow down when everything feels urgent."

References

1. Hasler RM, Exadaktylos AK, Bouamra O, Benneker LM, Clancy M, Lecky F. Epidemiology and predictors of spinal injury in adult major trauma patients. Eur Spine J. 2011;20(12):2174–80.
2. Singletary EM, Zideman DA, De Buck ED, et al. 2020 International Consensus on First Aid Science With Treatment Recommendations. Circulation. 2020;142:S284–334.
3. American College of Surgeons. Advanced Trauma Life Support (ATLS) Student Course Manual. 10th ed. Chicago: ACS; 2018.
4. Hewett Brumberg EK, Douma MJ, Alibertis K, Charlton NP, Goldman MP, Harper-Kirksey K, et al. 2024 American Heart Association and American Red Cross Guidelines for First Aid. Circulation. 2024;150:e519–e579.

Chapter 76: Musculoskeletal Injuries & Fractures

Musculoskeletal injuries

During a cricket match, a batsman twists his ankle while running. He collapses, unable to bear weight, and his joint rapidly swells. Teammates try to pull and massage the ankle. You step in, recognizing that this is not a sprain but could be a fracture or a ligament tear.

Introduction

Sprains, strains, and minor joint injuries are commonly seen in sports, road accidents, and falls. Generally not life-threatening, but improper handling can worsen damage and delay recovery. First aid aims to reduce pain, prevent further injury, and support immobilization until medical care is available. (1,2) Injury triggers inflammation and bleeding in peri-articular tissues. Unnecessary movement can increase vascular and nerve damage. Immobilization stabilizes broken fragments and reduces pain.

Recognition

Sprain: stretched or torn ligament, swelling, pain, bruising, and difficulty moving.

Strain: muscle or tendon injury, pain during movement, localized tenderness.

Joint injury: swelling, deformity, inability to bear weight, limited motion.

Red flags: gross deformity, open wounds, and severe pain could indicate a fracture or dislocation. (2,3)

First Aid Steps

RICE protocol: Rest, Ice, Compression, Elevate

Rest and Immobilize: Immediately stop all activity and refrain from bearing weight. Keep the injured limb in the same position it was found. Use splints, cardboard, or a firm bandage for support.

Cold Compress (Ice): Apply a cold pack for 15–20 minutes to reduce pain and swelling. Wrap the ice in a cloth, and avoid direct application to the skin. Cold application should be limited to 20 to 30 minutes per session, without direct contact with the skin, to avoid cold injury. (3)

Compression and Elevation: Use an elastic bandage as a compression wrap that isn't too tight and does not compromise circulation.

Elevate the limb above heart level to reduce swelling.

Pain relief: Paracetamol can be given if available and safe.

Transport: Refer for X-ray/orthopaedic evaluation to rule out fractures.

What NOT to Do

- Do not massage or attempt forceful pulling.
- Do not apply heat in the first 24 hours.
- Do not allow the patient to walk on the injured limb.

Outcome

With proper first aid (RICE and immobilization), most sprains and strains recover well. Delays or harmful practices (like massage) can worsen ligament damage or displace fractures. Definitive care includes imaging, casting, or surgical repair if needed.

Learning Points

- Musculoskeletal injuries require immobilization, not manipulation.
- RICE protocol is the cornerstone of care.
- Always exclude fractures before resuming activity.

Fractures & Dislocations

During a college sports day, a runner trips and lands awkwardly. His leg appears deformed. Friends try to straighten the limb while lifting him. He screams in pain. You step forward, realizing that careless movement could worsen the fracture and damage nerves or blood vessels.

Introduction

Dislocations involve bones being displaced from their joints while fractures are breaks in bones. It is commonly seen in injuries due to falls, road traffic accidents, and sports. First aid targets immobilization, pain relief, and preventing further damage until proper medical treatment is available. (2-4)

Recognition

Fracture: Pain, swelling, deformity, abnormal movement, loss of function, and bone protruding through the skin (open fracture).

Dislocation: Visible deformity at the joint, pain, immobility, swelling, and abnormal bony contour.

Red flags: absent pulse, pale and cold limb, uncontrolled bleeding suggesting vascular injury. (3,5)

First Aid Steps

1. Reassure and assess ABCs: Airway, breathing, and circulation always come first in polytrauma. Ensure ABCs are managed properly.

2. Control bleeding: Apply direct pressure around the wound (if it is an open fracture), not directly on the exposed bone. Cover it with a sterile or clean dressing.

3. Immobilize the limb: Use splints secured above and below the injury to reduce pain, reduce risk for further injury, and facilitate transport to a medical facility. In the absence of medical splints, you can use modified splints such as wood, cardboard or an umbrella. For suspected dislocations, immobilize 'as found' and do not attempt forceful repositioning. (3)

4. Support and elevate: Raise the injured limb if there is no suspicion of vascular compromise. Apply cold compresses to reduce pain and swelling.

5. Pain relief: Use paracetamol or ibuprofen if available and safe.

6. Urgent transport: Move carefully, keeping the limb immobilized. For a suspected spinal fracture, transfer on a firm board with full neck support.

What NOT to Do

- Do not massage or attempt to "straighten" the bone or joint.
- Do not delay referral by applying traditional splints or oils.
- Do not ignore an absent pulse; this is an emergency.

Outcome

Proper first aid prevents further damage to nerves and vessels. Definitive treatment involves reduction, casting, or surgery, depending on the type of fracture.

Learning Points

- Fractures and dislocations require immobilization; do not attempt to manipulate them.
- Always check circulation below the injury site.
- Open fractures need urgent sterile dressing and referral.

☕ Coffee Moment

At the hospital canteen, the student remembered the runner's leg bent in an unnatural way. "It felt like time froze until we splinted it," she said softly. Her senior responded: "Sometimes the best first aid is about holding things still—until advanced care can take over."

References

1. Bleakley CM, Glasgow P, MacAuley DC. PRICE needs updating, should we call the POLICE? Br J Sports Med. 2012;46(4):220–1.
2. Singletary EM, Zideman DA, De Buck ED, et al. 2020 International Consensus on First Aid Science With Treatment Recommendations. Circulation. 2020;142:S284–334.
3. Hewett Brumberg EK, Douma MJ, Alibertis K, Charlton NP, Goldman MP, Harper-Kirksey K, et al. 2024 American Heart Association and American Red Cross Guidelines for First Aid. Circulation. 2024;150:e519–e579.
4. American Academy of Orthopaedic Surgeons. First Aid for Fractures, Sprains, and Strains. Rosemont: AAOS; 2019.
5. American College of Surgeons. Advanced Trauma Life Support (ATLS) Student Course Manual. 10th ed. Chicago: ACS; 2018.

Chapter 77: Crush Injuries

After a building collapse during heavy rains, rescuers pulled out a factory worker trapped under rubble for over an hour. His legs are swollen, bruised, and cold. As people rush to lift him quickly, you remember that sudden release of pressure without preparation can inject toxins into the bloodstream that are potentially fatal without proper first aid.

Introduction

Crush injuries result from prolonged pressure on muscles and soft tissues, usually during building collapses, road traffic accidents, or industrial incidents. The main risk is crush syndrome, where muscle breakdown releases potassium, myoglobin, and toxins, causing kidney failure, arrhythmias, and death after freeing the trapped limb. (1,2)

Recognition

- History of entrapment under a heavy object or rubble.
- Swollen, bruised, or deformed limb.
- Loss of sensation or absent pulses in the limb.
- Systemic signs: shock, difficulty breathing, altered consciousness after release.

First Aid Steps

1. Ensure rescuer safety: Remove the patient only when the area is safe (no ongoing collapse or electrical hazard).

2. ABCs first: Airway, breathing, circulation stabilization. Provide oxygen if available.

3. Control bleeding: Apply direct pressure for external bleeding.

4. Immobilize the limb: Apply splints to the injured extremity. Before release, keep the limb at heart level, not elevated.

5. IV access if available: If trained and equipped, start IV fluids (preferably normal saline) before releasing compression, to prevent shock and kidney injury.

6. Release of compression: Should be done carefully with medical support if possible. Apply a tourniquet above the injured limb if a prolonged crush injury (>1 hour) and advanced care are delayed, to prevent sudden washout of toxins.

7. Transport urgently: All patients require hospital care, fluids, electrolytes, and dialysis support if needed.

What NOT to Do

- Avoid massaging or wrapping the crushed area with tight bandages.
- Do not delay referral; renal failure can occur within hours.

Outcome

Proper first aid, IV fluids, careful release of pressure, and urgent transfer can prevent death. Delay or mishandling often leads to shock, arrhythmias, or acute kidney injury. Definitive management requires IV fluids, dialysis, surgical debridement and critical care.

Learning Points

- Crush injury syndrome is more dangerous than the visible injury.
- IV fluids and careful release reduce systemic complications.
- Early hospital transfer is essential for survival.

☕ Coffee Moment

Later, with a hot cup of tea, the young doctor shares, It wasn't the rubble that scared me, it was the silence after we lifted him. Her senior added, crush injuries teach us that sometimes the real danger begins after rescue. First aid is about preparing for that hidden storm.

References

1. Sever MS, Vanholder R, Lameire N. Management of crush-related injuries after disasters. N Engl J Med. 2006;354(10):1052–63.
2. Singletary EM, Zideman DA, De Buck ED, et al. 2020 International Consensus on First Aid Science With Treatment Recommendations. Circulation. 2020;142:S284–334.
3. Better OS. The crush syndrome revisited (1940–1990). Nephron. 1990;55(2):97–103.

Chapter 78: Eye Injuries

In the biochemistry lab, a student accidentally splashes acid into his eye. He screams in pain and rubs his face; others panic. You remember that every second counts; this is a true ocular emergency.

Introduction

The eyes are delicate organs, and trauma can cause pain, vision loss, or permanent blindness. Common causes include chemical burns, blunt trauma, penetrating injuries, and foreign bodies. First aid can help protect vision and prevent complications before specialized care is received. (1,2) Foreign-body sensation is a common symptom caused by a loose foreign body (e.g., an eyelash or piece of dust or sand), a foreign body embedded on the surface of the cornea, superficial corneal abrasion, a penetrating eye injury, or other causes such as chemical injury, ultraviolet radiation exposure, eye inflammation, or infection. Ocular foreign bodies are a common workplace injury, too.

High-speed injuries can cause significant damage to the eye globe, ranging from simple corneal abrasions to penetrating injuries to the anterior or posterior chamber of the eye. Foreign bodies embedded in the cornea often require removal by a healthcare professional. The corneal epithelium is highly sensitive to chemical injury. Acids cause coagulative necrosis, whereas alkalis penetrate deeply, causing liquefactive necrosis. Rapid dilution is the cornerstone of care in chemical injuries.

Recognition

Chemical injury: sudden pain, redness, tearing, and difficulty opening the eye.
Foreign body: gritty sensation, excessive blinking, redness.
Blunt trauma: swelling, bruising, double vision, decreased vision.
Penetrating injury: laceration, visible object, severe pain, bleeding, loss of vision.

First Aid Steps

Chemical burns: Immediately irrigate the affected area with clean, running water or saline solution for 15–20 minutes. Keep eyelids open while flushing. Continue irrigation during transfer to the hospital.

Foreign body (dust/small particle): Ask the patient not to rub. Instruct to blink or wash with clean water or saline. If associated with a contact lens, remove it. If it persists, cover the area with a pad and seek immediate ophthalmology review. (1)

Blunt trauma: Gently apply a cold compress over the closed eyelid. Immediate medical attention is needed.

Penetrating injury: Do not try to remove the object. Cover both eyes with sterile pads to reduce movement. Keep the patient still and transfer urgently to the hospital.

Foreign body related to low-energy mechanism: If foreign body sensation is from a low-energy mechanism (e.g. dust, dirt, or other object blown into the eye or eyelash), it is reasonable to attempt to remove it by allowing natural tears to wash it out or by irrigating the eye with tap water or a commercial eye wash solution. (1) Over-the-counter oral acetaminophen or NSAIDs may be given to treat residual discomfort after ocular foreign-body removal. (1)

What NOT to Do

- Do not rub your eye or apply ointment or chemicals unless prescribed.
- Do not delay irrigation in chemical burns.
- Do not try to remove embedded objects.

Outcome

Early irrigation of chemical injuries and careful protection in trauma cases significantly enhance visual outcomes. Delay or improper handling leads to permanent vision loss.

Learning Points

- Chemical burns: Irrigate immediately; do not wait.
- Protect and immobilise injured eyes.

Coffee Moment

Later, sipping coffee, the student reflected: "It wasn't the acid that scared me most, it was the panic of waiting." The senior smiled: "With eyes, time is sight. Sometimes your first aid is the line between darkness and light."

References

1. Hewett Brumberg EK, Douma MJ, Alibertis K, Charlton NP, Goldman MP, Harper-Kirksey K, et al. 2024 American Heart Association and American Red Cross Guidelines for First Aid. Circulation. 2024;150:e519–e579.
2. Singh P, Tyagi M, Kumar Y, Gupta KK, Sharma PD. Ocular chemical injuries and their management. Oman J Ophthalmol. 2013;6(2):83–6.
3. Singletary EM, Zideman DA, De Buck ED, et al. 2020 International Consensus on First Aid Science With Treatment Recommendations. Circulation. 2020;142:S284–334.
4. American Academy of Ophthalmology. Eye Health and Safety: First Aid for Eye Injuries. San Francisco: AAO; 2019.

Chapter 79: Dental Avulsion and Epistaxis

In the hostel canteen, a classmate slips on spilt water and hits the edge of a table. His front tooth is knocked out completely, bleeding from the gum. Students scramble for tissues, and someone suggests throwing the tooth away. You recall that how the tooth is handled now can determine whether it is saved or lost.

Introduction

Dental emergencies are common among young people, especially due to sports injuries, falls, or road accidents. Avulsed teeth, fractured teeth, and uncontrolled dental bleeding require prompt and appropriate first aid. Proper handling of the tooth and early referral to a dentist can preserve function and appearance. (1,2)

The periodontal ligament cells on the root surface are highly sensitive to drying; the survival of these cells determines the success of reimplantation. Reimplantation is recommended for permanent teeth; primary teeth (deciduous teeth or baby teeth) are not typically reimplanted. (1)

Recognition

Avulsion (tooth knocked out): visible gap, bleeding socket, intact whole tooth.

Fracture: broken piece, sharp edges, pain, possible pulp exposure.

Bleeding: persistent gum bleeding after trauma or extraction.

Other signs: swelling, severe pain, and difficulty in chewing.

First Aid Steps

Control bleeding: Press firmly with clean gauze or cloth. Instruct the patient to bite down gently.

Handle the tooth properly (avulsion): Grip the tooth by the crown only (not the root). Avoid scrubbing or scraping the root surface. Remove visible debris from the tooth by brief rinsing with clean water (<10 seconds), taking care not to damage the tooth or attached tissue, and attempting to replant the tooth in the socket.

Immediate self-implantation: The chance of survival of the tooth is greatest if it can be replanted immediately. The injured person may be able to replant the tooth themselves with follow-up care delivered by a dentist.

Reimplantation (within 30 minutes): Gently reinsert the tooth into the socket and ask the patient to bite down on gauze. Seek dental or medical care immediately.

Store and bring: If onsite replantation is not possible, place the tooth in the storage media and immediately bring it to the dentist or physician.

Recommended storage media for avulsed tooth (1)

First choice (high success rate): Hanks Balanced Salt Solution, oral rehydration salt solutions, propolis solution (10%, 50%, or 100%), rice water (preprepared), wrapping in cling film.

Second choice: Cow's milk (any fat content), person's own saliva (inside cheek)

Third choice: Another person's saliva, probiotic media (eg, probiotic yoghurt, Lactobacillus reuteri solution), egg white, almond milk.

Pain relief and referral: Paracetamol or ibuprofen if available. Transport urgently to the dental unit for fixation and further care.

What NOT to Do

- Do not hold the tooth by root or scrub it.
- Do not store tooth in tap water.
- Do not attempt reimplantation of primary (milk) teeth.

Outcome

Teeth reimplanted or stored properly within the first hour have the highest chance of survival. Delays or improper handling (such as scrubbing or discarding) lead to permanent tooth loss and cosmetic or functional disabilities.

Learning Points

- Golden hour: tooth survival depends on the first 60 minutes.
- Always handle by the crown, never the root.
- Store in proper media.

Epistaxis (Nosebleed)

Epistaxis is bleeding from one or both nostrils. It usually happens from fragile vessels in the nasal septum (Kiesselbach's plexus). Most cases are mild and self-limiting, but they can alarm patients and bystanders.

Common triggers include digital trauma, dry air, allergic rhinitis, infection, or hypertension. The primary goal of first aid is to stop bleeding while maintaining a clear airway and preventing aspiration. Tilting the head forward (not backwards) prevents swallowed blood and nausea. (1)

First Aid Steps

- The patient should sit upright and slightly lean forward.
- Pinch the soft part of the nose firmly for 10–15 minutes without interruption.
- Encourage mouth breathing and spitting out blood rather than swallowing it.
- If bleeding persists >15–20 minutes, recurs, follows facial trauma, or the patient has light-headedness, refer for medical evaluation.
- If the patient is taking anticoagulants or antiplatelet medications or has a blood-clotting disorder, refer them for medical evaluation. (1)
- May apply a cold compress over the nasal bridge; however, the usefulness of cryotherapy (ice) for managing epistaxis in the first aid setting is unknown. (1)
- Discourage packing with tissues or the insertion of foreign material unless you are trained to use nasal tampons.

Coffee Moment

Over a late-night coffee, the student replayed the image of the boy's tooth lying on the floor. "I almost let them throw it away," she thought. Her friend replied, "You didn't just save a tooth, you saved his smile. That's first aid, too."

References

1. Hewett Brumberg EK, Douma MJ, Alibertis K, Charlton NP, Goldman MP, Harper-Kirksey K, et al. 2024 American Heart Association and American Red Cross Guidelines for First Aid. Circulation. 2024;150:e519–e579.
2. Andersson L, Andreasen JO, Day P, et al. International Association of Dental Traumatology guidelines for the management of avulsed permanent teeth. Dent Traumatol. 2012;28(2):88–96.
3. Singletary EM, Zideman DA, De Buck ED, et al. 2020 International Consensus on First Aid Science With Treatment Recommendations. Circulation. 2020;142:S284–334.

TEMPEST

When the Elements Test Us

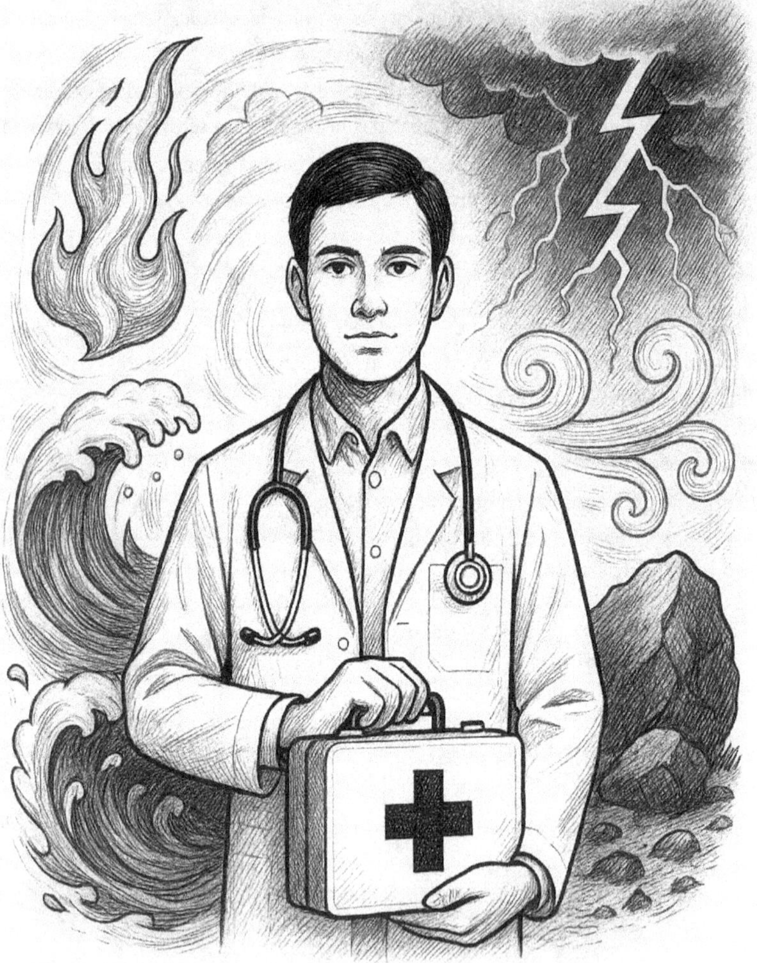

Tempest

When the Elements Test Us

There are moments in medicine when you face not just a patient, but the power of nature itself - a swollen river, a burning house, a stormy sky, the trembling ground.

These are not myths, but realities doctors confront in wards, villages, and disaster zones.

Ayurveda teaches that our body is a universe of *Panch Tatva*: Jal (water), Agni (fire), Vayu (air), Prithvi (earth), and Akash (sky). Modern science echoes this in its own way - water forms our cells, fire is a form of metabolism, air is our breath, earth is the foundation of structure, and the sky is the space where life unfolds.

When the harmony of the *Panch Tatva* is disturbed in the body, diseases arise, and when it is disturbed in the environment, disasters occur, and human life is threatened.
That is when the doctor must stand firm:
To triage amidst chaos,
To revive when breath falters,
To rescue from trauma or poison,
To restore balance when the elements rage.

S No.	Tempest: At a Glance
1.	**Chapter 80** Elemental Emergencies: Imbalance of Panch Tatva Understanding how disturbances of water, fire, air, earth, and sky translate into disasters. Principles of disaster management, triage, immediate care, and safe transport during mass casualty events.
2.	**Chapter 81** Drowning: When Water Takes Breath Away Recognition, rescue principles, resuscitation with early ventilations, and avoiding harmful myths.
3.	**Chapter 82** Heat Stroke: When Temperature Overpowers Body Life-threatening heat illness, rapid cooling strategies, prevention during Indian summers.
4.	**Chapter 83** Burns and Smoke Inhalation First aid for burns, airway vigilance in smoke inhalation, and debunking traditional remedies.
5.	**Chapter 84** Electrocution: The Invisible Current Scene safety, safe rescue, CPR and AED use, burn and trauma management after electrical injuries.
6.	**Chapter 85** Lightning, Flash Floods, and Landslides Combined-element disasters, recognition, CPR in lightning strikes, trauma and hypothermia in floods and landslides.
7.	**Chapter 86** High-Altitude Illness and Hypothermia Recognition of AMS, HAPE, HACE, principles of descent, oxygen, and rewarming strategies.

Chapter 80: Elemental Emergencies- Panch Tatva Imbalance

Introduction

Since ancient times, life has been described as a dance between the five great elements, known as the Panch Tatva: Jal (water), Agni (fire), Vayu (air), Prithvi (earth), and Akash (sky/space). Ayurveda sees our body as a miniature universe, sustained by the same elements that govern the cosmos. Modern physiology, though using different language, agrees: water forms our blood and cytoplasm, fire echoes in metabolism, air is respiration, earth is the minerals and structures of our body, and space is the cavities that allow organs to function. (1)

As long as these internal Panch Tatva (five elements) remain in balance, we enjoy health. When imbalance arises, disease follows - dehydration (loss of water), fever or hypermetabolism (excess fire), hypoxia (oxygen deficiency/air imbalance), bone or mineral deficiency (earth imbalance), or psychological stress and sensory overload (sky imbalance).

But imbalance also occurs outside us. When the Panch Tatva of nature are disturbed, the result is what we call disasters: floods and epidemics (water), fires and heatwaves (fire), storms and toxic gas leaks (air), earthquakes, landslides, and bites and stings from inhabitants like reptiles and insects (earth), lightning and extreme climates (sky). These disturbances may arise from a single element, such as burns from fire, drowning in water, or lightning from the sky, or from complex combinations. A flood may carry outbreaks of diarrheal disease with it. A landslide triggered by torrential rains and thunderstorms is a complex imbalance of water, earth, and sky. A lightning strike during a monsoon flood demonstrates the simultaneous fury of sky and water. Disasters are not mere elemental disruptions but also intersections where multiple natural forces converge, amplifying their impact on human life. Doctors and first responders rise to restore equilibrium.

Elemental Emergencies Leading to Potential Disasters

Water (Jal): Floods, drowning and waterborne infections.

Fire (Agni): Burns, smoke inhalation and heatstroke.

Air (Vayu): Airborne pandemics in communities, toxic gas exposure, blast injuries and altitude illness.

Earth (Prithvi): Crush injuries, snakebites, insects and contaminated soil wounds.

Sky (Akash): Lightning strikes, cold exposure and storms.

Each element is both life-giving and life-threatening. In harmony, they sustain life; in imbalance, they demand skilful intervention.

The Doctor's Role: Bridging Equilibrium

Your task as a young doctor is not to control the elements; no one can. Your role is to be a bridge between imbalance and equilibrium. With triage, rescue, medical stabilization, and trauma care, you give patients a fighting chance against forces larger than themselves.

As CPR revives a failing heart, elemental first aid or disaster management revives communities in crisis.

Disaster Management

Disasters are not defined only by collapsing buildings or rising waters. They are defined by imbalance: when the number of people needing urgent care suddenly overwhelms the available resources of healthcare, community, and system. The World Health Organization (WHO) defines a disaster as a serious disruption of the functioning of a community or a society, causing widespread human, material, economic or environmental losses that exceed the ability of the affected community or society to cope using its own resources. (2)

In India, the National Disaster Management Authority (NDMA) emphasizes preparedness, rapid response, and coordinated rehabilitation. (3,4) For the medical student, the key is to understand both the science and the humanity of disaster care: how to prioritize, how to act with limited resources, and how to bring calm to chaos.

Key Concepts

Principles of Disaster Management

Preparedness: Planning, drills, stockpiling supplies, training responders.

Mitigation: Measures to reduce impact (flood embankments, fire safety norms).

Response: Immediate lifesaving actions, rescue, triage, stabilization.

Recovery: Rehabilitation, psychological care, rebuilding systems.

Triage in Disasters

- Triage comes from the French word *trier,* meaning "to sort."
- It is the process of sorting patients by urgency, not arrival time.
- Goal: To do the greatest good for the greatest number.

Types of Triage

On-field / Pre-hospital Triage: Sorting at the disaster site.

Hospital Triage: Sorting as patients arrive at casualty/ED.

Re-triage: Ongoing reassessment as conditions change.

International Models

WHO & Sphere guidelines: Standard triage tags (Green, Yellow, Red, Black). (2)

START (Simple Triage and Rapid Treatment): Widely used for rapid field triage. (5)

NDMA India Guidelines: Align with global frameworks, emphasize coordination with community and hospital disaster plans. (3,4)

Triage Categories and Care

This is the crucible where your skills, learned in the revive, rescue, and impact sections, are tested in real-world situations. Assess scene safety, and recognize triage categories for individual victims. (2-5)

Red (Life-threatening and salvageable)

These patients require immediate interventions for revival and rescue. Examples include severe bleeding, tension pneumothorax, airway obstruction, and unresponsive victims with breathing or with a pulse.

CPR: Provide high-quality chest compressions for victims who are unresponsive and have abnormal breathing or gasping, or no pulse or pulse less than 60/min, with poor perfusion or no signs of life.

Airway: Open the airway using a head-tilt–chin-lift or jaw-thrust manoeuvre. Insert an airway adjunct if you are trained to do so.

Breathing: Provide ventilation (breaths) if apnoeic but with a pulse. Administer oxygen if available.

Circulation: Control severe external bleeding with direct pressure or a tourniquet. Get IV or IO access for further fluid resuscitation.

Shock: Lay patient flat, keep warm, and facilitate rapid evacuation.

Yellow (Serious but non-life-threatening for the moment)

These patients require hospital care but can wait safely while Red category patients are prioritized. Examples include stable abdominal injuries, long-bone fractures and burns without airway compromise.

Airway: Clear if obstructed. Monitor for any deterioration.

Breathing: Oxygen if available.

Circulation: Control moderate bleeding, splint fractures, and elevate injured limbs.

Analgesia: Provide pain relief if drugs are available.

Green (Minor)

Reassure, provide simple dressings, hydration and instructions to follow.

Black (Dead)

Provide comfort, cover the body respectfully and focus resources on salvageable victims.

Transportation Principles in Disaster Situations

Transport is not simply a 'first-come, first-served' act. It follows prioritization rules similar to those used in triage to maximize survival. (6)

1. Red-tagged (Immediate) Patients

Transported first, once stabilized.

Send to the nearest hospital with surgical facilities, ICU, and emergency capacity.

During transport, maintain the airway, control bleeding, monitor vital signs, and keep the patient warm.

Escort with trained personnel if possible.

2. Yellow-tagged (Delayed) Patients

Transport after Red patients.

They can be sent to secondary hospitals or facilities without advanced critical care, provided monitoring continues.

Splint fractures, cover wounds, and provide analgesia during transport.

3. Green-tagged (Minor) Patients

Transported last, often in groups or via non-medical vehicles.

Some may self-evacuate after basic care and instructions.

4. Black-tagged (Expectant or Dead)

Transport priority after alive and injured. Ensure respectful handling coordinated with disaster authorities.

Transport Guidance (WHO/NDMA)

- Do not overcrowd ambulances. Each vehicle should carry patients that match its capability (e.g., Red with oxygen-equipped ambulance).
- Mark destination hospitals clearly with advanced communication. Prevent "patient dumping" at already overwhelmed hospitals.

- Maintain communication between field command, the control centre, and hospitals (using mobile or satellite phones through the police or NMDA).
- Provide transfer documents, tags, basic vitals, interventions given and time of departure.

Case Snapshot

A bus accident on a highway leaves 40 injured. Responders apply triage:
10 Red: bleeding, chest trauma, unconscious but breathing.
15 Yellow: fractures, burns and abdominal pain.
12 Green: walking wounded with abrasions.
3 Black: pulseless, apnoeic despite attempt of CPR.
First ambulances take the 10 Red-tagged to a trauma centre. Patients in the yellow category are transported in the second wave to a district hospital. Green-tagged patients are reassured, treated for minor wounds, and later transported in non-medical vans. The triage system ensures that lives that can be salvaged with immediate care are prioritized.

Learning Points

- A disaster means an imbalance between needs and resources.
- Triage is the backbone. Red first, Yellow second, Green last.
- Red needs immediate care. Airway, breathing, bleeding control and shock prevention.
- Yellow care includes stabilize, splinting, pain relief and deferring advanced intervention.
- Transport decisions are as critical as treatment. Wrong evacuation can overwhelm hospitals and cost lives.
- The guiding principle remains greatest good for the greatest number.

Coffee Moment

After the drill, you sit on the hospital steps with your friends. Different colored triage tags are still in your pocket. You think of the difficult decision of marking someone Black, of sending Greens away, of seeing Red rushed off first. Your senior says quietly, "Disaster medicine isn't about doing everything for one. It's about doing enough for many." You sip your chai, and for the first time, the abstract word *triage* feels like a moral compass. (7)

References

1. Gupta S, Warner DS. Environmental emergencies. Miller's Anesthesia. 9th ed.

Philadelphia: Elsevier; 2020.

2. World Health Organization. Mass casualty management systems: strategies and guidelines for building health sector capacity. Geneva: WHO; 2007.
3. National Disaster Management Authority (NDMA). Guidelines on management of floods, heat wave, and lightning. Govt of India; 2020.
4. National Disaster Management Authority, Government of India. National Guidelines: Hospital Safety. New Delhi: NDMA; 2016.
5. Benson M, Koenig KL, Schultz CH. Disaster triage: START, then SAVE — a new method of dynamic triage for victims of a catastrophic earthquake. Prehosp Disaster Med. 1996;11(2):117–24.
6. Lerner EB, Schwartz RB, Coule PL, et al. Mass casualty triage: an evaluation of the data and development of a proposed national guideline. Disaster Med Public Health Prep. 2008;2(S1):S25–34.
7. Sphere Association. The Sphere Handbook: Humanitarian Charter and Minimum Standards in Humanitarian Response. 4th ed. Geneva: Sphere; 2018.

Chapter 81: Drowning

You are walking past a village pond when a 10-year-old boy is pulled out, limp and not breathing. There is no ambulance, but a crowd is gathered, shouting to "drain the water." You have seconds to act: open the airway, check breathing, and deliver two rescue breaths before starting compressions. (1)

Introduction

Drowning is a respiratory impairment caused by submersion or immersion in liquid and may lead to death or survival with or without morbidity. India bears a significant burden, primarily among children and young adults who are exposed to open water bodies and lack swimming skills. Rapid first aid significantly improves outcomes by quickly reversing hypoxia. (1,2)

The Drowning Chain of Survival was first developed in 2002 and then updated in 2014. (3) It refers to a series of interventions to reduce mortality associated with drowning, when put into action by trained or lay rescuers.

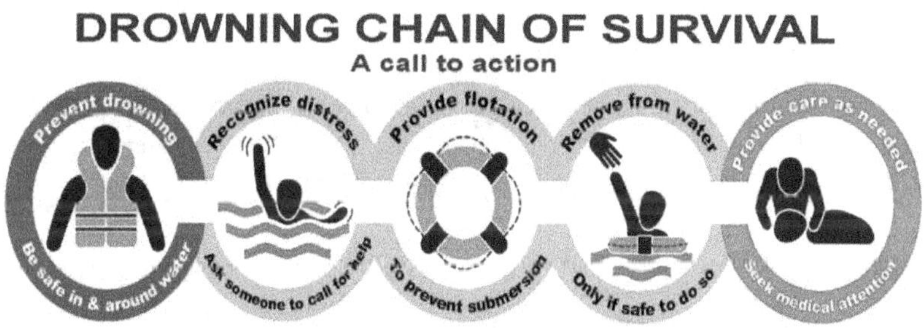
DROWNING CHAIN OF SURVIVAL
A call to action
Prevent drowning
Be safe in & around water
Recognize distress
Ask someone to call for help
Provide flotation
To prevent submersion
Remove from water
Only if safe to do so
Provide care as needed
Seek medical attention

Figure 81.1: Drowning Chain of Survival

Image is reproduced with permission from the International Life Saving Federation.

Recognition (what you'll see)

- Victim found in water; struggling, floating, or submerged
- Coughing/gasping; absent or abnormal breathing; cyanosis
- Unresponsiveness; possible cardiac arrest (2–4)

First Aid: What to do

Safe rescue (reach or throw, don't go): that means assist a drowning person from land, using available tools or flotation devices, without entering the water. (4) "Reach" means extending a pole, branch, towel, or any object to the victim to pull them to safety. "Throw" means tossing a buoyant aid such as a life ring, rope, or empty container that floats, to keep the victim afloat until trained rescuers arrive. Rescuers should only enter the water if professionally trained and equipped, following lifesaving protocols with flotation support.

Remove from water & assess ABCs immediately: On land, open the airway, and check breathing (≤10 seconds). If breathing is present, place the person in the recovery position, keep them warm (remove wet clothes, cover with a blanket), monitor their airway and breathing, and give oxygen if available. (3,4,6)

If not breathing or only gasping: give two breaths, then begin 30 compressions: 2 breaths (CAB with early ventilations in drowning). If the rescuer cannot give breaths, provide chest compressions.

Use a barrier device if available. Attach an AED as soon as it is accessible. Initiation of CPR and breathing should not be delayed to obtain or apply an AED. Continue until recovery or handover. (3-5)

Early transport: Even if the victim appears "better," there is still a risk of delayed lung injury. Refer for observation (aspiration, hypoxia-related complications). (2–4)

When respiratory arrest is addressed by rescue breathing that interrupts the drowning process, the death rate is lower (44%) than in those cases in which CPR (including chest compressions) is initiated (93%). (6)

In-water rescue breathing may be considered only in situations where an appropriately trained rescuer determines that the rescuer's safety, available equipment, and the distance to shore warrant its use. (6)

What NOT to do

- Do not attempt to "drain water" or hang the victim upside down.
- Don't delay ventilations/CPR while trying to expel water.
- Don't assume complete recovery if the victim awakens. (2–4)

Outcome

You provided rescue breaths, started chest compressions and ventilation, and ensured high-quality CPR because drowning is primarily a hypoxic event. Another bystander takes turns with you every two minutes to deliver chest compressions. The child began to move and cough after five minutes of high-quality CPR. An AED was not available, but you quickly transferred the child to a nearby hospital, where oxygen was administered, and the ER team provided further care.

Learning Points

- **Safety first:** Don't become a second victim. (4)
- **Ventilations matter:** In drowning, give rescue breaths with chest compressions

in a 30:2 ratio. (3,4)

- **Prompt first aid and transport:** Delays increase the risk of ARDS and poor neurologic outcomes. (2–5)
- **Hospital evaluation** is necessary even after apparent recovery. (2)

Drowning in Children: A Preventable Emergency

Introduction

Drowning is one of the leading causes of unintentional injury-related death in children worldwide. Unlike adults, drowning in children often occurs silently, rapidly, and in familiar environments such as homes, neighbourhoods, or school settings. In India, drowning-related deaths are frequently underreported, especially in rural areas. Open water bodies such as wells, ponds, canals, rivers, and floodwaters pose significant risks.

Environmental risks

- **At home:** buckets, bathtubs, water storage drums, overhead tanks, open toilets
- **Swimming pools:** lack of four-sided fencing, inadequate supervision, absence of trained lifeguards
- **Community settings:** open wells, ponds, canals, rivers, and construction sites
- **Seasonal risks:** flooded streets and overflowing water bodies during monsoon

Most childhood drowning events occur during brief lapses in supervision, often when caregivers believe the child is safe.

Prevention: The Most Effective Intervention

Supervision: Close, constant, and attentive supervision ("touch supervision") is essential for infants and toddlers near water. During group activities, a designated adult should be responsible solely for water supervision.

Environmental modification:

- Four-sided fencing with self-closing gates around swimming pools
- Covering wells, tanks, and buckets
- Emptying water containers after use
- Ensuring safe bathroom and household water practices

Management: How Pediatric Drowning Differs from Adults

While basic resuscitation principles are similar, important distinctions are-

- Hypoxia is the primary insult; cardiac disease is rarely the initiating event.
- Children deteriorate rapidly but may recover well with early rescue and CPR.

Immediate management:

- Rapid removal from water and early airway opening.
- Prompt breaths and ventilation are critical, as hypoxia precedes cardiac arrest.
- CPR should prioritise oxygenation.
- Hypothermia is common; rewarming should be gentle and controlled.
- All children with significant submersion should be observed in hospital, even if initially asymptomatic, due to the risk of delayed respiratory complications

☕ Coffee Moment

After the handover, you sit on a wall with a paper cup of chai, hands still shaking. You feel the compressions in your forearms and hear the rescue breaths. Someone mutters, "Good thing you were there." You shake your head. Good thing we acted. The chai is steady, like breath returning to a chest that almost forgot how to breathe.

References

1. World Health Organization. Global report on drowning: preventing a leading killer. Geneva: WHO; 2014.
2. Szpilman D, Bierens JJLM, Handley AJ, Orlowski JP. Drowning. N Engl J Med. 2012;366(22):2102–10.
3. Szpilman D, Webber J, Quan L, Bierens J, Morizot-Leite L, Langendorfer SJ, et al. Creating a drowning chain of survival. Resuscitation. 2014;85:1149–1152.
4. Singletary EM, Zideman DA, De Buck ED, et al. 2020 International Consensus on First Aid Science With Treatment Recommendations. Circulation. 2020;142(16_suppl_1):S284–S334.
5. Tiwari L. Drowning: IAP Textbook of Tropical Diseases. First edition. Jaypee Brothers Medical Publishers, New Delhi/ London. 2020 ISBN 978-93-89776-33-1: 617-22.
6. Dezfulian C, McCallin TE, Bierens J, Dunne CL, Idris AH, Kiragu A, et al. 2024 American Heart Association and American Academy of Pediatrics Focused Update on Special Circumstances: Resuscitation Following Drowning: An Update to the American Heart Association Guidelines for Cardiopulmonary Resuscitation and Emergency Cardiovascular Care. Circulation. 2024;150:e501–e516

Chapter 82: Heat-Related Emergencies

In mid-May, a 40-year-old farmer collapses unconscious under the sun during a health camp. His skin is hot; bystanders pour water on him and fan him. Someone suggests giving tea with salt. As a medical student with seconds to act, you must decide how to cool, hydrate, and prevent brain damage.

Introduction

Heat-related emergencies are common in India and other tropical and temperate countries, especially among farmers, children, athletes, outdoor workers, and crowd attendees. The spectrum of heat-related illnesses ranges from heat cramps or exhaustion to life-threatening hyperthermia or heat stroke. Etiologies include environmental exposure, exertion and medication. Prolonged temperature elevation leads to multiorgan failure that resembles septic shock. (1,2) Temperature and duration are critical determinants of survival. It is a preventable cause of cardiac arrest.

Pathophysiology: Prolonged heat exposure leads to dehydration, resulting in low intravascular volume (hypovolemia) and increased core body temperature. In hypovolemia, the body's natural physiological reflex is to reduce peripheral (skin) perfusion and maintain vital organ perfusion by facilitating peripheral vasoconstriction, thereby allowing the oxygen demand of vital organs to be met. In hyperthermia, evaporative cooling through sweating and cutaneous vasodilation normally dissipates heat. In heat illness, dehydration, inadequate acclimatization, or drugs that impair sweating overwhelm these defences. In a combined situation of hyperthermia and hypovolemia, the body faces contrasting needs: maintaining vital organ perfusion while facilitating heat loss through peripheral vasodilation, resulting in significant strain on the cardiovascular system. Core body hyperthermia causes protein denaturation, endothelial injury, and multiorgan dysfunction.

Children are at higher risk of hyperthermia compared to adults. They are at a higher risk for heat gain due to their larger ratios of body surface area to body mass, increased metabolic heat production, and ineffective sweat glands that fail to dissipate heat effectively. They are also unable to self-extricate from hyperthermic environments.

Heat Exhaustion

A mild heat-related illness due to prolonged exposure to high temperatures and inadequate water or salt replacement, leading to dehydration and strain on the cardiovascular system. Thermoregulatory mechanisms of the body are still intact, but the cardiovascular system cannot meet the combined demands of thermoregulation and volume loss. (3)

Clinical Features: Core body temperature < 40°C (104°F); Profuse sweating and pale, clammy skin; weakness, dizziness, headache, nausea and vomiting; tachycardia and hypotension. Mental status is still intact.

Management: Move to a cool location, remove excess clothing, administer oral or IV fluids, and encourage rest. Recovery is typically rapid when treatment is initiated early.

Life-threatening hyperthermia and Heat stroke

Heat stroke is characterized by a core body temperature ≥ 40°C and central nervous system dysfunction (such as altered mental status, delirium, seizures, or coma) due to failure of the thermoregulatory mechanism. In the transitional state of **life-threatening hyperthermia,** body temperature is ≥40°C, thermoregulatory failure is imminent, and systemic inflammatory response syndrome (SIRS) is triggered, but central nervous system function is preserved. Unlike heat exhaustion, it involves a core temperature over 40°C and CNS dysfunction. (1-4)

Recognition (Clinical Features)

- High body temperature (≥ 40°C)
- Confusion, delirium, seizures, unconsciousness
- Hot, flushed, dry skin or profuse sweating
- Rapid pulse and shallow breathing
- Headache, dizziness, nausea, or vomiting
- Multiorgan failure (hepatic, renal, cardiac, and coagulopathy) may develop rapidly. (2,3)

First Aid Steps

Ensure Safety & Call for Help: Move the victim to a cool, shaded area and call emergency services immediately. Position the victim on their side (recovery position).

Airway, Breathing, Circulation (ABCs): Assess responsiveness, airway patency, breathing, and pulse. If absent → begin CPR.

Critical skill is aggressive cooling:

- Cool first, transport immediately.
- Active cooling is recommended to be initiated concurrently with standard resuscitation with life-threatening hyperthermia. (3,4)
- Immersion in ice water (1–5 °C) is the most preferred method for cooling.
- If ice water immersion is not available, immersion in tepid water (8–17 °C) or tarp-assisted ice water cooling may be used as an alternative. (3,4)

- Cool as rapidly as possible with a decrease of at least 0.15 °C/min until the core temperature reaches 38.6 °C (101.5 °F). (3,4)
- Immerse the patient (torso and limbs, ideally up to the neck) in cold water and agitate the water for rapid heat transfer. Keep clothing minimal, protect the airway. (4-6)
- If a tub isn't available, use vigorous evaporative cooling by continuous water spraying and strong fanning, with ice or wet towels on the neck, axillae, and groin.
- Do not give antipyretics (they don't work in heat stroke)
- Dantrolene is not useful to treat life-threatening hyperthermia from causes other than malignant hyperthermia.
- Avoid alcohol rubs. Start cooling before transport if feasible. (1,6).

Supportive Care: Maintain the airway and monitor closely (5). If conscious and able to swallow, give sips of cool water or oral rehydration solution (ORS). If unconscious, keep the person in the recovery position and do not administer fluids orally. Check glucose if readily available, as hypoglycemia can mimic or worsen symptoms. Avoid antipyretics, as hyperthermia is not cytokine-mediated.

Outcome

With timely cooling and hospitalization, most victims recover. Delay leads to multi-organ failure, coma, or death. Prevention (acclimatisation, hydration, shaded rest breaks) is important, but when heat stroke occurs, rapid active cooling can be life-saving (1,2).

Learning Points

- Heat stroke is preventable. Stay hydrated and avoid prolonged sun exposure.
- First aid includes quick cooling and safe transfer.
- Every minute is critical; mortality doubles if cooling is delayed by more than 30 minutes.
- Community awareness in rural India can play a major role in reducing deaths during summer heatwaves.

Coffee Moment

After the farmer's revival, the medical student was discussing with his senior over tea in the camp tent. It felt like life returned with each splash, he said. The senior smiled, "That's first aid, simple acts, profound impact." The tea tasted warmer that day, flavoured with relief and learning.

References

1. Barletta JF, Palmieri TL, Toomey SA, et al. Guideline for the treatment of heat stroke. Crit Care Med. 2025;53(2):e490–e500.
2. Sorensen C. Treatment and prevention of heat-related illness. N Engl J Med. 2022;387(25):2370–9.
3. Cao D, Arens AM, Chow SL, Easter SR, Hoffman RS, Lagina AT III, et al. Part 10: adult and pediatric special circumstances of resuscitation: 2025 American Heart Association Guidelines for Cardiopulmonary Resuscitation and Emergency Cardiovascular Care. Circulation. 2025;152(suppl 2):S578–S672.
4. Hewett Brumberg EK, Douma MJ, Alibertis K, Charlton NP, Goldman MP, Harper-Kirksey K, et al. 2024 American Heart Association and American Red Cross Guidelines for First Aid. Circulation. 2024;150:e519–e579.
5. Morris A. Heat Stroke. In: StatPearls [Internet]. Treasure Island (FL): StatPearls Publishing; 2023.
6. International Liaison Committee on Resuscitation (ILCOR). First-aid cooling techniques for heat stroke and exertional hyperthermia—CoSTR [Internet]. 2019 Nov 28 [cited 2025 Sep 1]. Available from: https://costr.ilcor.org/

Chapter 83: Burns and Smoke Inhalation

You're on duty at a health centre when a villager rushes in with his 7-year-old son, whose shirt has caught fire while he was near a chulha. The child's arms and chest are blistered, and he's coughing. The father shouts, "Put ghee and turmeric on it!". You have minutes to cool the burns, secure the airway, and prevent damage.

Introduction

Burns and smoke inhalation are common in India due to open flames, unsafe stoves, electrical faults, and house fires. Thermal injury can occur from flames, liquids, surfaces, or gases. Burns can be classified as superficial, partial-thickness, or full-thickness. Smoke inhalation is particularly dangerous, often leading to airway compromise, hypoxia, and carbon monoxide (CO) poisoning. First aid can reduce mortality and long-term disability, but incorrect folk remedies are still widely practiced. (1,2)

Recognition

Burn injury signs: Pain, redness, blistering, charred skin, swelling, loss of sensation in deeper burns.
Smoke inhalation signs: Soot around nose or mouth, cough, hoarseness, stridor, shortness of breath, confusion, drowsiness (possible CO poisoning). (2,3)

First Aid Steps

1. Ensure safety: Remove the victim from the fire or smoke area. The rescuer should avoid inhaling smoke.
2. Stop the burning process: Extinguish flames with water, blanket, or "stop, drop, and roll.". Remove smouldering clothes, jewellery, and belts to prevent constriction.
3. Cool the burn: Immediately irrigate with cool (not ice-cold) running water for 20 minutes. In preadolescent children, monitor for hypothermia during active cooling. If no water, ice wrapped in cloth for superficial intact-skin burns may be reasonable; limit to ≤10 min to avoid frostbite. Avoid butter, oil, toothpaste, etc. (3,4)
4. Cover the burn: Use a clean, dry cloth, cling film, or sterile dressing. Do not break blisters.
5. Manage airway and breathing (for smoke inhalation): Assess airway-hoarseness and stridor indicate risk of obstruction. Suspect CO poisoning in all enclosed-space fires and provide 100% oxygen if available.
6. Circulation & fluids: Large burns have a high risk of shock due to fluid loss. Keep the victim supine, elevate their legs if possible, and provide oral fluids if they are alert and not vomiting. (3,4)
7. Pain relief & transfer: Give simple analgesics if available. Urgently transfer to the hospital for IV fluids, advanced airway care, and burn management. (1,3,4)

What NOT to Do

Do not apply ghee, butter, toothpaste, or turmeric. Do not pop blisters. Do not cover with cotton wool (it sticks to the wound). Do not delay transfer to the hospital.

Outcome

Early cooling and airway protection improve survival. Delayed or harmful treatments increase the risk of infection and complications. Hospital management involves respiratory support, fluids (Parkland formula), wound debridement, and grafting. (5)

Learning Points

First aid for burns- cool, cover, and transfer.
Airway vigilance is crucial in smoke inhalation.
Traditional remedies cause more harm than good.
All significant burns require hospital care, even if they look minor.

☕ Coffee Moment

Later that evening, the student sat in the canteen, sipping lukewarm coffee. "I kept hearing the father say ghee and turmeric… but all I did was water and cloth," he thought. The senior smiled: "Sometimes the best medicine is the simplest, and the hardest part is convincing others to believe it." The coffee soothed deeper scars.

References

1. Peck MD. Epidemiology of burns throughout the world. Part I: Distribution and risk factors. *Burns*. 2011;37(7):1087–100.
2. Singletary EM, Zideman DA, De Buck ED, et al. 2020 International Consensus on First Aid Science With Treatment Recommendations. *Circulation*. 2020;142(16_suppl_1):S284–S334.
3. Cao D, Arens AM, Chow SL, Easter SR, Hoffman RS, Lagina AT III, et al. Part 10: adult and pediatric special circumstances of resuscitation: 2025 American Heart Association Guidelines for Cardiopulmonary Resuscitation and Emergency Cardiovascular Care. Circulation. 2025;152(suppl 2):S578–S672.
4. Hewett Brumberg EK, Douma MJ, Alibertis K, Charlton NP, Goldman MP, Harper-Kirksey K, et al. 2024 American Heart Association and American Red Cross Guidelines for First Aid. Circulation. 2024;150:e519–e579.
5. Tiwari L. Smoke inhalation: "Synopsis of Pediatric Emergency", Editors – Sunit Singhi, J Surpure. Peepee Publication India. 2014. ISBN 81-8445-076-1

Chapter 84: Lightning, Flash Flood and Landslide

During a monsoon thunderstorm in Motihari, Bihar, villagers hear a deafening sound. A farmer collapses in the field after a lightning strike. He is unresponsive, with shallow breathing. Everyone hesitates to touch him, fearing they too will get an electric shock. At the same time, in Dharali, Uttarakhand, a landslide accompanied by a flash flood sweeps away houses and vehicles, and buries part of a bus. Survivors are pulled out, some with fractures, others shivering and gasping after near-drowning in floodwaters.

Introduction

Lightning strikes, flash floods, and landslides are common natural disasters in India, often resulting in multiple casualties. Lightning delivers a massive electric current within milliseconds, which can cause cardiac arrest or burns. Floods and landslides lead to trauma, drowning, hypothermia, and crush injuries. First aid emphasizes rapid rescue, resuscitation, and preventing secondary injuries. (1,2)

Recognition

- **Lightning injury:** unconsciousness, cardiac arrest, burns with feathering patterns, hearing loss, confusion, fractures from muscle spasm.
- **Flood and landslide victims:** drowning signs (coughing, frothing, respiratory distress), hypothermia, fractures, entrapment injuries, shock.

First Aid Steps

Lightning injury

- **Scene safety:** It is safe to touch the victim; the current does not stay in the body.
- **Check ABCs:** If there is no breathing or pulse, start CPR immediately. Survival is possible with prolonged resuscitation.
- **Treat burns:** Cover the affected area with a clean cloth and avoid using ointments.
- **Fracture and spine care:** Immobilize as needed.

Flash flood/landslide injuries

- **Rescue carefully:** Avoid further landslide risk.
- **Airway and breathing:** Ensure the airway is clear, and administer breaths if the person isn't breathing.
- **Hypothermia prevention:** Remove wet clothes and wrap in blankets.

- Fracture or crush injuries: splint the affected area, control bleeding, and initiate fluid replacement if trained and available.
- **Psychological support:** Victims may be in severe shock or panic; calm, reassuring words are essential.

What NOT to Do

- Do not delay resuscitation in lightning victims; success is possible even after prolonged arrest.
- Do not light fires too close to hypothermia (risk of burns).
- Do not rush into unstable landslide zones without proper safety precautions.

Outcome

Quick CPR and hypothermia management improve survival. Improper handling or delayed rescue in floods or landslides results in high mortality. Definitive care involves hospital treatment for burns, trauma, and kidney protection after crush injuries.

Learning Points

- Lightning victims are safe to touch; start CPR without delay.
- Flood or landslide victims may have multiple simultaneous problems (trauma, hypothermia, drowning).
- Safety of rescuers is critical; do not become the second victim.

☕ Coffee Moment

Over a warm cup of tea after the rescue, the young doctor reflected: "He looked gone, but after CPR, he gasped." A colleague added: "Disasters remind us, sometimes, survival rests on hands that refuse to give up, even in the storm."

References

1. Cooper MA, Holle RL, Andrews CJ. Lightning injuries. In: Auerbach PS, editor. Wilderness Medicine. 7th ed. Philadelphia: Elsevier; 2017. p. 71–108.
2. Singletary EM, Zideman DA, De Buck ED, et al. 2020 International Consensus on First Aid Science With Treatment Recommendations. Circulation. 2020;142:S284–334.
3. Collins AJ, et al. Disaster management and response in landslides and floods. Disaster Med Public Health Prep. 2016;10(1):59–67.

Chapter 85: High-Altitude Illness and Hypothermia

During a trek in Ladakh, a 21-year-old medical student starts experiencing severe headaches, nausea, and trouble sleeping on the second night at 3,600 meters. The group thinks it is fatigue. By the next day, he is breathless even at rest and stumbles while walking. You realize this could be high-altitude illness, potentially life-threatening if untreated.

Introduction

At altitudes above 2,500 meters, lower oxygen pressure increases the risk of Acute Mountain Sickness (AMS), High-Altitude Pulmonary Edema (HAPE), and High-Altitude Cerebral Edema (HACE). These conditions are life-threatening but can be prevented through awareness, gradual ascent, and prompt first aid. (1,2)

Recognition

- **AMS:** Headache, nausea, fatigue, poor sleep, loss of appetite.
- **HAPE:** Breathlessness at rest, cough with frothy sputum, rapid heartbeat, blue lips.
- **HACE:** Severe headache, confusion, ataxia, altered consciousness, coma. (2,3)

First Aid Steps

1. **Stop ascent immediately**: Do not climb higher if symptomatic.

2. **Rest and monitor**: Rest, hydration, light diet, paracetamol for headache.

3. **Oxygen therapy**: Give supplemental oxygen if available.

4. **Descent** (most effective treatment): descend at least 500–1000 meters if symptoms worsen or if HAPE is HACE is suspected.

5. **Medications** (if trained and available)

Acetazolamide: accelerates acclimatization (125–250 mg twice daily).

Dexamethasone: for severe AMS or HACE.

Nifedipine: can be used in HAPE.

6. **Portable hyperbaric bag** (if available in expeditions): temporary relief until descent is possible.

What NOT to Do

- Do not ignore early symptoms or continue climbing.

- Do not give alcohol or sedatives (worsen hypoxia).
- Do not rely on medicines alone; descent is key.

Outcome

Most AMS cases resolve with rest or descent. Untreated HAPE or HACE are often fatal. With early recognition and proper first aid, the prognosis is excellent.

Hypothermia

During a winter health camp in the Himalayas, villagers bring in a shepherd found unconscious after a night in the open. His skin is pale and cold, his pulse slow and weak. Some suggest rubbing him vigorously or giving him alcohol to "warm him up." You know that mishandling could worsen his condition.

Hypothermia is an involuntary drop in core body temperature below 35°C, caused by prolonged exposure to cold environments, wet clothing, or immersion in cold water. Frostbite is a condition characterised by localised tissue freezing, most commonly affecting the digits, ears, or nose. Hypothermia is often overlooked but occurs in high-altitude regions, disaster situations (floods/landslides), or in newborns. Severe hypothermia can cause arrhythmias, unconsciousness, and death. (4,5)

Pathophysiology: When environmental heat loss exceeds metabolic heat production, peripheral vasoconstriction and shivering attempt to conserve body temperature. Below 32 °C, both fail, leading to bradycardia, coagulopathy, and reduced consciousness. Ice crystal formation in tissues during frostbite causes microvascular thrombosis and necrosis.

Table 85.1: Stages of hypothermia

Stage of hypothermia Temp °C	Signs and Symptoms
Cold stress, 35–37 °C	Alert, ± shivering
Mild 32–35 °C	Altered level of responsiveness, shivering
Moderate 28–32 °C	Decreased responsiveness, ±shivering, ± slow heart rate, pale, non-blanching exposed skin, frozen tissue/frostbite
Severe <28 °C	Unresponsive, may appear lifeless, no shivering, slow heart rate and breathing, High risk for arrythmia and cardiac arrest.
Profound <24 °C	

Mechanisms of heat loss

- **Conduction:** Heat is transferred directly from warmer to cooler objects that touch each other.

- **Convection**: Heat transferred to or from a gas or liquid that is in motion.
- **Radiation** Heat is released into the air from the body.
- **Evaporation**: Heat is lost from the vaporization of liquid on the skin.

Recognition

Signs and symptoms depend on the stage of hypothermia. (5,6)

First Aid Steps

Ensure safety and get the patient out of the cold: Move them to a warm, dry shelter. Remove wet clothes and replace them with dry, layered clothing.

If a person cannot be immediately moved to a warm area, prevent further heat loss by insulating from the ground, covering of head and neck, and shielding from wind with a plastic or foil layer over a dry insulating layer. (4)

Activate emergency response while starting rewarming with any available method if patients have decreased responsiveness, pallor, cyanosis or frostbite.

Passive rewarming: Wrap the individual in blankets, cover their head, and utilise body heat from another person to maintain their temperature. Insulate from the cold ground with mats or blankets. (4)

Active external rewarming (if available): Use warm packs on the groin, armpits, and neck (avoid direct hot water). Offer warm, sweet fluids if alert. Place insulation between the heat source and skin, and frequently monitor for burns and pressure injury. Body-to-body rewarming is not beneficial for active rewarming. (4)

Monitor ABCs: If no breathing or pulse → start CPR. Continue resuscitation longer than usual; recovery is possible even after prolonged cardiac arrest in cold conditions.

Urgent referral: Severe cases require hospital care, including warm IV fluids, heated oxygen, and rewarming devices.

Alert patients in cold stress or mild hypothermia who can safely consume oral food or fluids should be provided with high-calorie foods or drinks.

What NOT to Do

- Small glove or boot insert chemical heat packs are not useful as the sole or primary means of rewarming. (4)
- Heat sources, rubbing, and massage should not be applied to the extremities. Rough movement may trigger ventricular fibrillation. (4)
- Use of a warm shower or warm water immersion is harmful if the victim has a decreased level of responsiveness because of the risk of core temperature after-drop, hypotension, falls, and drowning. (4)

- Do not give alcohol or sedatives (increase heat loss).

Outcome

Most cases of mild to moderate hypothermia recover with proper rewarming. Severe hypothermia requires specialized care, but survival is possible even in prolonged cases with correct management.

☕ Coffee Moment

Later, warming his hands around a cup of steaming coffee, the student thought: "The mountain doesn't forgive haste, and the cold can steal life so quietly." His mentor added, "First aid at altitude is not only about oxygen—it's about patience and knowing when to turn back."

References

1. Basnyat B, Murdoch DR. High-altitude illness. Lancet. 2003;361(9373):1967–74.
2. Hackett PH, Roach RC. High-altitude illness. N Engl J Med. 2001;345:107–14.
3. Imray C, Wright A, Subudhi A, Roach R. Acute mountain sickness: pathophysiology, prevention, and treatment. Prog Cardiovasc Dis. 2010;52(6):467–84.
4. Hewett Brumberg EK, Douma MJ, Alibertis K, Charlton NP, Goldman MP, Harper-Kirksey K, et al. 2024 American Heart Association and American Red Cross Guidelines for First Aid. Circulation. 2024;150:e519–e579.
5. Brown DJA, Brugger H, Boyd J, Paal P. Accidental hypothermia. N Engl J Med. 2012;367:1930–8.
6. Singletary EM, Zideman DA, De Buck ED, et al. 2020 International Consensus on First Aid Science With Treatment Recommendations. Circulation. 2020;142:S284–334.

Chapter 86: Electrocution

It is a hot summer afternoon when you hear a scream near a construction site. A 25-year-old worker is lying on the ground, unconscious, his hand still in contact with a live electric wire. People are shouting, "Pull him away!" A few attempt to approach, but you know that one wrong move could make you the next victim. You have seconds to act safely; cut the current, protect yourself, and then begin resuscitation.

Introduction

Electrocution is an injury caused by contact with electrical energy. Electricity causes various injuries depending on the voltage, duration of contact, type of current (alternating or direct), and pathway of current travelling through the body. Patients may experience significant burns, traumatic injuries, arrhythmias or cardiac arrest. It is a common occupational hazard among construction workers, farmers, and children exposed to unprotected wires or faulty appliances. Mortality remains high because bystander CPR is often delayed or not performed.

Recognition

The victim found near an electrical source or wire, collapse during electrical work/exposure, and burns at entry/exit points (hand, foot) are common indicators. Victim may have secondary trauma (falls from ladders, roofs) or cardiac arrest. (1,3)

First Aid Steps

- **Ensure rescuer safety first:** Do not touch the victim until the power is switched off, stand on a dry, insulated surface, turn off the mains, unplug the device, or push the wire away using a dry wooden stick, plastic, or cloth.
- **Remove from source & Assess ABCs:** Once the victim is free from electrical hazards, assess responsiveness, airway, breathing, and circulation.
- **Resuscitation:** If no breathing or pulse → start CPR immediately following standard CPR algorithm, use an AED early if available as arrhythmias are common after electrocution. (3,4) If the victim is breathing, place them in the recovery position.
- **Treat burns and injuries:** Look for entry/exit wounds, do not apply butter, oil, or paste and manage associated trauma due to falls.
- **Transport to the hospital urgently:** Even if the victim appears recovered, arrhythmias and other complications may develop later (2,5).

What NOT to Do

- Do not touch the victim before switching off the current.
- Do not pour water on the person (risk of further conduction).

- Do not ignore external burns; internal injuries are serious.
- Do not delay transfer after apparent recovery.

Outcome

With safe removal, immediate CPR, and early hospital transfer, survival improves. Delay or unsafe rescue often leads to death or injury to multiple rescuers.

Learning Points

- Safety first: protect the rescuer before helping the victim.
- If cardiac arrest occurs, CPR and AED are lifesaving.
- Burns and trauma are frequent companions.
- Even "normal-looking" victims need hospital evaluation for delayed complications.

☕ Coffee Moment

Later, with shaking hands wrapped around a cup of coffee, the student replayed the moment when everyone else had hesitated. "The hardest part wasn't starting compressions, it was forcing myself to wait until the power was off", she said. Her mentor nodded, that is the paradox; sometimes doing nothing for a second saves the victim as well as a prompt rescuer. The coffee tasted strong, with the realization that safety is the first step.

References

1. Koumbourlis AC. Electrical injuries. Crit Care Med. 2002;30(11 Suppl):S424–30.
2. Arnoldo BD, Purdue GF, Kowalske K, Helm PA, Burris A. Electrical injuries: a 20-year review. J Burn Care Rehabil. 2004;25(6):479–84.
3. Singletary EM, Zideman DA, De Buck ED, et al. 2020 International Consensus on First Aid Science With Treatment Recommendations. Circulation. 2020;142(16_suppl_1):S284–S334.
4. Cao D, Arens AM, Chow SL, Easter SR, Hoffman RS, Lagina AT III, et al. Part 10: adult and pediatric special circumstances of resuscitation: 2025 American Heart Association Guidelines for Cardiopulmonary Resuscitation and Emergency Cardiovascular Care. Circulation. 2025;152(suppl 2):S578–S672.
5. Cooper MA. Electrical and lightning injuries. Emerg Med Clin North Am. 1992;10(2):211–29.

Illumination

When Knowledge Lights the Way

Medicine is not only about resuscitation and response. It is also about understanding, learning to see patterns, weighing evidence, asking questions, and making choices that heal wisely.

Light (*Tejas*) or knowledge is the force of clarity. ***Illumination*** is about the light that guides practice, the skills of communication, research, evidence, and public health that turn scattered facts into wisdom.

Here, you learn how to speak with patients, listen with intent, build trust, read and conduct research, and place every action on the firm foundation of evidence.

Illumination does not happen in an instant. It grows: one conversation, one ethical choice, one careful observation at a time. Facts are fuel, but understanding is flame.

Illumination is not only about knowing, but about seeing - clearly, calmly, and compassionately.

S No.	Illumination: At a Glance
1.	**Chapter 87** Foundation of Clinical Communication How to listen, how to speak, and how to connect. A structured, humane way to deliver difficult truths while supporting patients and families.
2.	**Chapter 88** Introduction to Medical Research From curiosity to question to study design: learning how doctors create new knowledge.
3.	**Chapter 89** Evidence-Based Medicine The art of blending best research, clinical skill, and patient values to make sound decisions.
4.	**Chapter 90** Accessing Online Resources This is your gateway to evidence and research explaining how to use online learning and research resources.
5.	**Chapter 91** Vaccination and the National Immunization Schedule Understanding vaccines, schedules, myths, and the science of prevention in India and beyond.
6.	**Chapter 92** Biomedical Waste Management Safe handling of hospital waste to protect patients, staff, and the environment.
7.	**Chapter 93** Hand Hygiene, Universal Precautions and PPE From the simple act of hand washing to the larger vision of family-centred, community-based care.

Chapter 87: Foundation of Clinical Communication

Introduction

A physician's technical expertise has a limited impact without effective communication. Patients judge the quality of their care by clinical outcomes and how respected, understood, and supported they feel. The AETCOM curriculum revisits communication skills in each professional year. This chapter provides a stepwise approach to developing competence in patient-centred communication. (1,2)

Principles of effective communication

Communication is a fundamental prerequisite in the medical profession, and it involves a structured process with identifiable skills. Active listening, verbal and non-verbal skills and creating respect in patient encounters are essential to master communication. Students should learn to:

- **Prepare yourself:** Introduce, ensure privacy and minimize distractions.
- **Engage with the patient:** Ask open-ended questions and avoid medical jargon. Maintain eye contact, nod, and lean forward to signal attention.
- **Empathize and validate feelings:** Acknowledge emotions without judgment.
- **Summarise and educate:** Reflect on what the patient has said to confirm understanding, explain the plan, and check comprehension.

Active listening and data gathering

In initial interactions with patients and their families, such as taking histories, identifying patient concerns, and summarizing information, focus on establishing open communication, active listening, and gathering relevant data. (3) In a study published in JAMA, the mean uninterrupted speaking time of patients was 92 seconds (median 59 s), and in 80% of visits, patients finished presenting all concerns within 2 minutes if uninterrupted. (4)

- **Open the discussion:** Start with questions such as "How can I help you ?" and "What concerns do you have?"; avoid directing the agenda too quickly.
- **Listen without interruption:** Give the patient space to tell their story. Most patients speak for less than two minutes when allowed.
- **Elicit psychosocial context:** Ask about lifestyle, family, work and emotional factors that may influence health.

Dealing with emotions

Once you are adept at basic skills, begin learning to address emotional responses. Practice recognizing verbal and non-verbal cues of anger, fear, sadness and denial, and respond with empathic statements such as 'That sounds very upsetting' or 'I can see this is difficult for you.' (5)

Administering informed consent

Obtaining informed consent is a medicolegal and ethical requirement. It needs professional communication skills. Explain procedures, risks and alternatives clearly and answer patient queries. Ask patients to restate their understanding, to ensure comprehension. Document in a language that the patient can understand and take a signature. Put your signature, name, time and date.

Communicating Bad News: The SPIKES Protocol

Delivering bad news is a challenging and essential component of medical care. It requires understanding the technical aspects of treatment and the ability to communicate sensitive information in a compassionate and clear manner. The SPIKES protocol is a structured approach for delivering bad news. (6,7)

S - Setting up the Interview

Before delivering bad news, ensure that the conversation occurs in a quiet, private space with an environment of trust and security. Communication should occur without unnecessary interruptions. Body language, eye contact and an open posture are important in conveying empathy and support.

P - Perception

Understand the patient's perspective before jumping into the bad news. Understand what they already know and what their fears or misconceptions are. Ask, "Can you tell me what you understand about your condition so far?" Build rapport based on their emotional state and knowledge to guide the conversation. This helps in tailoring the information to the patient's needs.

I - Invitation

Develop a rapport and understand how much information they can process. Respect their autonomy and understand their readiness to hear the news so that they are active participant in their healthcare.

K - Knowledge

Now it is time to share the information clearly and honestly, without overwhelming the patient. Break the news gently but directly. Use simple language to ensure patients understand. 'The tests show the tumour is malignant' does not make sense to the patient; a better sentence is 'The results indicate that there is a cancerous growth in your body, and we need to discuss a treatment plan.' Pause and allow the patient to process the information, and be ready for their emotional response.

E - Emotions

Emotions of shock, anger, sadness, or denial are common when they hear bad news. Acknowledge these emotions without judgment. A brief silence gives them time to process at their own pace. Allow them to express their feelings, maintain comforting gestures and offer tissues or a glass of water.

S - Strategy and Summary

Discuss the treatment plan and other options, such as referrals, a second opinion, and additional tests. It helps them regain a sense of control over their situation. Summarize the conversation by restating the key points to ensure a common understanding. Allow them to ask questions and offer other professional support. Ensure that patients feel heard, respected, and supported during one of the most challenging moments in their lives.

Reflection

Effective communication is not an innate ability; it needs practice and refinement. Use this framework in increasingly complex contexts such as dealing with strong emotions, obtaining consent, breaking bad news and negotiating treatment plans.

Case Scenario: "Two Faces of a Consultation"

Case A- The Distracted Doctor: Mrs Kaur, a 45-year-old schoolteacher, visits her family physician with complaints of fatigue and palpitations. The doctor, glancing at his computer screen, asks abruptly, 'So what is the problem?' Before she completes, he interrupts, 'It is probably stress.' While she tries to speak, he answers a phone call, keeps typing, and finally hands her a prescription without making eye contact. Mrs Kaur leaves the clinic feeling unheard, anxious, and unsure about the tests.

Case B- The Attentive Doctor: Mrs Kaur now consults Dr Kulshreshtha. He greets her warmly: 'How can I help you today, Mrs Kaur?' Sitting face-to-face, he maintains eye contact and allows her to speak uninterrupted. 'Can you tell me more about the palpitations? When do they occur?' He acknowledges her stress at work and home, summarises her concerns, explains possible causes in simple terms and plans for counselling and investigations if symptoms persist. Finally, he invites her to ask questions and answers patiently. Mrs Kaur leaves reassured and respected.

Core Concept

Patient-Centred Communication: Physicians listen actively, respect patients' perspectives, and provide clear information in simple language. It improves trust, adherence, and satisfaction and minimizes errors related to poor communication.

Approach

- Active listening and empathy.
- Clear, jargon-free explanation of diagnosis and plan.
- Patient or family participation and shared decision-making.
- Professional etiquette, maintaining eye contact, minimising distractions, and exhibiting respectful body language.

Outcome

Case A reflects poor communication, which erodes trust and increases anxiety. Case B shows effective communication, confidence, and better compliance.

Learning Points

- Good communication is as important as clinical skills.
- Emotional support is also part of overall management with medical treatment.
- Respect, attention, and clarity make it professional.

☕ Coffee Moment

Imagine Mrs Kaur sipping tea at home. In one version, she feels helpless and ignored; with Dr Kulshreshth, she feels hopeful and valued. The same cup of tea tastes very different depending on how the listener perceives it. Small behavioural changes profoundly influence the patient's experience.

References

1. Silverman J, Kurtz S, Draper J. Skills for communicating with patients. 3rd ed. CRC Press; 2013.
2. National Medical Commission. AETCOM: Attitude, Ethics and Communication Module for the Undergraduate Medical Curriculum. NMC; 2019.
3. Ha JF, Longnecker N. Doctor-patient communication: a review. Ochsner J. 2010;10(1):38–43.
4. Marvel MK, Epstein RM, Flowers K, Beckman HB. Soliciting the patient's agenda: Have we improved? JAMA. 1999;281(3):283-287.
5. Levinson W, Lesser CS, Epstein RM. Developing physician communication skills for patient-centred care. Health Aff. 2010;29(7):1310–8.
6. Buckman R. Breaking Bad News: A Guide for Health Care Professionals. Baltimore: Johns Hopkins University Press; 1992. p. 15.
7. Baile WF, Buckman R, Lenzi R, Glober G, Beale EA, Kudelka AP. SPIKES—A six-step protocol for delivering bad news: Application to the patient with cancer. Oncologist. 2000;5(4):302–11.

Chapter 88: Introduction to Medical Research

Introduction

Research is disciplined curiosity with a purpose. For a young doctor, it is a habit to turn everyday doubts into structured questions and use data, ethics, and compassion to find better answers for patients and communities.

Key Concepts

Research: A systematic way to generate reliable knowledge.

Common pathways:

- Basic science describes cells, molecules, interactions, and genetics.
- Clinical research is primarily focused on case series, cohorts, and trials.
- Epidemiology to understand who gets sick, where, and why.
- Qualitative research includes interviews, focus groups, and patient experience.
- Health-systems research (how services are organized and improved)
- Evidence-based medicine: critically review studies for applicability in safe clinical practice.
- Ethics first: Respect, consent, privacy, fairness, and correct reporting. No project is "too small" to ignore ethics.

Micro Skills

Crisp question (PICO if clinical): "In first-year MBBS students (P), does a structured sleep-hygiene handout (I) compared with usual advice (C) reduce daytime sleepiness at 4 weeks (O)?" PICO is a tool to frame a structured research question that includes **P**opulation, **I**ntervention, **C**omparison and **O**utcome. (2)

Literature review: Search PubMed/Google Scholar to refine the idea and avoid duplication.

Study design: Begin with a simple design. A mini-survey, clinical audit, case series, or a small cohort. Keep it feasible in terms of time and scope.

Study protocol: Write a 2-3 page protocol including objectives, methods, input and outcome variables, a basic statistical analysis outline (percentages, means, chi-square/t-test), and a consent plan.

Research guide: Find a mentor and obtain IEC approval. Even surveys involving people or identifiable data need oversight.

Piloting: Test the form with a few records or participants; revise unclear items.

Analyze: Focus on effect sizes and confidence intervals; state any deviations from the plan.

Share and discuss: Present a poster, write for a student journal, or submit to ICMR-STS during vacations. Understand, what will we do differently next time? (3)

Explain to study participants in plain language:

"This study aims to understand X. If you join, we will do Y. Participants may not benefit directly, but the findings may help future patients. Participation is voluntary, information remains confidential, and participants can withdraw anytime."

Essential Medical Statistics

Statistics is not just formulas; it turns observations into valid conclusions. We use statistical formulas and tests to analyze and validate every guideline, investigation, and risk score before implementing them. A few core ideas help learners confidently read papers, ask more effective questions, and contribute responsibly to the science that informs patient care.

Mean, Median, Mode: Mean, median, and mode are three different ways to determine the central value of a dataset. These are also referred to as measures of central tendency. The mean is the arithmetic average. The median is the middle value in a dataset ordered from smallest to largest. The mode is the number that appears most frequently in the dataset.

Spread of data: Standard deviation (SD) and interquartile range (IQR) describe the spread or variation of data, indicating how tightly or loosely the data clusters. SD measures the distance of each data point from the mean, providing a comprehensive measure of spread for data with normal or symmetrical distributions. IQR (Q1-Q3), which measures the spread of the middle 50% of the data, is a more robust tool for asymmetrical data or a dataset with a skewed distribution.

Null Hypothesis: When comparing two groups (e.g., mean BP fall with Drug A vs Drug B), there is a question whether the observed difference is a random chance or it is real. We assume (hypothesize) there is no real difference, and the observed difference is just a random chance. This is called the **null hypothesis**. We apply different statistical tests to examine whether the observed difference can reject the null hypothesis. This is to rule out the possibility that the result is due to chance. We cannot eliminate the chance element, but conventionally, if the probability of 'no difference' (observed difference being 'by chance') is less than 5%, the difference is considered statistically significant enough to reject the null hypothesis.

P-value: We calculate the difference between the two groups using statistical tests. The p-value is the probability of 'no difference' between the two groups. A p-value of 0.05 indicates a 5% probability that this result could be due to chance.

Conventionally, if the p-value is <0.05, you have evidence against the null, or the difference is statistically significant. If p is large (>0.05), your data are compatible with 'no difference', or the observed difference is not statistically significant.

Sample size: P-values depend on the number of participants included in the study (sample size). Large samples can make tiny, trivial differences 'significant,' while small samples can miss real effects. So the p-value is reliable (or the study is valid) only if the study sample includes a certain number of participants. This number can be calculated and is called the sample size, a prerequisite for your study proposal.

Mean or median gives a point estimate of the average for the population based on your study sample. There is uncertainty since it is a sample, not the whole population. This estimate might be slightly off from the actual average for the whole population. Always report confidence interval (CI) and effect size (e.g., mean difference) to make it meaningful.

A confidence interval (CI) is a range of values that indicates the level of certainty we have in our estimate. For example, suppose we calculate the average height of students to be 164 cm and find a 95% CI from 160 to 170 cm. It means we are reasonably confident that the true average height of all students in the population lies somewhere between 160 and 170 cm. The "95%" comes from the method we used: if we repeated this whole study many times, about 95 out of 100 such intervals would capture the true average. The CI does not mean that 95% of students are between 160 and 170 cm, or that the sample mean will fall in that range. It only means we are confident that the true population mean is in that interval.

Think of a CI like fishing with a net - sometimes the net (CI) will catch the true fish (the real mean), sometimes it will not. However, if the net is designed to succeed 95% of the time, we can trust it.

Effect Size: Effect size indicates the 'size' or 'magnitude' of a result - how large the difference is between groups or how strong the relationship is between variables. The p-value only indicates whether an effect is statistically significant (unlikely by chance phenomenon), but the effect size shows whether that effect is practically meaningful in the real world. A larger effect size indicates a greater impact or a stronger relationship. Different measures of effect size include relative risk, odds ratio, correlation, and Pearson coefficient.

Relative Risk (RR) and Odds Ratio (OR) are standard measures of effect size and association between an exposure and an outcome. RR is the ratio of the risk (probability) of an event in an exposed group to that in a non-exposed group, commonly used for prospective and cohort studies. Odds ratio is the ratio of the odds of the event in the exposed group to those in the non-exposed group, commonly used for retrospective or case-control studies where exposure has already happened. Both help quantify how much an exposure changes risk. Always pair them with CIs.

Diagnostic Accuracy: Sensitivity is a diagnostic test's ability to correctly identify individuals with a disease (true positives), minimizing false negatives. Specificity is a test's ability to correctly identify individuals without the disease (true negatives), minimizing false positives. There is often a trade-off, where increasing one measure decreases the other, and choosing a test's cutoff point impacts both. **Positive Predictive Value (PPV)** is the probability that a person actually has a disease, given a positive test result. **Negative Predictive Value (NPV)** is the probability that a person does not have the disease, given a negative test result. PPV and NPV are important measures of diagnostic test performance that depend on the disease's prevalence in the population, unlike sensitivity and specificity, which are properties of the test itself. This means they must be recalculated if you apply the same test to a different population with a different disease prevalence.

How to Read a Paper

Research question: How clear is the research question on the population, intervention/exposure, comparator and outcomes (PICO) framework?

Check the design: RCT, cohort, case-control, cross-sectional, or diagnostic accuracy? Is the design fit for the question?

Sampling & flow: Information about inclusion and exclusion criteria, losses to follow-up, and whether the sample represents the patients coming to the hospital.

Outcomes: Identify the primary outcome and when and how it was measured.

Effect and precision: Look for RR, OR, mean difference and CI. Interpret clinical importance, not only p-values.

Harms & subgroup analyses: Are adverse events measured? Check if subgroups are pre-specified and adequately powered, or if they are an afterthought based on observations.

Ethics and Applicability: Note approval by the ethics committee and obtain patient consent. Consider feasibility, costs, and patient values as well as applicability of study findings in different settings. (4)

Starting First Project

Ask a focused question: "What proportion of upper respiratory tract infection patients coming to our OPD are prescribed at least one antibiotic?"

Select a design: Start with simple studies such as an audit or quality improvement (QI) project, survey, case series, or a small cohort.

Plan methods: Define variables, decide data sheet, and a statistical analysis plan, such as proportions with 95% CIs; chi-square for pre-post change.

Permissions: Discuss with a mentor beforehand. Obtain ethics approval, anonymize data and ensure secure storage.

Analyze simply: Prepare descriptive summaries (mean/median, percentages), analytic reports. Run basic tests as applicable for the type of data (t-test, chi-square), plots (bar/box). Include effect sizes and CIs.

Tools: Prepare clean data in spreadsheets. Utilise freely available tools or library subscriptions. R, Jamovi, or SPSS are a few examples.

Write and share: Write in a structured format with an abstract, background, method, results, discussion and conclusion. Present your work locally for feedback before submitting it for publication. Maintain authorship transparency and data integrity.

Learning Points

- Statistics help ask sharper questions, read evidence wisely, and change practice responsibly.
- Precision (CI) and magnitude (effect size) speak louder than p-values alone.
- Good design up front prevents most analytic headaches later.
- Ethical approval, data privacy, and honest reporting are non-negotiable.
- Audits, surveys, case series, and small student projects are excellent, achievable entry points.

Case Snapshot: A Small Audit, A Big Change

A student team audits hand-hygiene compliance against the WHO's five moments in the paediatric OPD over one week. Baseline compliance is 48%. After a 10-minute reminder huddle each morning and placing an alcohol rub at every desk, a repeat audit shows 71% compliance (a 23% difference, 95% CI 14-32). The team presents to the hospital infection-control committee; the huddles become a standing practice.

Why this works: It had a specific question, measurable outcome, simple, attainable and reproducible methods, minimal risk, and clinical relevance.

Coffee Moment

When numbers start to blur, remember: every data point began as a person who trusted the system to learn and do better. Let curiosity and humility guide you, and integrity protect your patients. Start small, think clearly, and keep returning to the question: Does this help us provide better care?

References

1. Hulley SB, Cummings SR, Browner WS, Grady DG, Newman TB. Designing

clinical research. 4th ed. Lippincott Williams & Wilkins; 2013.
2. Straus SE, Glasziou P, Richardson WS, Haynes RB. Evidence-Based Medicine: How to Practice and Teach EBM. 5th ed. Elsevier; 2019.
3. ICMR. National Ethical Guidelines for Biomedical and Health Research Involving Human Participants. New Delhi: ICMR; 2017.
4. Greenhalgh T. How to read a paper: the basics of evidence-based medicine. 6th ed. Wiley; 2019.

Chapter 89: Evidence-Based Medicine

Introduction

Evidence-based medicine (EBM) is not research for researchers. It is a practical way of thinking that helps us answer a daily question, such as what is the best next step for this patient? EBM combines the best current evidence, clinical expertise, and the patient's values and context to make scientifically sound and humane decisions. (1)

The 5 Steps of EBM

- **Ask** a focused question (PICO: Patient/Problem, Intervention, Comparator, Outcome). (2)
- **Acquire** the most reliable evidence promptly (summaries, guidelines, systematic reviews).
- **Appraise** for quality: risk of bias, precision (CI), effect size, and applicability.
- **Apply** to patients, weighing benefits, harms, costs, and preferences.
- **Assess** the outcome and process; incorporate learning into practice (audit/QI).

Reading Evidence Without Getting Lost

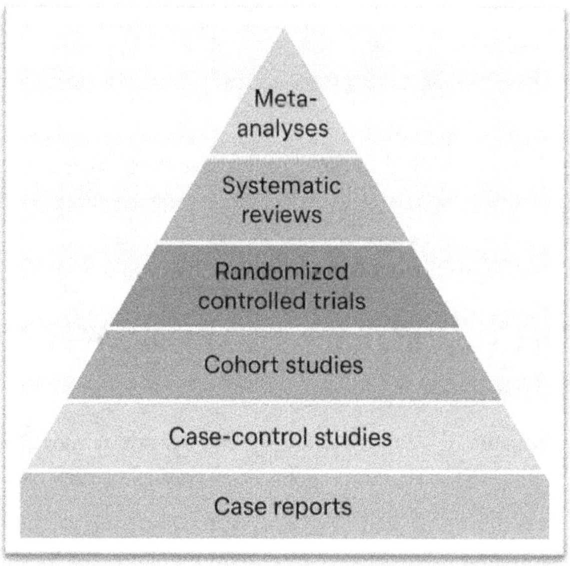

Figure 89.1: Hierarchy of Evidence Pyramid.

Hierarchy of evidence: Systematic reviews & meta-analyses → RCTs → cohort → case-control → cross-sectional → case series/reports → expert opinion. Quality still matters at every level. (3)

Effect sizes beat p-values: Look for absolute risk reduction (ARR), relative risk (RR/OR), number needed to treat (NNT) or harm (NNH), and their confidence intervals.

Internal validity: Were randomization, concealment and blinding adequate? Were the groups similar? Were outcomes predefined?

External validity: Are the patients, setting, and resources similar to your setting?

GRADE basics

Clinical practice guidelines commonly employ the GRADE (Grading of Recommendations, Assessment, Development, and Evaluation) approach to communicate the level of confidence in the available evidence and the strength of a recommendation.

The level of confidence is classified as **high, moderate, low, or very low**, reflecting the likelihood that future research may alter our confidence in the estimated effect of an intervention. High-certainty evidence means we are very confident in the results, whereas low or very low certainty indicates substantial uncertainty.

The strength of recommendation is described as **strong or conditional (weak)**. A strong recommendation suggests that most informed patients would choose the recommended action and that clinicians can generally apply it to most situations. A conditional or weak recommendation suggests that the best course of action may vary depending on the patient's values, clinical context, resource availability, or feasibility.

Therefore, guideline recommendations are **not rigid rules**. Clinicians must interpret them in light of the individual patient's condition, preferences, risks, benefits, and the local healthcare setting before deciding how closely to follow a recommendation. This approach supports evidence-based yet patient-centred care. (4)

Shared Decision-Making: EBM and AETCOM

EBM is an ethical practice for patient-centred care.

Patient involvement in decision making: Discuss available options. 'This one works better but is costlier and needs daily visits; this one is cheaper and available in our pharmacy. What matters most to you?'

Use precise language: Option A vs Option B. Employ teach-back methods like 'can you tell me in your own words what we decided?'. Record the discussion, especially if care is limited by availability or cost.

EBM in the Local Context

- **Adapt to resources:** A "gold-standard" imaging test may be unavailable or unaffordable; use clinical criteria or point-of-care alternatives.

- **Equity perspective:** Weigh factors like travel distance, follow-up feasibility, and cost, essential for adherence and results.
- **Legal and ethical care:** Document the reasoning behind the treatment option selected, supporting evidence, other options discussed, and consent or refusal. Proper documentation is important for the safety of patients and the treating team.

Case Snapshot

A 6-month-old presents with cough and increased work of breathing; SpO_2 is 89% in room air, chest is full of wheezes. A colleague suggests a nebulized bronchodilator and steroids "to be safe."

Ask (PICO): In infants with bronchiolitis (P), do bronchodilators (I) versus supportive care (C) improve clinical outcomes (O)?

Acquire: A quick search of systematic reviews and guidelines reveals high-quality evidence that the routine use of bronchodilators and systemic steroids does not improve length of stay or reduce the need for oxygen; supportive care remains essential.

Appraise: Multiple RCTs and meta-analyses show consistent findings, low risk of bias, and strong recommendations against routine use of bronchodilators.

Apply: Start oxygen to maintain $SpO_2 \geq 92\%$, perform nasal suction, ensure hydration, and educate caregivers. Consider a single trial of bronchodilator to identify if there is a clear, immediate clinical response. Do not use steroids.

Assess: Monitor respiratory rate, feeding, and SpO_2; re-evaluate every 2-4 hours. Document the evidence included and the shared decision with parents.

Outcome: Infant stabilizes with supportive care, and respiratory distress improved over the next 2 days. No routine steroids or bronchodilators are administered. Parents understand warning signs at home and follow up.

Why this is EBM: Clear question, rapid retrieval, critical appraisal, context-sensitive application, respectful communication, and documentation.

☕ Coffee Moment

EBM is not about being perfectly "textbook." It is about being honest with uncertainty, curious about better answers, and inclusive in involving the person (or family) whose life is in front of you. Ask in a structured way, acquire and appraise the evidence, decide together, and let each patient interaction start teaching you how science becomes care.

References

1. Sackett DL, Rosenberg WM, Gray JA, Haynes RB, Richardson WS. Evidence based medicine: what it is and what it isn't. BMJ. 1996;312(7023):71–2.
2. Guyatt G, Rennie D, Meade MO, Cook DJ. Users' guides to the medical literature: a manual for evidence-based clinical practice. 3rd ed. McGraw-Hill; 2015.
3. Murad MH, Asi N, Alsawas M, Alahdab F. New evidence pyramid. Evid Based Med. 2016;21(4):125–7.
4. Schünemann HJ, Brożek J, Guyatt G, Oxman AD, eds. GRADE handbook. The GRADE Working Group; 2013.

Chapter 90: Accessing Online Resources

Introduction

Medicine never stands still. What was true last decade may be obsolete today. A good doctor, therefore, does not memorize everything but knows where to look and how to judge what is reliable. Accessing authentic online resources is an important professional skill. Whether you're clarifying a rare diagnosis, exploring the latest guideline, or preparing your research project, the best evidence is a few clicks away. This chapter will help you navigate this with clarity and confidence.

Evidence-based medicine (EBM) rests on three pillars: The best available research evidence, clinical expertise, and patient values. To apply evidence, you must learn to find it. Searching effectively saves time, prevents misinformation, and ensures that every clinical or research decision is based on reliable data. This skill lays the foundation for a lifetime of scientific curiosity and responsible practice. (1,2)

Your Gateway to Evidence and Research

The Core Databases Every Medical Student Should Know are listed below

Table 90.1: List of resources for evidence search

Resource	What It Offers	How to Use It Effectively
PubMed pubmed	The largest biomedical literature database by the U.S. National Library of Medicine.	Use Medical Subject Headings (MeSH with Boolean operators (AND, OR, NOT) for precise search. Apply filters for date, age group, article type. (3)
Cochrane Library Cochrane	Evidence-based systematic reviews and meta-analyses.	Summary of multiple trials into one high-quality synthesis for treatment recommendations. (4)
Embase **embase.com**	Biomedical and pharmacological literature.	Use Emtree terms. Often used for systematic reviews along with PubMed.
UpToDate **uptodate.com**	Point-of-care clinical summaries written by global experts, updated daily.	Ideal for quick clinical queries, protocols, and management updates. Widely available in institutions.
ClinicalTrials Link	Global Registry of ongoing & completed clinical trials.	Explore interventions under investigation, methodology, and outcomes.
Google Scholar Link	Academic search engine.	Useful for finding grey literature, and cross-disciplinary works.

Toolkit Beyond Databases

Once you have retrieved reliable evidence, the next step is to manage, analyse, and present it. The following tools are helpful.

Table 90.2: List of resources for evidence analysis and referencing

Purpose	Tool	Why It's Useful
Reference Management	Zotero, Mendeley	Save PDFs, insert citations in Word, and auto-generate bibliographies.
Statistical Analysis	SPSS, R, Prism GraphPad	For descriptive and inferential statistics in research projects.
Meta-analysis	RevMan, JASP	Used for pooling data from multiple studies; Cochrane reviews use RevMan.
Plagiarism & Writing Support	Grammarly, Turnitin, QuillBot	Maintain clarity, grammar, and originality in writing.
Data Visualization	Tableau, Power BI, Google Data Studio	Create infographics and dashboards for presentations or publications.

Step-by-Step: How to Search for Evidence

Frame your question using the PICO model

P – Patient or Problem

I – Intervention

C – Comparison

O – Outcome

Example: In children with pneumonia (**P**), does oral amoxicillin (**I**) compared to IV ceftriaxone (**C**) reduce hospital stay (**O**)?

Select the right database

- Use PubMed or Embase for primary studies.
- Use Cochrane for high-quality systematic reviews.
- Use UpToDate for clinical summaries.

Use search strategies wisely

Combine keywords with Boolean operators:
pneumonia AND (amoxicillin OR azithromycin)
Apply filters such as 'human', 'English', 'last 5 years', and 'RCT'.

Read abstracts critically

Review the study design, sample size, outcome measures, and methods for controlling bias.

Appraise quality

Prefer RCTs, meta-analyses, and cohort studies over case reports or editorials. Learn to interpret p-values, confidence intervals, and effect sizes.

Store and cite correctly

- Save full-text articles in Zotero/Mendeley.
- Generate citations in Vancouver or APA format.
- Keep a separate "Evidence Logbook" for reference.

Reflect and apply

Ask: How does this evidence change my understanding or my next clinical step?
Ethical and Practical Guidelines
Use institutional subscriptions; avoid pirated PDFs.
Cite the sources using acceptable citation style with no plagiarism.
Beware of predatory journals, check indexing (PubMed, Scopus).
Ensure data privacy, do not upload patient information to online tools.
Balance technology with thinking: Databases assist you, but clinical judgment is yours alone.

Case Scenario

A 2-year-old child presents with recurrent wheezing. You recall reading conflicting management guidelines for bronchiolitis. Instead of relying on hearsay, you open PubMed, use "bronchiolitis AND nebulized hypertonic saline AND randomized controlled trial" as your search phrase.
Within minutes, you find recent meta-analyses showing limited benefit.
You discuss this evidence with your faculty, that's the moment you realize: research literacy saves real lives.

Learning Points

- Accessing authentic databases is a professional responsibility.
- Learn to use MeSH and Boolean search techniques early.
- Evaluate the level of evidence: not all studies are equal.
- Use citation managers to stay organized.

☕Coffee Moment

The next time you open PubMed, don't just look for a quick answer. Look for understanding. Each search is a small step toward becoming the kind of doctor who heals with both science and soul.

References

1. Guyatt GH, Rennie D, Meade MO, Cook DJ, editors. Users' Guides to the Medical Literature: A Manual for Evidence-Based Clinical Practice. 3rd ed. New York: McGraw-Hill Education; 2015.
2. Greenhalgh T. How to Read a Paper: The Basics of Evidence-Based Medicine and Healthcare. 6th ed. Hoboken (NJ): Wiley-Blackwell; 2019.
3. U.S. National Library of Medicine. PubMed Overview. Bethesda (MD): National Center for Biotechnology Information; 2024 [cited 2025 Oct 10]. Available from: https://pubmed.ncbi.nlm.nih.gov
4. Higgins JPT, Thomas J, Chandler J, Cumpston M, Li T, Page MJ, Welch VA, editors. Cochrane Handbook for Systematic Reviews of Interventions. Version 6.3. London: The Cochrane Collaboration; 2022.

Chapter 91: Vaccination and Immunization Schedule

Introduction

Immunization is one of the most powerful tools in medicine. It is not a timetable to remember but a complete patient-safety system to prevent disability, death, and outbreaks. Before you heal others, you must protect yourself. This chapter orients you to your immunization requirement, post-exposure prophylaxis related to occupational risks, the National Immunization Schedule (NIS/UIP) for children, and the vaccine requirement for international travel. (1)

Immunization for Healthcare Professionals

As a healthcare professional, you are at increased risk of exposure to infectious diseases. Immunization is not only personal protection; it's a duty to patients, colleagues, and your own family. (2-3)

Table 91.1: List of vaccines for healthcare workers

Vaccine	Schedule / Dose	Remarks / Notes
Hepatitis B	3 doses at 0, 1, and 6 months if unimmunized; antibody titre to guide	Booster if anti-HBs <10 mIU/mL after 5 years
Tetanus, Diphtheria	One booster every 10 years (Td/Tdap)	Tdap preferred if not received earlier
Influenza (Seasonal)	Single dose annually (before flu season)	For ICU, pediatric, and elderly care areas
Varicella (Chickenpox)	If no prior infection: 2 doses, 4 - 8 weeks apart	Check history or IgG antibody status
COVID-19	As per national schedule and booster policy	Mandatory for clinical postings during outbreak
Optional (as per risk)	Hepatitis A, Typhoid, Rabies, Japanese Encephalitis	For specific high-risk exposures or areas

Why It Matters

Occupational Exposure: Healthcare professionals, including doctors, nurses, and students, frequently encounter blood, body fluids, and airborne pathogens that can transmit infections.

Preventing Transmission: Vaccination prevents healthcare workers from becoming carriers of infectious diseases to vulnerable patients.

Outbreak Control: Immunized staff help prevent hospital-based outbreaks (nosocomial infections).

Professional Responsibility: Many institutions and councils now require proof of vaccination upon entry or prior to posting.

Post-Exposure Prophylaxis

In hospitals, accidents happen: a needle prick, a blood splash, a torn glove. It can transmit infections like Hepatitis B, Hepatitis C, or HIV. Post-Exposure Prophylaxis (PEP) is the emergency protocol to prevent infection after exposure. The key is speed and accuracy: act within minutes. (4,5)

Step 1: What to Do Immediately

Table 91.2: Immediate actions after exposure

Type of Exposure	Immediate Action
Needle-stick or cut	Wash the area thoroughly with soap and running water (do not scrub or squeeze). Do not use antiseptics like spirit or bleach.
Mucous membrane exposure (eyes, mouth)	Rinse with copious amounts of clean water or saline.
Broken skin or splash	Wash gently with soap and water; avoid harsh rubbing.

Report the incident immediately to the infection control nurse, your supervising resident, and the institutional PEP officer.

Step 2: Assess the Risk

Source status: Is the patient known or suspected to have HIV, HBV, or HCV?

Type of exposure: Hollow-bore needle (high risk), superficial scratch (low risk), mucosal splash, etc.

Vaccination status: Are you vaccinated for Hepatitis B, and what is your antibody titre level?

Step 3: Disease-Specific PEP

HIV: Start antiretroviral therapy (TDF + 3TC + DTG) or equivalent 3-drug regimen within 2 hours (maximum 72 hours), and continue for 28 days. Baseline and follow-up HIV testing should be done at 6 weeks, 3 months, and 6 months.

Hepatitis B: If vaccinated and anti-HBs titre is ≥10 mIU/mL, no action needed. If vaccinated but titer <10 mIU/mL, a booster dose is needed. If unvaccinated, administer HBIG (0.06 mL/kg IM) and initiate the vaccine series (0, 1, 6 months) within 24 hours. Check the HBsAg status of the source.

Hepatitis C: No approved PEP protocol. Monitor for HCV RNA and LFTs at baseline, 4-6 weeks, and 3 months. Early detection will ensure prompt treatment.

Step 4: Documentation and Follow-up

Record exposure details (date, time, nature, source, site, and actions taken).

Obtain consent for source testing if possible.

Report to the institutional infection control / PEP register.

Attend follow-up testing as per protocol.

Prevention

Use gloves and eye protection goggles. Ensure safe disposal of sharps.

Never recap used needles.

Know the location of your PEP kit in every posting area.

Maintain full Hepatitis B immunization and annual antibody check.

The National Immunization Schedule

- **At birth:** BCG, Hepatitis-B birth dose and OPV-0 (zero dose).
- **Infancy (at 6, 10, and 14 weeks):** Pentavalent 1–3 (DPT + Hep-B + Hib); OPV 1–3, IPV 1–2 (usually at 6 and 14 weeks); Rotavirus 1–3 (oral); PCV 1–2 (in UIP districts/states).
- **9–12 months:** MR-1 (Measles-Rubella); PCV booster (where PCV is implemented) and JE-1 (in identified endemic districts).
- **16–24 months:** DPT 1st booster, OPV booster, MR-2, JE-2 (endemic areas).
- **5–6 years:** DPT 2nd booster.
- **Adolescents:** Td at 10 years and 16 years.
- **Pregnancy:** Td (2-dose schedule or one booster if previously vaccinated).
- **Vitamin A supplementation:** It is part of child health programs given from 9 months of age, but it is not a vaccine. (1)

Principles that keep the schedule safe and effective

Cold chain: Vaccines are protected if their storage is maintained correctly according to cold chain requirements. Observe vaccine vial monitors (VVMs) for efficacy, store them at a temperature of 2–8 °C, and never refreeze. (6)

Right child, right vaccine and right time: Verify identity of the child, check contraindications, and ensure age-appropriate dose, route, and site.

AEFI readiness: Ensure an anaphylaxis kit is available, observe the child for 30 minutes after vaccination, and be familiar with the reporting pathway.

Documentation and reminder systems: Update the vaccination record card and schedule the next visit before the family departs.

Communication: Use simple language 'fever and pain at vaccination site are common and settle with paracetamol; revisit if…".

Vaccine Counselling

Risk-benefit analysis: This prevents severe diseases, including TB meningitis, diphtheria, pertussis, and measles complications, among others. Mild fever can occur, but severe reactions are rare and manageable.

Equity & access: All vaccines in the national schedule are available free of charge in government facilities.

Myths: Vaccines do not cause autism, infertility, or weaken immunity. Breastfeeding and mild respiratory illness are not contraindications. (7)

Vaccines for International Travel

Travel medicine is an essential component of safe practice. Advise students and their families to plan 4-6 weeks in advance of departure.

Yellow Fever (YF): Required for entry into many African/South American countries (and re-entry into India from those areas) and administered at an authorized centre ≥10 days before travel. The International Certificate is valid for life.

Meningococcal (Against serogroups ACWY): Required for Hajj/Umrah pilgrimages and frequently advised for travel to dormitories or large gatherings.

Polio (IPV/OPV): Some countries require proof of polio vaccination for travellers arriving from or passing through polio-affected regions; check current advisories.

Hepatitis A and Typhoid vaccines: Highly recommended for numerous destinations in Asia and Africa; also beneficial within India for travellers who are not immunized.

MMR & Varicella: Ensure two documented doses or serologic immunity.

Influenza (seasonal): Particularly for elderly, pregnant travellers, and those with chronic disease.

Japanese Encephalitis: For extended rural stays in endemic parts.

Other region-specific recommendations: Rabies PrEP for adventure or animal-exposed travel; **Cholera** in rare, high-risk situations, as advised. (8)

Always check the latest IHR and consular requirements.

Vaccine Industry

The global vaccine industry is dominated by a few multinational giants such as Pfizer, Moderna, Sanofi, and GlaxoSmithKline, with advanced R&D ecosystems and strong regulatory frameworks. These companies have historically led innovation in novel platforms like mRNA and conjugate vaccines. In contrast, the Indian vaccine industry has emerged as the world's largest supplier by volume, led by institutions like the Serum Institute of India, Bharat Biotech, and Biological E. India plays a pivotal role in manufacturing affordable vaccines for global immunization programs, especially through partnerships with WHO, GAVI, and UNICEF. India produces 60% of the world's vaccine doses, largely through cost-effective manufacturing and WHO-prequalified facilities. While global players focus on cutting-edge innovation, Indian manufacturers are increasingly bridging this gap with cost-effective innovation, rapid scalability, and robust public-private collaboration, as seen during the COVID-19 pandemic.

Table 91.3: Examples of Indian Vaccines

Vaccine	Target Disease	Developer/ Manufacturer	Remarks
COVAXIN	COVID-19	Bharat Biotech	India's first indigenous COVID-19 vaccine; inactivated virus platform.
COVISHIELD	COVID 19	Serum Institute of India (SII)	Indian-manufactured version of Oxford–AstraZeneca vaccine.
Rotavac	Rotavirus (diarrhea)	Bharat Biotech	WHO prequalified; low-cost rotavirus vaccine used globally.
RUBYVAX	Measles-Rubella	Serum Institute of India	Widely used in India's MR immunization campaign.
TT and DT Vaccines	Tetanus, Diphtheria	Biological E, SII, Bharat Biotech	Used in India's Universal Immunization Programme (UIP).
Typhivax/ Tybar	Typhoid conjugate vaccine	Bharat Biotech / Biological E	WHO prequalified typhoid vaccines exported globally.
JENVAC	Japanese Encephalitis	Bharat Biotech	India's first indigenous JE vaccine.
iNCOVACC	COVID-19 (intranasal)	Bharat Biotech	World's first intranasal COVID-19 vaccine (non-invasive delivery).

Case Snapshot: The Missed Booster

An 18-month-old child is brought in with a cough. The record indicates that infant doses are complete, but there is no mention of the MR-2 or DPT booster. The mother assumed "all vaccines are complete." Action: Treat the cough and take the opportunity for catch-up vaccination. Administer MR-2, DPT and OPV boosters if due and schedule JE-2 if in an endemic district.

Why it matters: Opportunistic immunization prevents gaps that can lead to outbreaks.

Learning Points

- The NIS protects against serious infections from birth to adolescence. It maintains a vaccination chart by age groups.
- Document, counsel, and observe. These habits help prevent errors, ease anxiety, and foster trust.
- If some doses are missed, create a catch-up plan; do not restart the series.
- Healthcare workers require additional protection.
- Travel may require specific vaccines (e.g., YF, ACWY, polio, Hep A/Typhoid); plan accordingly.

☕ Coffee Moment

Each small drop in a vial holds decades of science and a parent's hope. When you open the immunization card, you are not simply ticking boxes but helping protect against diseases that once filled hospital wards. Learn the schedule, speak kindly, and use every clinic visit to keep a child and the community safer.

References

1. Government of India. National Immunization Schedule for Infants, Children and Pregnant Women. Ministry of Health and Family Welfare; 2022.
2. World Health Organization. Immunization of Health Workers: WHO Position Paper. Wkly Epidemiol Rec. 2022;97(15):185–208.
3. Ministry of Health and Family Welfare. National Immunization Schedule for Health Care Workers. Government of India; 2023.
4. World Health Organization. Post-Exposure Prophylaxis to Prevent HIV Infection: Guidelines. WHO Press; 2021.
5. National AIDS Control Organisation (NACO). Guidelines for HIV Post-Exposure Prophylaxis. Government of India; 2021.
6. World Health Organization. Immunization in practice: A practical guide for health staff. 2015 update. Geneva: WHO; 2015.
7. MacDonald NE, SAGE Working Group on Vaccine Hesitancy. Vaccine hesitancy: Definition, scope and determinants. Vaccine. 2015;33(34):4161–4.
8. Plotkin SA, Orenstein WA, Offit PA, Edwards KM. Plotkin's Vaccines. 7th ed. Elsevier; 2018.

Chapter 92: Biomedical Waste Management

Introduction

Biomedical waste (BMW) is not "someone else's job." Every bandage you remove, cannula you cut, or slide you prepare generates waste that can harm staff, patients, and the environment if mishandled. Knowing the colour codes and adhering to safe practices at the bedside is part of being a responsible doctor. (1)

Principles

- **Segregate at the source:** Dispose of waste in the correct container where it is generated, not later at the nursing station.
- **Four-colour system:** Yellow, Red, Blue, and White. Memorize what goes in each; do not mix.
- **3/4th rule:** Close and replace bags or containers when they are three-quarters full. Never overfill.
- **No recapping or hand-passing sharps:** Dispose of them immediately in a sharps container within arm's reach.
- Label & barcode as per hospital policy: Store for less than 48 hours.
- **Personal safety:** Hand hygiene, gloves or appropriate PPE, immunization (Hep-B, Td/Tdap, influenza), and immediate reporting of exposures.
- **Respect the team:** Avoid leaving risks for housekeeping staff; safety is everyone's responsibility.

BMW Colour Codes

Yellow (incineration or deep burial as per policy): Human and animal anatomical waste (such as placenta, tissue, and body parts), soiled waste (including blood-soaked dressings, cotton, and plaster casts), microbiology and culture plates, expired or contaminated medicines (for antibiotics and some cytotoxic drugs, follow your centre's specific guidance), and contaminated linen. Never put plastics or sharps here.

Red (autoclave, microwave or chemical disinfection → shred → recycle): Contaminated, recyclable plastic items include IV tubing and sets, catheters, cannula (without needle), syringes without fixed needles, gloves, urine bags, and suction tubing. No sharps. No glass. No paper.

White (Puncture, leak and tamper-proof, Translucent bin for sharps): Needles, blades, scalpels, syringes with fixed needles, and metal stylets. Do not recap; discard immediately after use. Treated through sterilization or encapsulation as per policy.

Blue (disinfection or autoclave → recycling): Glassware (broken vials and ampoules without medication residues), slides, and metallic implants removed from patients. Medicine vials with residual drugs typically follow the Yellow per local SOP.

Black (General Non-BMW for municipal stream): Paper wrappers, food waste, and kitchen waste should never be mixed with BMW. Hospitals may use black or green bins for disposal.

If you are unsure, ask the nurse-in-charge or check the ward poster before dropping off the item. Mixing at source is the leading cause of injuries and regulatory non-compliance. (1,2)

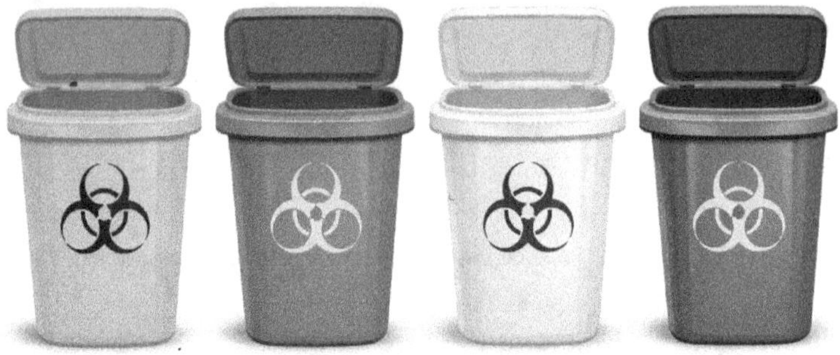

Figure 92.1: BMW Colour Codes Yellow, Red, White and Blue

Exposure & Spill: What to Do Now

Needle-stick or mucocutaneous exposure

- **Wash immediately** with soap and water; do not squeeze or use bleach.
- **Report** the incident immediately to designated officer and document the details.
- **Assess** the risk and immunization status.
- **Post-exposure prophylaxis (PEP)**: Initiate HIV PEP according to protocol (preferably within 2 hours). Check HBsAg and anti-HBs levels, and administer a booster or HBIG as needed. Update tetanus vaccination if necessary.
- **Conduct follow-up** testing and counselling as scheduled. (3)

Blood or body fluid spill

Restrict area → PPE → absorb → disinfect with approved agent and contact time → discard materials in correct colour bins → document.

Sharps Injury During Waste Handling

- Stop work immediately; encourage gentle bleeding without squeezing.
- Wash with soap and water; apply antiseptic.
- Report and document the incident promptly.

- Risk assessment and PEP as per needle-stick protocol.
- Reinforce no manual sorting or recapping of sharps.

Broken Glassware or Ampoule Injury

- Do not pick up fragments with your bare hands.
- Use forceps or scoop; discard into Blue or White bin as appropriate.
- Clean the area with disinfectant if contaminated.
- Manage cuts as per the sharps injury protocol if skin is breached.

Chemical Spill (Disinfectants, Laboratory Reagents)

- Evacuate and restrict the area.
- Use appropriate PPE (gloves, mask, eye protection).
- Neutralize or absorb using spill kit materials.
- Dispose of waste as per the chemical waste SOP.
- Report the spill; seek medical care if skin or eye exposure occurs.

Cytotoxic Drug Spill (Oncology Areas)

- Restrict access immediately.
- Use cytotoxic spill kit only; full PPE required and avoid aerosolization.
- Dispose of waste strictly in accordance with the cytotoxic waste protocol.
- Document and report to the pharmacy/oncology safety officer.

Exposure to Aerosol-Generating Procedures

(Suctioning, intubation, bronchoscopy)

- Ensure appropriate mask/respirator use.
- Follow hand hygiene and PPE doffing protocol after exposure.
- Report if unprotected exposure occurred.
- Risk assessment for TB, COVID-19, or other airborne infections.

Exposure During Transport of Biomedical Waste

- Stop transport immediately.
- Contain the spill; use PPE and absorbent materials.
- Decontaminate the trolley or transport container.
- Report to the Infection Control/Waste Management team.

Splash to Eyes, Nose, or Mouth

- Rinse immediately with clean water or saline for at least 10–15 minutes.

- Do not use disinfectants or irritants.
- Report exposure and assess need for PEP.
- Document and follow institutional protocol.

Case Snapshot: The Red Bag Mistake

A student drops a needle into the red BMW bag after IV cannulation. Later, a housekeeping worker sustains a finger prick while handling the bag. The incident triggers PEP, counselling, and an internal audit. (4)

What changed: Sharps boxes were placed on every bedside trolley; students received a quick refresher on the four-colour system and the 3/4th rule. Over the next month, incidents of mixed waste decreased by 70%.

Lesson: One moment of inattention can endanger colleagues; systems help, but habits protect.

☕ Coffee Moment

When we use the correct bin, we protect a person we may never meet, such as the worker who keeps our ward clean, the child living near the landfill, or the colleague who trusts our habits. BMW management is committed to upholding ethics in its daily practices.

References

1. Ministry of Environment, Forest and Climate Change. Biomedical Waste Management Rules. New Delhi: Govt of India; 2016 (amended 2018).
2. Central Pollution Control Board (CPCB). Guidelines for management of healthcare waste as per BMW Rules. 2020.
3. World Health Organization. Safe management of wastes from health-care activities. 2nd ed. Geneva: WHO; 2014.
4. Chartier Y, Emmanuel J, Pieper U, Prüss A, Rushbrook P, Stringer R, et al. Safe management of wastes from health-care activities. Geneva: WHO; 2014.

Chapter 93: Hand Hygiene, Universal Precautions and PPE

Introduction

Some habits save many lives. Hand hygiene is a simple and cost-effective measure to prevent hospital-acquired infections. According to WHO estimates, hand hygiene can reduce healthcare-associated infections by up to 50%. (1,2) It reflects respect for patients, colleagues, and us. Each time we clean our hands, we uphold the principle of *"do no harm." (1)* Every patient deserves safe care, and every doctor deserves safety while giving it. Universal precautions are the golden rules of infection control, while personal protective equipment (PPE) serves as your shield against risk.

Universal precautions

Universal precautions are the golden rules of infection control: simple actions that protect both healthcare workers and patients from infections that spread through blood, body fluids, and secretions. They are called universal because they must be followed for every patient, every time, regardless of diagnosis or appearance. (3,4)

Hand Hygiene

WHO recommends the five moments for hand hygiene.

- Before touching a patient.
- Before clean/aseptic procedures.
- After body fluid exposure.
- After touching a patient.
- After touching the patient's surroundings. (1)

Steps of Handwashing

Wash with soap and water or alcohol-based hand rub. It takes 20–30 seconds with sanitizer and about 40–60 seconds with soap and water.

- Rub palms together.
- Rub the back of each hand with the other palm.
- Interlace fingers and rub.
- Interlock fingers and rub the backs of fingers.
- Rub each thumb in a rotating manner.
- Rub the tips of fingers in the opposite palm.
- Rub wrists and let them air-dry. (1,5)

Core Principles

- Treat all blood and body fluids as potentially infectious.
- Hand hygiene is the single most effective measure for preventing infections.
- Use appropriate PPE (gloves, masks, gowns, eye protection).
- Handle sharps safely: no recapping, bending, or overfilling bins.

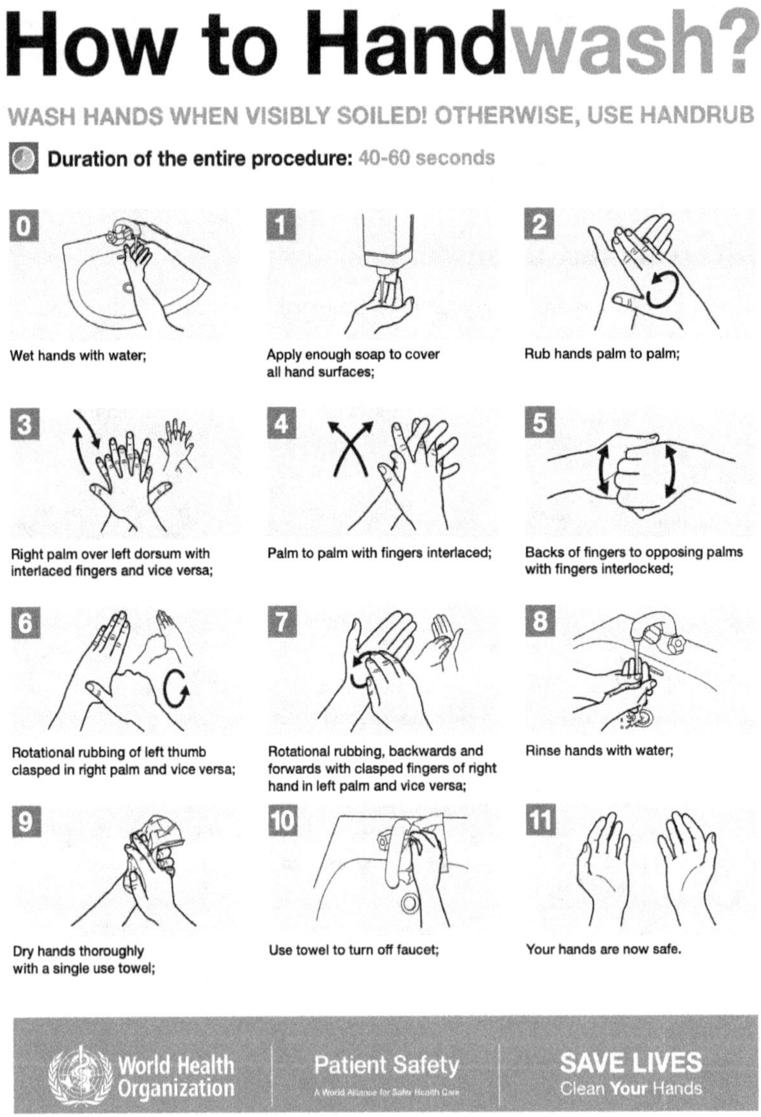

Figure 93.1: Steps for Hand Wash

(Used with permission from WHO)

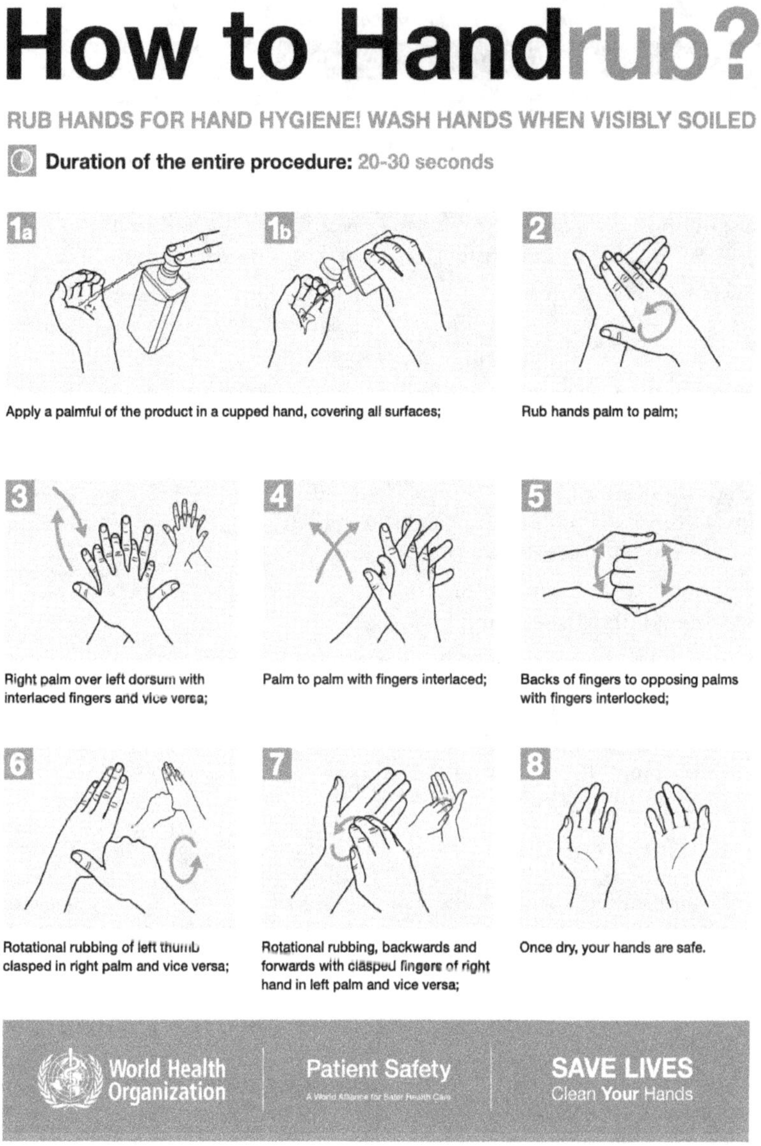

Figure 93.2: Steps for Hand Rub

(Used with permission from WHO)

- Follow the safe disposal of biomedical waste as per the colour-coded bins.
- Disinfect surfaces and equipment after each use.
- Ensure proper vaccination (especially Hepatitis B).
- Report and manage exposures promptly (follow PEP protocol).
- Personal Protective Equipment (PPE): Your Safety Shield

Table 93.1: Use of different personal protective equipment

PPE Item	Purpose	When to Use	Key Points
Gloves	Protects hands from contact with blood/body fluids	All patient contact, blood draws, procedures	Change between patients; do not reuse
Mask / Respirator	Protects from droplets or airborne pathogens	Aerosol-generating procedures, respiratory patients	Fit snugly; N95 for TB/COVID care
Gown / Apron	Prevents contamination of clothing and skin	Handling fluids, wound dressings, surgery	Remove before leaving patient area
Eye protection (goggles/face shield)	Shields from splashes	Suctioning, surgery, deliveries	Clean and disinfect after use
Head cap / Shoe covers	Prevents contamination in sterile areas	OT, delivery rooms, ICUs	Dispose as per BMW guidelines

Case Snapshot: Missed Step

During her internship in the pediatric ward, Dr Aarti examined a child with diarrhoea. She put on gloves but forgot to wash her hands. The next day, two more children developed diarrhoea in the same ward. Aarti realized that gloves are *not* a substitute for handwashing.

☕ Coffee Moment

Over a quick coffee, a senior tells: "You will forget formulas, you will Google drug doses, but your patients will remember if you touched them with clean hands or not. Every handshake with a patient begins with hand hygiene."

References

1. World Health Organization. WHO guidelines on hand hygiene in health care. Geneva: WHO; 2009.
2. Pittet D, Allegranzi B, Boyce J. The World Health Organization Guidelines on Hand Hygiene in Health Care and their consensus recommendations. Infect Control Hosp Epidemiol. 2009;30(7):611–22.
3. World Health Organization. Practical Guidelines for Infection Prevention and Control in Health Care Facilities. WHO; 2021.
4. Ministry of Health and Family Welfare. National Guidelines for Infection Prevention and Control in Healthcare Facilities. Government of India; 2020.
5. Allegranzi B, Pittet D. Role of hand hygiene in healthcare-associated infection prevention. J Hosp Infect. 2009;73(4):305–15.

Resonance

Resonance is the echo that lingers after a sound - the vibration that connects hearts. In medicine, it is the human connection: empathy, listening, communication, and leadership without authority.

This section teaches you the art of soft skills, where your words, gestures, and silences become instruments of healing that resonate far beyond the clinic. These are not skills you'll find on your final exam. But they may be the ones that save a life, mend a heart, or bring you peace after a long shift.

They are soft only in name; in truth, they are the steel threads of a doctor's soul.

Before you learn to hold a scalpel, learn to hold a hand. Before you cure the illness, listen to the pain.

Never forget the quiet language of kindness in the noise of beeping monitors and ticking charts.

S No.	Resonance: At a Glance
	Part 1 **Professional Soft Skills**
1.	**Chapter 94** Empathy: How to Win Hearts in a Hospital Beyond sympathy: stepping into the patient's shoes and making presence itself a treatment.
2.	**Chapter 95** The Listener's Touch: Doctor Who Hears Active listening as clinical work: how silence, nods, and summaries can uncover the truth behind symptoms.
3.	**Chapter 96** Remembering Names & Faces: Building Connection Names restore dignity, prevent errors, and build bridges of trust between patients and colleagues.
4.	**Chapter 97** Power of Appreciation The medicine of gratitude: how timely, specific thanks can energize teams and prevent burnout.
5.	**Chapter 98** Building Trust: The Golden Bridge Trust as the hidden currency of medicine: the foundation of safety, learning, and collaboration.
6.	**Chapter 99** Situational Awareness: Seeing the Whole Picture From scattered details to safe action: developing the sharp eye that prevents harm before it happens.
7.	**Chapter 100** Doctoring with Diplomacy: Criticism, Conflict, and Conversations Grace under fire: scripts and strategies to turn tension into teamwork and criticism into growth.

Chapter 94: Empathy- How to Win Hearts in a Hospital

Introduction

Medicine is more than tests and treatments; it's the art of being present when someone is frightened, in pain, or alone. Empathy transforms clinical knowledge into compassionate care, and patients can feel the difference.(1)

Key Concepts

Empathy ≠ Sympathy: Sympathy means 'I feel bad for you.' Empathy means 'I am with you and I am listening.' (2)

Presence over performance: Attention is at eye level, and short silences are signals that show care.

Dignity first: View the person beyond the diagnosis, safeguard privacy, modesty, and boundaries.

Cultural humility: Ask, don't assume about language, beliefs, decision-makers, and affordability.

Clinical impact: Empathy enhances adherence, decreases conflicts and complaints, and can lead to better outcomes, particularly in chronic and palliative care.

Micro Skills

- **Begin with identity & consent**: Namaste, Ashish ji. I am Riya, a medical student with Dr Jaiman. May I sit and talk for a minute?
- **Open and wait**: 'What worries you most right now?' Pause. Let them speak.
- **Show you're listening**: Sit at eye level, use gentle nods. Summarise: So the swelling and breathlessness worsen at night, and confirm - did I get that right?
- **Validate feelings**: It's understandable to feel scared. Anyone would.
- **Explain in plain language**: We will start medication to remove excess fluid that will help with breathing. I will return after the tests to review the next steps.
- **Check understanding (teach-back)**: 'To be sure I explained it well, please tell me how you will take this tablet?'
- **Close the loop & document**: 'Thank you for all the information. Do you have any questions?' Write in notes: plan discussed, addressed fears, teach-back done.
- **Avoid**: 'Don't worry,' jokes about illness, rushing the door handle, or discussing sensitive issues in the presence of others. (2,3)

Case Snapshot

Ravi, a second-year MBBS student, entered the pediatric ward during his clinical posting. He noticed a 5-year-old boy receiving chemotherapy for leukaemia and his mother sitting beside. The child's frail frame and the tears in the mother's eyes made Ravi unsettled. Unsure of what to say, he blurted, 'I am so sorry for you. It must be so hard. I don't know how you manage.' The mother gave a faint smile but looked away, her grief untouched.

Later, his senior resident, Dr Shreya, walked over and gently sat beside the mother. 'This is a tough time for you. Would you like to share how he is doing now? I can sit with you for a few minutes.' Hearing these words, the mother's tears flowed freely, and she opened her heart about her child's illness, her fears, and the exhaustion of caregiving. Ravi was puzzled by the different response and asked Dr Shreya why his words did not help. She explained, 'Sympathy is when we feel for someone from a distance, but empathy is when we step into their shoes and feel with them. They don't need pity, they need presence, understanding, and a genuine connection.'

Core Concept: Empathy

This scenario highlights the importance of empathy as a vital professional skill in patient care. Ravi's statement, though well-intentioned, placed the mother in a position of helplessness by expressing pity. On the other hand, Dr Shreya validated the mother's emotions, invited dialogue, and offered presence without judgment.

Learning Points

Empathy strengthens trust and improves communication in the doctor–patient relationship. Patients value attentive presence more than sympathy. Medical students must practice active listening and compassionate language as part of their professional behaviour.

Coffee Moment

Sipping coffee, Ravi thought, 'Being a doctor goes beyond medical knowledge; it involves having compassion, ethical integrity, and effective communication.'

References

1. Mercer SW, Reynolds WJ. Empathy and quality of care. Br J Gen Pract. 2002;52(Suppl):S9–12.
2. Hojat M, Louis DZ, Markham FW, et al. Physicians' empathy and clinical outcomes for diabetic patients. Acad Med. 2011;86(3):359–64.
3. Neumann M, Bensing J, Mercer S, et al. Analyzing the "nature" and "specific effectiveness" of clinical empathy: A theoretical overview and contribution towards a theory-based research agenda. Patient Educ Couns. 2009;74(3):339–446

Chapter 95: The Listener's Touch- Doctor Who Hears

Introduction

Medicine begins when a patient feels safe enough to share their true story, long before the prescription. Listening is an active clinical skill that fosters trust, enhances diagnosis, and alleviates fear. In busy wards, your quiet attention is the first treatment you provide to a suffering patient. (1)

Listening to the Patient's World

A patient's story is more than a list of symptoms. It's a window into their home, habits, fears, and surroundings. Understanding how environment, lifestyle, and social context influence health is crucial for providing compassionate, community-based medicine. (2)

Key Concepts

- Environment and diseases: Air pollution, housing, hygiene, water quality, and occupation directly affect disease patterns.
- Social determinants: Poverty, education, gender, and culture influence when and how people seek healthcare. Careful listening uncovers social barriers, such as cost, caregiving issues, and transportation, that textbooks often overlook.
- Family perspective: Understanding family structure helps doctors see the emotional and caregiving ecosystem around a patient.
- Trust and empathy: Listening builds rapport, reduces anxiety, and improves adherence. Patients share crucial details only when they feel heard and safe.
- Therapeutic effect: Acknowledging emotions builds trust, reduces anxiety, and improves adherence. It translates into fewer tests, fewer complaints, and better patient care.

Micro Skills

Set the scene

Prioritize privacy and sit at eye level. Namaste, I'm a medical student with Dr Sharma. May I speak with you for a few minutes?

Open and wait

What are the problems you have? Wait and resist the urge to interrupt; let the silence work.

Show you're listening

Gentle nods, open posture, eye contact and minimal typing. Summarise at the end what you understand. (1)

Name the emotion (NURS tool):

- **N**ame - You seem anxious.
- **U**nderstand - Anyone would feel this way.
- **R**espect – You have managed it well so far.
- **S**upport - We'll plan this together.

Explain & check understanding

Teach-back- 'So how will you take your inhalers?'

Close the loop & document

Record chief complaints and worries, management plan, actions taken, and any safety-net advice.

Avoid saying 'don't worry,' rushed discussions, discussing confidential issues openly, or judging lifestyles and beliefs. (3,4)

Table 95.1: Communication tools in different clinical scenarios

Clinical Setting	Activity	Analyze
Hospital	Interview a patient and family member to understand daily challenges and living conditions.	Connect disease with environment and lifestyle.
Community: field visit or home visit	Observe sanitation, water source, cooking methods, and living conditions.	Recognize links between environment and illness.
Group discussion and debrief scenarios	Discuss how housing, pollution, or stigma affect health-seeking behaviors.	Strengthen understanding of social determinants.

Practices that improve interpersonal relationships

Practice active listening with friends. Look at their eyes, not your mobile screen, when talking.

- Ask: How can I help? Not What should I do?
- Celebrate others' wins loudly and sincerely. It brings warmth to relationships.
- Check in on your introverted peer; they are waiting for a friend.
- With family, schedule at least 10 minutes of daily communication. Share your joys and sorrows, even insignificant ones!

Safety & Professional Boundaries

Zero tolerance for abuse or threats. If a conversation becomes unsafe, exit and report it to a senior, warden or security personnel. (2)

- **Maintain confidentiality:** avoid discussing patient care in public areas or open messaging groups.
- **Safety protocol:** In cases involving patient safety disputes, follow the hospital's chain of command and document a brief factual note including date, time, personnel involved, issue, and actions taken.
- **Respect the hierarchy and your voice:** speaking up about safety is a duty, not a sign of disrespect.

Practice Box

- **One-line acceptance:** That's fair feedback; I will re-check fluids and antibiotics now.
- **Boundary phrase:** I want to help, but this tone isn't productive. Let's revisit after rounds.
- **De-escalator to relatives:** I understand why you're upset. Let's sit for two minutes, I'll explain what we've done and what comes next.

Case Snapshot

A 56-year-old woman is readmitted with uncontrolled diabetes. She does not speak much about her illness until you ask, 'What has been hardest about your sugar control? She whispers, 'I am alone, meals are irregular, and I forget tablets.' You acknowledge her loneliness, arrange a simple meal plan, shift her metformin dosing to fit her routine, set phone reminders, and connect her with a local health worker. You teach back the plan and schedule a follow-up call.

Outcome: Her HbA1c improves, and she maintains follow-ups because the plan fits her life.
Why it worked: Listening uncovered the true barrier (isolation), enabling a humane, effective plan.

Learning Points

- Listening is a clinical skill that can be observed, taught, learned and assessed.
- Utilize names, seek permission, ask open questions, use silence, provide summaries, and employ teach-back methods.
- Name feelings respectfully; it calms patients and clarifies priorities.
- Document concerns and agreements, beneficial for care and correct on the medico-legal ground.

- Teams are more efficient and recover effectively when they feel heard.

Coffee Moment

One busy evening, I could not go for a walk with Bruno; struggling to take both of us as always, he finally settled on going out with Jyoti alone. L evening I was still working at my d surrounded by open textbooks, no and half-marked, deadlines. Acr the table, Bruno climbed onto chair and settled himself in front me as if he was reading an open bo His gaze fixed not on the room, l on me. He wasn't demand attention. He wasn't restless. simply stayed. As I turned pages, leaned forward as if studying with - silent, attentive, completely prese And in that stillness, I reali something profound: empathy d not always speak. It sits. It waits. shares the weight without trying solve it.

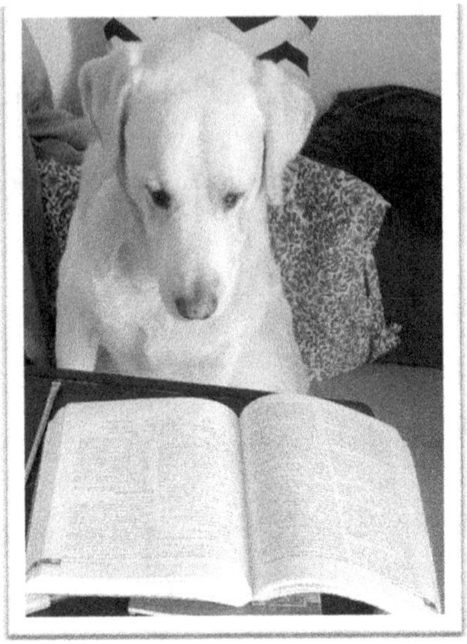

Figure 95.1: Bruno Teaching a Lesson on Empathy

In medicine, we are trained to inte it patients often need what Bruno offered that evening: an undistracted presence. A quiet assurance that someone is there, not to fix anything immediately, but to understand the space they are in.

Empathy is not dramatic. It does not always come with perfect words. Sometimes, it is simply the courage to stay at the table. That night, my most sincere lesson in empathy did not come from a textbook. It came from a white Angel who understood that being present is sometimes the highest form of care.

References

1. Levinson W, Roter DL, Mullooly JP, et al. Physician–patient communication: The relationship with malpractice claims among primary care physicians and surgeons. JAMA. 1997;277(7):553–9.
2. Ha JF, Longnecker N. Doctor–patient communication: A review. Ochsner J. 2010;10(1):38–43.
3. World Health Organization. *Social Determinants of Health: The Solid Facts.* 2nd ed. WHO Press; 2003.
4. Charon R. Narrative Medicine: Honoring the Stories of Illness. Oxford University Press; 2006.

Chapter 96: Connection- Remembering Names & Faces

Introduction

Hospitals act quickly, but trust develops through slow, human moments. Remembering someone's name is the fastest way to say, "I know you well." It restores dignity to patients, enhances teamwork, and helps you understand the stories behind symptoms. (1) Let's explore how to convert that good intention into a habitual professional practice.

Key Concepts

Why Names Matter

- **Dignity:** "Mr Rao" carries more dignity than "bed 14." It affirm personhood.
- **Rapport & adherence:** Patients are more likely to open up and follow plans when they feel understood. (2)
- **Team glue:** Recognizing nurses, technicians, and support staff by name fosters a respectful, high-reliability culture.
- **Safety:** Precise identification with two identifiers prevents errors and mix-ups.

Micro Skills

- **Ask & verify**: "Namaste, I'm Siddharth, a medical student with Dr Rajgopal. "Please tell me your full name and how you prefer to be addressed?" Confirm with the wristband or record for two identifiers.
- **Repeat immediately**: "Thanks, Shreya. I will send some blood investigation for you now." Early repetition cements memory.
- **Create a quick link**: Form a respectful connection by including a feature and a fact (e.g., "Shreya-blue hairband, loves drawing"). Keep it as a personal note; never joke about appearance.
- **Spell it correctly**: If unsure, ask: "Is it Sharma with an 'r' or Shama?" Proper spelling demonstrates attention and helps prevent mistakes. (3)
- **Use the name naturally**: "Vishwas, thanks for flagging the increasing heart rate of Raman on bed 7." Associate the name with a specific behaviour; people remember that you noticed.
- **Name-maps for wards**: Sketch a bed layout during rounds and record the first names or initials of the patients. This helps with handovers and reduces mistakes.
- **When you forget**: Acknowledge, 'I'm sorry, I have met many patients today. Could you remind me of your name once more?" Better to ask than guess.
- **Cultural respect**: Use titles appropriately (e.g., Mr./Ms./Master, Dr., Sister).

Ask for preferred names and pronouns; avoid nicknames that may be disrespectful. "Ramesh bhaiya" is acceptable if used in a respectful manner.

Case Snapshot: The Missed Name, the Missed Clue

Second-week posting. A child smiles, but you can't recall her name. I apologise, could you please remind me of your name? "Roshni," her mother says. Kneeling, you ask, "Roshni, what's hardest about your injections?" She whispers, "They hurt more when I am hungry." That cue leads you to coordinate her meals and snacks with insulin injections at the right times. No hypoglycaemic dip, better glucose control, and a happier child who now waves when you enter the ward.

Why it worked: Name → rapport → honest detail → tailored plan.

Professional Boundaries & Safety

- Use names kindly, never to compel or shame.
- Keep patient identifiers off WhatsApp or personal notes; adhere to privacy rules.
- Document full, correct names in the record.
- For paediatrics, learn both the child's and caregiver's names.

Learning Points

Remembering names is a clinical behaviour that improves dignity, trust, and safety. Pair a person's name with respectful repetition, a quick association, and a secure note. Ask, verify, and spell correctly. These small steps leave big impact on identification errors. When you forget, apologise and ask again. Honesty preserves rapport.
The ward runs on mutual respect.

☕ Coffee Moment

Between cases, you hand over a cup and say, "Ramesh, thank you for keeping the floor dry. It helps with hygiene and safety." He smiles; the environment softens. Names are tiny bridges. Cross them often.

References

1. Makoul G. Essential elements of communication in medical encounters: The Kalamazoo consensus statement. Acad Med. 2001;76(4):390–3.
2. Beach MC, Roter DL, Wang NY, et al. Are physicians' attitudes of respect accurately perceived by patients and associated with more positive communication behaviors? Patient Educ Couns. 2006;62(3):347–54.
3. WHO. Patient identification. Patient safety solutions. Geneva: World Health Organization; 2007.

Chapter 97: Power of Appreciation

Introduction

Hospitals rely on protocols and staff. In high-pressure wards, a brief, sincere "thank you" is not just for show; it's fuel for hard work. Appreciation boosts morale, reduces conflict, and reinforces the small human connections that keep patients safe. (1,2)

Key Concepts

- **Be specific, not generic:** "Thanks for catching that potassium of 2.8 before rounds" lands; "good job" fades.
- **Timely and public (when safe):** Share appreciation promptly, and if appropriate, so that others can learn from it.
- **360° gratitude:** Upward (to seniors), sideways (peers), downward (juniors), and outward (nurses, technicians, sanitation, security).(3)
- **No flattery:** Be honest, fair, and based on actions; steer clear of favourites or superficial praise.

Micro Skills

- **Open rounds with thanks:** Before we start, thanks, Sister Nirmala, for flagging low urine output at 2 AM.
- **Name the behaviour plus impact:** Your careful review of prescribed medicines prevented a duplicate dose of anticoagulant.
- **Use 'thank-then-coach':** Thank you for escalating early. Next time, also inform the anaesthesia team while we are en route.
- **Write it down:** Add one appreciative line in the progress note or handover; copy the person and their supervisor in a brief message.
- **Include the 'invisible work':** Porters, housekeeping, security, dietetics and many, invisible to you play significant role in patient care. Acknowledge their quiet reliability in patient management.
- **Peer-to-peer messages:** 30-second text-note after duty "You kept the code calm, it really helped all"; small efforts give big morale boost.
- **Self-appreciation (quietly):** 'I managed the angry relative with patience.' It builds resilience without arrogance. (2)
- **Avoid:** Backhanded praise like 'you finally did it right', public comparisons, and praise that overlooks others contributions.

Case Snapshot: Appreciation that Averted an Error

During a busy evening in the Surgery ward, a junior nurse alerts the team that a patient scheduled for a laparoscopic cholecystectomy is labelled with a penicillin allergy, yet piperacillin-tazobactam has been prescribed. The resident pauses, reconfirms that it was a mild reaction, not anaphylaxis and says, "Thank you for catching that; let's switch to cefuroxime," and notes her name on the OT whiteboard as "Safety Star of the Day."

What changed: Others begin voicing small concerns sooner. Near-miss reports increase (in a good way), and antibiotic errors drop on the next audit.

Why it worked: Immediate, specific appreciation normalised speaking up and converted a near-miss into a system fix.

Professional Boundaries & Equity

- Keep praise behaviour-focused, not appearance-based.
- Distribute recognition fairly; track who gets appreciated to avoid blind spots.
- Respect privacy and always seek consent before mentioning individuals publicly; never disclose patient identifiers in messages.

☕ Coffee Moment

After a heavy round, you say hello to the housekeeping staff, "Thank you Sudhir, you are keeping the floor and equipment surfaces dry and clean, it prevents a lot of hospital-acquired infections." He smiles, surprised. The ward feels lighter. Sometimes the smallest recognition is the strongest medicine you give all day.

References

1. Maslach C, Leiter MP. The truth about burnout: How organizations cause personal stress and what to do about it. San Francisco: Jossey-Bass; 1997.
2. Fredrickson BL. The broaden-and-build theory of positive emotions. Am Psychol. 2001;56(3):218–26.
3. Shanafelt TD, Noseworthy JH. Executive leadership and physician well-being: Nine organizational strategies to promote engagement and reduce burnout. Mayo Clin Proc. 2017;92(1):129–46.

Chapter 98: Building Trust - The Golden Bridge

Introduction

When you walk onto a ward, you enter a living ecosystem. Your daily life is filled with people, patients, peers, professors, nurses, technicians, mentors, and family who keep the system moving. Every interaction, every word you speak or don't, adds up to define who you are. Your scientific knowledge matters, but your ability to develop healthy interpersonal relationships and earn trust is what opens doors to learning and care. The ability to build meaningful relationships isn't 'extra,' it is essential. It is a trail of small, consistent behaviours. (1,2)

Key Concepts

The Beauty of Human Connection

Think of the patients who remember your kindness but forget your diagnosis. Think of the peer who became your support system during a difficult rotation. Think of the teacher whose single encouraging sentence changed how you saw yourself.

Real and Relatable Challenges

Despite living in a crowd, many medical students feel alone. In a recent study from India, students were found to have some degree of anxiety (63%), stress (53%) and depression (36%) within 6 months of admission to medical college. (3) Intense competition breeds isolation, and time pressure (deadlines to complete a task) limits real human conversations. Cultural taboos around emotional vulnerability add to this, and a person starts feeling relatively safe in emotional isolation. Many students feel awkward initiating friendships beyond academic or professional discussions.

Additionally, misunderstandings among clinical team members, inadequate information and lack of transparency with seniors can quickly erode confidence. When hierarchy is misunderstood as superiority, the problem gets multiplied. Personal relationships often suffer due to professional commitments.

Why Trust Matters

Building interpersonal trust enhances communication, collaboration, and overall effectiveness. This is not a soft skill; it is a survival skill.

- **Learning:** Seniors invest more in students who listen, prepare, and follow through.
- **Safety:** Nurses and staff will warn you about risks only if they expect respect in return.

- **Flow:** Cooperation reduces delays, facilitates smooth handovers, and eases tension.
- **Culture:** Your behaviour influences the team's attitude either positively or negatively.

Doctors who communicate well have

- Higher patient satisfaction rates
- Lower rates of malpractice claims
- Better treatment adherence among patients (3,4)

Micro-Skills

Ward Etiquette: First Principles

- **Introduce yourself and your role:** I'm a first-year student with Dr. Sharma; I'm here to observe and help where appropriate.
- **Observe the rhythm:** Each unit has a flow and culture. Watch before you speak up.
- **Ask, do not assume:** Sister, where should I discard this soaked dressing?
- **Two ears, one mouth:** Listen twice as much as you talk, especially in the initial days.
- **Mind the space:** Do not block the path, do not lean on the bed-rails touching it with your coat, and do not touch equipment without permission and unnecessarily.

With mentors

- **Be teachable:** Present yourself for learning and follow the class-rules. Thank for the feedback. Read and present again next day.
- **Close the loop:** When a senior provides guidance, respond with, "I used your advice on fluid balance; it made the plan clearer."
- **Respect others' time:** Take appointment in advance or confirm if it is good time to discuss before any out of schedule discussion.
- **Hierarchy with respect:** Question ideas, not people. If you see a safety risk, speak up: 'May I confirm the dose? The chart says 5 mg.'

With nurses and support staff

- **Acknowledge expertise:** Sister Lalita, could you demonstrate the dressing protocol for me?
- **Closed-loop communication:** Sister, I took blood samples for bed 12 and sent at 9:15.

- **Pitch in:** Fetch the sharps box, label tubes correctly. Small acts earn great trust.
- **See the person:** Remember names and express gratitude.
- **Share responsibility:** Avoid passing hazardous disposal tasks to others.
- **Express appreciation:** Offer it for specific actions rather than generic praise. For example, 'Thank you for flagging the low urine output.'

Redefine Leadership

- Leadership is not a position. It's how you show up in every room.
- You don't have to wait to be a senior. You lead every time you help a peer through burnout, ask a question others are afraid to ask, or stand up for a patient's dignity.

Professional Boundaries & Communication

- **Confidentiality:** Avoid discussing cases and sharing identifiers on open WhatsApp groups.
- **Documentation:** If you promise to do something, do it on time. Reliability is remembered.
- **Clean handovers:** "Bed 14, bloods drawn 9:10; sent; no complications."
- **Help invisibly:** Keep files organised, print reports; no announcements are necessary.
- **Own your mistakes:** Report, repair, learn, and avoid blame shifting.
- **Credit publicly, correct privately:** Praise in the group; raise concerns one to one.

Case Snapshots

Aarav forgets to sign a lab form; the nurse notices and corrects it. Because he usually communicates clearly, she quietly informs him and shows the correct workflow. **Why it worked:** The trust you build makes people believe you will learn and improve.

☕ Coffee Moment

After a long call and back-to-back duties, I reached home completely exhausted. I opened the door to find Bruno waiting—tail wagging, eyes shining, no questions asked. In a world that measures you by deadlines and degrees, here was a soul who celebrated just your return. Medicine teaches us to heal others, but sometimes it's we who come home needing healing. And sometimes, healing looks like a wagging tail and a heart that never stopped waiting. It is trust and connection.

Trust is like a golden bridge; it takes time and care to construct, but once built, it carries both patient and doctor safely across uncertainty.

References

1. Thom DH, Hall MA, Pawlson LG. Measuring patients' trust in physicians when assessing quality of care. Health Aff. 2004;23(4):124–32.
2. O'Donovan R, van Dun D, McAuliffe E. Measuring trust in healthcare: A systematic review. Patient Educ Couns. 2020;103(10):1873–92.
3. Mallaram GK, Gopalakrishnan U, Mathews DA, Mudamala DS, Gangavarappagari H, Modi U, et al. Stress, Anxiety, and Depression in the First-year Students of Medical Education: A Prospective Cohort Study from a Women's Medical College in South India. Indian J Psychol Med. 2024 Nov 19:02537176241282100.
4. Ranjan P, Kumari A, Chakrawarty A. How can doctors build trust with their patients? J Clin Diagn Res. 2015;9(3):JE01–4.

Chapter 99: Situational Awareness- Seeing the Whole Picture

Introduction

Hospitals are dynamic environments; patients change, alarms beep, teams rotate, and orders update. Situational awareness (SA) is the clinical habit of noticing what is happening, understanding its meaning, and anticipating what might happen next. (1) For medical students, SA transforms scattered details into safe action and helps avoid "I didn't realise" moments.

Key Concepts

SA is a three-step loop (Endsley model): Perceive the elements → Comprehend their meaning → Project what comes next, act and repeat. (1)

How SA is lost: Tunnel vision on one task, fatigue, interruptions, noisy environments, poor handovers, hierarchy (hesitating to speak up), and alarm fatigue.

Why it matters: Early recognition of deterioration, fewer errors, and faster recovery from surprises such as oxygen running out, wrong patient on the procedure table or missing consent. (2,3)

Micro Skills

The 30-second SCAN when you walk to a bedside

- Signs: vital trends, monitor limits, and early warning score.
- Cannula/catheters, lines, airway, and oxygen.
- Active orders & allergies: check charts and boards.
- Near risks: wet floor, misplaced sharps, and a patient without bed rails.

Perceive → Comprehend → Project → Act and Inform

- **Perceive:** Gather information and key cues, such as patient appearance, vital signs, monitor trends, and equipment function.
- **Comprehend:** Integrate and interpret the significance and pattern (risk of sudden hypoxia, worsening ventilation).
- **Project:** Anticipate what will happen next if no intervention is made.
- **Act and Inform:** Intervene early and communicate clearly with the team. (1)

DOPE check

SpO_2 dropped from 96 to 88; perform a quick DOPE check. Take the patient off the ventilator and onto the bag, then check for

Displacement of tube

Obstruction

Pneumothorax, and

Equipment failure.

You find, tube is displaced and reposition it. Saturation improves, and an impending cardiac arrest is averted.

ABCDE mini-check for any "not right" feeling

Airway, Breathing, Circulation, Disability, Exposure: 60 seconds first, details later.

Post-round huddle (1 min)

Diuresis for bed 12, bloods for bed 14, discharge for bed 9. Risks - low K in bed 12.

Closed-loop communication

Aarav, please draw blood and send for LFT for bed 12. Aarav closes the communication loop by confirming, Yes, drawing blood for LFT for bed 12 now.

Read-back

For critical values and orders. Nurse- The patient's arterial pH is 7.15; You- the arterial pH is 7.15. Correct? Nurse- correct. Avoid assumptions, seek clarification if you have any doubts, and ensure documentation, even if it is a telephonic discussion.

Advocacy-inquiry

To express the concern about a situation someone is handling and understand their viewpoint on the situation and the expected outcome. It encourages two-way communication and shared problem-solving. If concern persists, state it more assertively in a graded manner.

Graded assertiveness to escalate concerns

PACE

- **P**robe: Doctor, I'm concerned about rising RR.
- **A**lert: RR 40, SpO_2 falling despite 4 L/min.
- **C**hallenge: We need a senior review now.
- **E**mergency: Calling code/PICU SR.

CUSS

- **Concern:** I am concerned that Ritu's blood pressure is falling after starting blood transfusion.
- **Uncomfortable:** I am uncomfortable with the trend; HR is also high.
- **Safety:** This is a safety issue; we need to re-evaluate her in detail immediately.
- **Stop:** STOP blood transfusion, I am calling a SR here now.

Reset during chaos: 10-for-10

Take 10 seconds to plan the next 10 minutes: Start with the airway first. Riya bag mask; Kabir monitor; I'll call the senior. Quiet for 30 seconds, everyone on the delegated task.

Protect your own SA: I'M SAFE self-check

- **I**llness
- **M**edication
- **S**tress
- **A**lcohol
- **F**atigue
- **E**motion

Are you safe for your patients? If you find yourself in any of the above situations, you are compromised. Inform your lead, pair up with a colleague and double-check immediate tasks.

Micro-debrief

What went well, what will we change? 2-minute debriefs turn surprises into learning.

Case Snapshot: A Hypoxic Patient

Medicine ward, evening rush. A student reaches Bed 14 for a routine exam. The **SCAN** habit kicks in: SpO_2 shows 91% (down from 96% an hour ago), the patient is breathing faster, and the oxygen cylinder gauge is nearing empty.

Action: Sister Lalita, cylinder for Bed 14 is red, need to shift to the wall oxygen now. You assist her in switching the patient to wall oxygen, confirm the flow, and recheck the SpO_2; it is now 96%. Closed-loop- wall oxygen running at 4 L/min, cylinder removed for replacement.

Why it worked: Perceive (gauge + vitals), comprehend (risk of sudden hypoxia), project (imminent failure), act and inform. The team trusts the student; learning continues.

Coffee Moment

You step into the ward, perform your quiet 30-second safety huddle, and address two small risks before anyone notices: an obstruction alarm on the infusion pump and a wet patch by the bed. No applause follows, but a calmer ward and a safer patient. That is situational awareness: invisible work that prevents visible harm.

References

1. Endsley MR. Toward a theory of situation awareness in dynamic systems. Hum Factors. 1995;37(1):32–64.
2. Schulz CM, Endsley MR, Kochs EF, et al. Situation awareness in anesthesia: Concept and research. Anesthesiology. 2013;118(3):729–42.
3. Wright MC, Taekman JM, Endsley MR. Objective measures of situation awareness in a simulated medical environment. Qual Saf Health Care. 2004;13(suppl 1):i65–71.

Chapter 100: Doctoring with Diplomacy

Introduction

Hospitals are places with an emotionally charged environment. You encounter strong opinions, tense tempers, and difficult questions. Diplomacy is the crucial skill that maintains uninterrupted service with preserved dignity of yourself and others. (1,2)

Criticism, Conflict, and Conversations

Key Concepts

- **Differentiate message from tone:** Even poor delivery of words can contain valuable messages. Extract the learning with effort.
- **Be hard on the problem but gentle with the person:** Focus on processes, procedures and behaviours, not individuals.
- **Intent does not equal impact:** If harm happened, recognize it, even if your intentions were good.
- **Follow escalation ladder:** Wait for self-management → do private discussion → take to mentor or faculty → follow formal process as per policy.
- **Documentation safeguards all:** Put brief, factual notes of important interactions, particularly when safety or medico-legal risk is involved.

Micro Skills

When feedback pinches: S.T.O.P.

- Stop: breathe, make eye contact.
- Thank: Thank you for pointing that out.
- Open: Could you please provide an example to clarify your explanation?
- Plan: I will read and present again tomorrow.

Avoid arguing in public; follow up later with your suggestions for improvement.

Team motivation (D.E.S.C. script)

- Describe situation: In the research project, reports were late twice this month.
- Express concern: I felt stressed working on the data entry alone.
- Specify task: Can we split tasks among the 3 of us and set a 6 PM meeting?
- Consequences expected: We will submit on time and share credit.(3)

Difficult conversations with patients (SPIKES-lite)

- Setting: Sit in a private space, switch off or silence your phone.
- Perception: What have you understood so far?

- **I**nvitation: Can we discuss all the details now?
- **K**nowledge: Present in clear, small sentences: The surgery was more complex. The next 24 hours are critical.
- **E**mpathy: Pause and name the emotion: I can see that this is frightening for anyone in this situation.
- **S**trategy/Summary: This is our plan for the night. Our team will update at 8 am. Keep empathy and document the discussion. (1)

Case Snapshot

Aman's case presentation is criticized during rounds. He resists the urge to defend himself and says, Thank you, Sir. Could you suggest one key paper? That evening, he revises the pathophysiology, emails a five-line summary to the professor, and presents the next day. The professor notices the improvement and appreciates.

S.T.O.P. turned a tough moment into a growth opportunity and demonstrated professionalism to peers.

Learning Points

- Diplomacy is deliberate: pause, clarify, and respond, not react.
- Scripts (STOP, DESC, SPIKES-lite) make difficult moments manageable.
- Private conversations protect dignity, documentation protects care.
- Escalate early when safety or fairness is at risk.
- The goal is not to "win" the exchange but to maintain relationships.

Coffee Moment

After a tense moment, you thank the nurse who challenged a dosing error. She smiles, we are on the same team. A quiet diplomatic reward, the work goes on, and it goes on together.

References

1. Baile WF, Buckman R, Lenzi R, et al. SPIKES—a six-step protocol for delivering bad news: Application to the patient with cancer. Oncologist. 2000;5(4):302–11.
2. Rosenstein AH. Nurse–physician relationships: Impact on nurse satisfaction and retention. Am J Nurs. 2002;102(6):26–34.
3. Thomas EJ, Sexton JB, Helmreich RL. Discrepant attitudes about teamwork among critical care nurses and physicians. Crit Care Med. 2003;31(3):956–9.

The Hidden Curriculum

Skills That Keep You Grounded and Growing

There is a side of medicine that no timetable will reveal. It does not appear on your exam sheet, yet it decides how long you last, how deeply you love this work, and how gracefully you live through it.

This is the hidden curriculum, the unspoken lessons learned in hostel corridors, midnight wards, viva halls, and in friendships. Here, you meet your fears, doubts, and triumphs.

You will explore what it means to:

Survive and thrive in the storms of MBBS, guard your most precious assets - time, energy, and focus; ask for help when it matters, and offer it when it's needed; stay calm in chaos; build bonds that uplift, not break and face exams without letting them define your worth.

It is about the inner scaffolding that holds you up and shapes not only the doctor you are becoming, but also the human you remain.

S No.	The Hidden Curriculum: At a Glance
1.	**Chapter 101** Surviving in MBBS When the storm of medical college hits: imposter syndrome, stress, and finding your anchors.
2.	**Chapter 102** Thriving in MBBS Beyond survival: building resilience, meaning, and purpose in the journey of becoming.
3.	**Chapter 103** Time, Energy, and Focus: Mastering the Trio Not just hours on the clock: the invisible balance of stamina, attention, and priorities.
4.	**Chapter 104** Seeking Help: The Power of Asking Why asking is not weakness but wisdom: the skill that protects patients and builds professionals.
5.	**Chapter 105** Doctor, Heal Thyself: Self-Compassion Turning the inner critic into an inner coach; learning to care for yourself while caring for others.
6.	**Chapter 106** The Art and Science of Facing Exams Composure and calm as a clinical drug during exams.
7.	**Chapter 107** Respectful Bonds: From Ragging to Mentorship Replacing coercion with culture: dignity, mentorship, and traditions worth keeping.

Chapter 101: Surviving in MBBS

Introduction

Stepping into medical college is like stepping into a process that will completely reshape you. Here, every student arrives with medals of past achievements, only to discover that the level of playing field has changed. You will quickly realize that it's not about knowing everything; it's about learning how to keep learning when nothing looks familiar.

Anatomy labs echo with nervous laughter. Your white coat feels a size too big. You see the corridors full of faces, some as dazed as yours, and some moving with confidence.

Finding Your Footing

Many students feel moments of self-doubt. They wonder if they belong, questioning their abilities, or fearing they will never match up to their peers. This is not a weakness; it is a common phenomenon called 'imposter syndrome' (1). With awareness, you can overcome it and thrive.

Imposter Syndrome

Imposter syndrome or Imposter phenomenon is the subjective experience of perceived self-doubt in one's abilities and accomplishments compared with others, despite evidence to suggest the contrary. (2) It is a persistent feeling that your own success is undeserved, or that you have somehow "fooled" others into believing you are capable. It may manifest as:

- Thinking that peers are smarter, faster, or more deserving.
- Dismissing own hard work as "luck" or "chance."
- Fear of being 'exposed' as inadequate.

These thoughts can lower morale, affect further learning, and lead to burnout. (3)

Adaptation Techniques: Turning Doubt into Growth

- **Acknowledge and Normalize:** You are not alone; more than half of medical students experience the imposter phenomenon. Naming the feeling reduces its power and impact on you.
- **Focus on Growth, Not Perfection:** Medicine is too vast for anyone to master. Celebrate progress, not perfection. Each clinical skill learned and each patient history taken is a step forward. (2)
- **Peer and Mentor Support:** Share your struggles and victories with classmates and seniors. You will find others have similar fears. Mentors can normalize

challenges and guide you through the path.

- **Reframe Mistakes as Learning:** Every error is a lesson; reflect on it, correct it, and move ahead. That's how you keep growing.
- **Self-Care and Balance:** Sleep, exercise, eat, and make time for your organic hobbies. Maintaining a slow pace is fuel for resilience.

Case Snapshot: "Am I Good Enough?"

Riya, a first-year student, found herself exhausted from the long hours of anatomy dissection. She felt that others grasped structures faster and began to think she wasn't good enough for medicine. She sought an advice from a senior, who reminded 'it's not about knowing everything today, it is an ongoing journey of learning.' With study groups and regular discussions, Riya not only improved her knowledge but also began mentoring peers. Naming the struggle, seeking support, and breaking tasks into achievable steps turns anxiety into confidence.

Learning Points

- Imposter syndrome is common; it doesn't mean you are unfit for medicine.
- A positive mindset and resilience practices can help reduce self-doubt.
- Sharing struggles with mentors and peers makes you strong.
- Balance and self-care are essential for steady growth.

Emotional Rollercoaster

No one prepares you for the emotional rollercoaster of medical college. You witness it when you see a child gasp in the emergency ward, fail a practical despite your efforts, feel lonely even among classmates, or experience a silent guilt of wanting a break. (3) Emotions can manifest as

- Shock, fear, or helplessness (after emergencies).
- Anxiety or dread (before rounds, exams).
- Sadness or grief (after a poor outcome).
- Frustration, anger, or irritability (when systems fail).
- Guilt or shame (after a mistake or needing rest).
- Self-doubt or impostor feelings ("Maybe I'm not cut out for this").
- Loneliness or homesickness (even in a crowd).
- Overwhelm or mental fatigue (too many demands).
- Numbness or detachment (compassion fatigue).
- Moral distress (knowing the right thing but unable to do it).
- Hopelessness or low mood (when setbacks pile up).

…and at times relief, pride, gratitude, awe, and hope.

No one writes it on the timetable, but it's there - behind every viva, every missed mark, every sleepless night. It whispers:

- You're not doing enough.
- Everyone else is ahead.
- You'll never catch up.

This silent storm is called stress, and left unchecked, it creeps into your breath, relationships, and ability to care - even your reason for being here. But stress is not the villain. How we relate to it is what matters.

Stress is the body–mind response to a demand or threat, such as exams, night duty, or family issues. It can be acute or chronic and sometimes helpful (eustress) by sharpening focus. It involves physiological arousal (adrenaline, faster pulse) and psychological tension.

Emotional fatigue is a state of feeling drained, numb, or lacking empathy after prolonged emotional stress, common in caregiving roles and frequent exposure to loss or trauma. It is a key component of burnout.

Ride the rollercoaster gracefully

Emotional mastery isn't about ignoring emotions. It's about honouring, understanding, and navigating them with grace. No state of mind is final. Anxiety, anger or frustration, it feels like it will never end. But every emotion is like a wave; it rises, peaks, and passes. Let the wave pass.

Coping With the Tough Days

There will be days you doubt yourself deeply. You'll blank out in the viva. You'll watch someone else score better and wonder if you belong here at all. You'll feel like you're sprinting, only to stay behind.

And on those days, your lifelines appear.

Sometimes, it is your roommate who leaves sticky notes on your desk: "Drink water. You're doing okay." Sometimes, it is someone you keep bumping into in the college corridor, who shares the same fatigue and glitter in their eyes. Sometimes, it is just yourself, not giving up on small obstacles and ready to show up each morning.

☕ Coffee Moment

You're in the Dissection Hall, gloves on, heart racing. You are fumbling with nerves when a quiet voice beside you says,

We have got this tibial nerve.

Such a clear nerve it is.

You are impressed, like all other tablemates and appreciate the discovery. Your group shows it proudly to the professor, who smiles and says,

This is not the tibial nerve,

but it is the 'fresher's nerve.

You all are confused.

He further explains that this is the tendon of the plantaris muscle, and most fresh anatomists, like you, confuse it for a nerve. Everybody laughs about anatomy, not fitting in yet, and maybe surviving this together.

You begin to lean into your friendships, your study group, and your support system. You start asking for help and offering it too.

References

1. Villwock JA, Sobin LB, Koester LA, Harris TM. Impostor syndrome and burnout among American medical students: A pilot study. Int J Med Educ. 2016;7:364–9.
2. Mak KKL, Kleitman S, Abbott MJ. Impostor Phenomenon Measurement Scales: A Systematic Review. Front Psychol. 2019 Apr 5;10:671.
3. Henning K, Ey S, Shaw D. Perfectionism, the impostor phenomenon and psychological adjustment in medical, dental, nursing and pharmacy students. Med Educ. 1998;32(5):456–64.
4. Tempski P, Martins MA, Paro HB. Teaching and learning resilience: a new agenda in medical education. Med Educ. 2012;46(4):345–6.

Chapter 102: Thriving in MBBS

Introduction

Surviving in MBBS is like learning to navigate long hours of training, managing different types of exams and keeping your head above water. Thriving is beyond survival. It needs to find balance, joy, and purpose within challenges and use them as a means for further growth. It requires developing coping mechanisms that turn stress into strength. Thriving does not mean that you never feel pressure or self-doubt; rather, it means that you learn how to respond to it with perspective and resilience. (1,2) Explore the secret in this chapter.

Reacting vs Responding: Choosing Wisely

A trigger for a complex emotion can be as simple as a word, a person, or a situation. How we deal with them can either drain us or help us grow. If you act during the wave, you often regret it. The key lies in reacting versus responding to a trigger. Responding builds trust, strengthens relationships, and protects your energy. In high-stakes settings, such as the wards or family life, the difference between a reaction and a response can mean conflict versus connection.

- **Reaction:** Quick, automatic, and emotion-driven. It often originates from the amygdala, the brain's alarm system. It can escalate conflict or cause regret. Example: Confrontation when criticized.
- **Response:** It is thoughtful, deliberate, and aligned with goals. It comes from our prefrontal cortex, the thinking brain, allowing us to weigh the consequences and act wisely. Example: Pause, listen, and reply calmly to criticism.

Train Yourself to Respond

- **Pause:** Take a deep breath before acting. Pause is power, and it buys you time. You can practice the 90-second rule. When triggered, breathe for 90 seconds and drink some water before speaking or acting.
- **Listen actively:** Hear the other person fully before forming your words.
- **Reflect and ask:** What outcome do I want? Is my response helpful in achieving that outcome?
- **Identify your triggers:** Awareness reduces the power of surprise. The more precisely you identify a trigger, the better control you have to work through it.
- **Use 'I statements':** Say "I feel hurt…" instead of "You always hurt me…" to prevent blame.

Micro-Presence Moments

Your presence in a moment is your power source. You need 30 seconds of full awareness, multiple times a day. (3) While washing your hands, feel the water; while eating, feel the taste, and while strolling outside, feel the breeze.

Before entering a ward, take a conscious breath and be aware. Between topics, close your eyes for 3 breaths. Unplug to recharge!

Mind Like Water

The phrase comes from martial arts and mindfulness. A still body of water clearly reflects everything around it. Throw a pebble into it, and it ripples—then returns to calm. Now compare that to your mind after a surprise viva or negative feedback. Does it reflect? Or does it react? It doesn't mean you're always calm. It means you respond appropriately, effectively, and then return to the centre.

Name It to Tame It

Name your emotion as precisely as possible. 'I feel tight in my chest.' This is anxiety. Naming your emotion decreases its power. You learn to observe it instead of drowning in it. Don't say: 'I'm not okay.' Say: 'I'm tired.' 'I'm grieving.'

Expand beyond 'sad' and 'happy' into words like restless, disappointed, guilty, content, and hopeful. The more precisely you name an emotion, the more control you have to work through it.

Process, Don't Suppress

Crying is not a sign of weakness. Journaling is not 'too intellectual'. Speaking to a mentor or therapist is not indulgent. Processing emotions helps develop empathy without emotional exhaustion, the very skill that makes great doctors.

Ask yourself, What am I feeling right now? What is this emotion trying to tell me? Be kind to yourself and use self-talk as you would with a good friend, acknowledging how you feel.

Ask for help

Instead of resisting anxiety, try saying- I allow this feeling to be here. I trust it will pass. If it does not pass, seek professional help. Asking for help is a sign of strength.

Look Beyond: Creator in Chaos

The first few weeks of medical college can feel like being dropped into a river already in flood. There's too much to read, too many expectations, too many voices, faculty, parents, peers, and that ever-critical one in your own head. Some days feel like you're just reacting…Wake up.. Rush.. Study.. Survive.. Repeat..

Take Control

You should choose your role, not as a passenger, but as the driver of your journey. This requires bringing your knowledge into practice, from information to transformation. It's moving from helplessness to ownership, from noise to clarity.

To achieve this clarity, you need to clear your mind of debris. If something is bothering you, such as a misunderstanding with a friend, a missed deadline, a messy desk, or even responding to an email, take a moment to complete or close it. Completion doesn't always mean perfection; it means closure, so that mind and heart are free to focus forward. Clear your physical space, let go of grudges about difficult conversations, forgive yourself for the missed lecture, and start again fresh.

Honour Your Words

When you honour your word to yourself, something magical happens to your confidence. You start trusting yourself. Whether it is reading one page a day, sleeping on time, or watching the daily sunrise, each small promise kept becomes an anchor in the storm. Make one simple promise: 'I will read this book daily for 30 minutes, or I will read physiology notes daily for 20 minutes before I sleep.' Take it and own it. When you stop blaming and start choosing, you gain energy, and your vision clears. That is power, and life becomes something you lead, not something you chase.

Growing as a Doctor

There comes a moment when you feel worthy. During your first ward posting, when a professor trusts you to suture or when a patient says, "Thank you, doctor," even though you're a student, something shifts inside. You realize you're no longer surviving. You're becoming. You fall in love not with a person, but with a purpose.

With medicine, with service, with the privilege of being allowed into the rawest moments of human lives and maybe, with that face in the corridor, it will become part of your routine.

Letter to Self

Here is a letter from your future self to your present self.

Dear me,

You will not always get it right. You will forget drug names, mix up nerves, and doubt yourself. But remember, your worth is not in being perfect, it is in how you stand. Tired, afraid and still willing.

You'll cry. You'll break. But you'll also laugh until your stomach aches. You'll find meaning in the smile of a patient. You'll understand what kind of doctor and human being you want to be. Fall in love with the mess, the journey and the people. You will survive MBBS. You'll stumble through night shifts, anatomy nightmares, and impossible exams, and you'll also dance in hostel corridors.

You'll meet people who become your anchors, friends who feel like family, the ones who'll hold your hand after a failed viva, share notes before exams, and sit with you in the mess of hostel nights. These friendships will last a lifetime. You will find the most cherished moments in their company, when you will meet with them at some airport, in a conference, in your alumni meet, or on a random rendezvous.

They'll become your strongest professional network, too. And maybe, you'll find someone who feels like home - a person who becomes your anchor in your personal life, your confidant, your partner, perhaps even your future spouse. Don't force it; let life surprise you in its own quiet way.

And when you're standing in a white coat one day, tired but proud, look back. See this version of you. The one who survived, stumbled, and still believed. Thank that version, because of that, you made it today!

Yours own

Me, my current version!

Coffee Moment

Think of MBBS as batting in cricket. Every ball is a fresh challenge, some easy to play, some demand your complete focus. You can't walk away from the deliveries if you want to stay in the game. The art lies not in avoiding problems, but in facing each one with patience and skill. You will defend some balls, leave some balls, and convert some balls into runs. No ball, no runs. Over time, you will realize that it is about building innings, gradually but consistently.

References

1. Sood A, Sharma V. Resilience and thriving in medical education: Evidence and strategies. Med Teach. 2020;42(9):1007–15.
2. Epstein RM, Krasner MS. Physician resilience: What it means, why it matters, and how to promote it. Acad Med. 2013;88(3):301–3.
3. Wald HS, Haramati A, Bachner YG, et al. Promoting resilience in medical education: Curriculum development with mindfulness and mind–body approaches. Acad Med. 2016;91(3):350–9.

Chapter 103: Time, Energy, and Focus-Mastering the Trio

Introduction

Time is always ticking in medicine, with countdowns to exams, submission deadlines, lecture bells, and clinical slots.

You plan your day… but distractions creep in.
You create a timetable, but you can't follow it.
You feel guilty for resting… and burnt out from working.

The real issue? Time management isn't only about time. It is about focus, energy, and time. We all have 24 hours, but how we use them shapes who we are becoming. Some students get overwhelmed by to-do lists; others float gracefully between wards, the library, and coffee breaks. (1)

What's the secret?

The difference between the overwhelmed and the steady isn't a better timetable; it's the quiet mastery of time, energy, and focus. (1-3)

Key Concepts

Time (visible): Hours you can block and plan.
Energy (variable): Physical, emotional, and mental stamina fluctuate throughout the day.
Focus (valuable): Ability to give full attention to one thing that matters now. (2)
Thumbrule: Protect focus, fuel energy, then plan time. The sequence holds the key.

Micro-Skills

Realign your invisible trio as Focus - Energy – Time.

Focus

- **Commitment:** Keep it brief, but own your words. I am in a 30-min sprint until 7:30.
- **Clean start with specific target:** "In this self-study session, I will complete…"
- **Digital boundaries:** Mute groups; uninstall one distraction app for a week.
- **Deep-work sprints:** 25 min study followed by a 5 min essential break. Drink water, hydrate, walk, and stretch, but avoid using your mobile or screen during this break. Increase the maximum to 50 min study sprint – 10 min break.

Energy: manage the battery, not the clock (3)

- **Sleep is non-negotiable:** Aim for a stable sleep cycle and preserve the post-night-duty day for recovery.
- **Unplug hourly for a small recharge:** Take a few conscious deep breaths, drink water and take a 5-minute walk or stretch after every 50 minutes.
- **Food is first aid:** Take breakfast on time, include fruits and nuts in meals and avoid caffeine spikes.
- **Audit People:** Spend time with power boosters and limit your exposure to time suckers.

Table 103.1: Fixing focus, energy and time

Element	Description	Common Leak	Fix
Focus	Your ability to stay present	Multitasking, social media	Deep work, single-tasking, digital boundaries
Energy	Your physical, emotional, mental stamina	Toxic people, no rest, poor diet	Sleep, exercise, meaningful breaks
Time	Hours in a day	Procrastination, poor planning	Time-blocking, calendars

Time

- **Rule of 3:** Decide and write your top three priorities in the morning and stick to them. Everything means nothing in the priority list. (4)
- **Time blocks like OT slots:** Create focused time blocks for study, rest, and physical activity.
- **Buffer bands:** Leave 10 - 15 minutes between blocks; life (and wards) spill over.
- **Energy-Based Scheduling:** Don't manage time. Manage your rhythms. Some students are sharp in the morning, while others are sharp at night. Identify your most alert 90-minute period and schedule your most challenging task during that time block.
- **Say No to Say Yes:** Every 'yes' is a 'no' to something else. If you say yes to every group, event, or late-night binge, you'll say no to rest, focus, and well-being.
- **Create your 'Not-To-Do List'** of activities, such as scrolling through social media during breaks, multitasking during focused study time, consuming alcohol or drugs, and adding more to it. Your 'yes' to productivity will naturally start flowing.

Friendship Factor

Focus doesn't mean isolation. Studying with good friends can boost your energy and help you stay on track with your schedule. Move in harmony with those who uplift you and gently steer clear of those who drain your time or energy and divert your focus. A trusted friend:

Can pull you back when you're drifting.

Can walk beside you when you're breaking down.

Can remind you to rest when you keep pushing too hard.

When You Fall Behind

You will miss deadlines, and you will have low-energy days. That's not failure; it's a signal to pause, reset, and recalibrate. (5)

- Name it, don't shame it: I'm behind on X.
- Narrow the task: Break it into small sub-tasks, achieve and celebrate.
- Start with two minutes: Momentum beats motivation.
- Ask for a tow: Can we do one sprint together at 7 pm?
- Reset tonight: Get an early sleep, avoid midnight panic, and start afresh in the morning.
- Clearly define the boundaries: No phones on the desk, honest behaviour and freedom to correct each other if they drift.
- Self-talk: I am not lazy, and I'm learning to manage things better.

Case Snapshot: The Pulse Group

Pooja, Sandeep, and Manish are getting exhausted in ward postings and exams. Frustrated with distractions and overwhelmed schedules, they create a group and make a deal. Daily two-hour deep study schedule in the library, phones off, 15-minute non-medical break after each hour, and a rule of sharing 3 top priorities each morning in the group. After two weeks, they have already finished their pending notes, are going to sleep earlier, and are feeling less irritable during ward postings. They report better recall and more laughter.

Why it worked: They protected focus, recharged energy, and organized time, simply together.

☕ Coffee Moment

After a long day of clinics, calls, and conversations that drained both mind and spirit, thinking about a Zoom meeting I planned to attend late in the evening, I reached home. As I approached my door, I heard the soft rising whimper from inside, the unmistakable sound of recognition. Not sight. Not proof. Just knowing. Even before I knocked, Aryan opened the door, and Bruno was almost on my chest, unable to contain the surge of energy. Boys were giggling, and Bruno's tail swept the floor like a metronome of joy, steady and rhythmic, announcing my return with a language older than words. His eyes were bright and fully alive in that one moment, as if the entire day had narrowed into a single, undivided welcome. He did not ask how many patients I saw, and the boys did not care how productive the day had been. They celebrated only one thing: I was home.

We often think mastery of time means squeezing more into the day. We think managing energy means pushing through fatigue. We think focus means narrowing our world to the next urgent task.

But the trio of boys and Bruno teach a different equation. They are not distracted by yesterday's absence. They are not anxious about tomorrow's walk. The energy gathers completely around the present moment, focus is undivided, and the joy is wholehearted.

- Time is not just to be managed - it is to be honoured.
- Energy is not just to be spent - it must be restored.
- Focus is not just about intensity - it is about presence.

As we sat down for the evening tea, we realised: mastery of the trio is not about control. It is about rhythm. Work deeply, Return fully, and Be where you are. Sometimes, the most powerful reset does not come from a planner or a productivity app. It comes from the giggling of children or a wagging tail that reminds you:

When you are here, be here completely.

No need to tell, I forgot to attend that Zoom meeting and I was happy about it.

References

1. Baethge C, Müller K, Rigotti T. Working conditions, work–family conflict, and well-being of German hospital physicians: Psychosocial and organizational predictors of work stress. Int Arch Occup Environ Health. 2006;79(5):395–402.
2. MeSHackett RD, Matthews G. Attention and Performance. Handbook of Human Factors and Ergonomics. 2006;3:189–219.
3. van der Meer D, Bakker AB, Demerouti E. Daily job crafting and momentary work engagement: The moderating role of day demands. J Vocat Behav. 2017;100:188–200.
4. Macan TH. Time management: Test of a process model. J Appl Psychol. 1994;79(3):381–91.
5. Dyrbye LN, Shanafelt TD. A narrative review on burnout experienced by medical students and residents. Med Educ. 2016;50(1):132–49.

Chapter 104: Seeking Help- The Power of Asking

Introduction

Medical college can feel like climbing a mountain. The quickest way to climb the path is not by being bold in actions but by having the courage to ask for help. Asking for help is not a sign of weakness; it is a professional skill that protects patients, accelerates learning, and preserves own well-being. (1)

Why Do We Hesitate

Fear of looking incompetent, pressure to manage alone, worry about burdening others, and cultural norms that equate asking with failure.
Rewire it: Leader, pilots, surgeons, and ICU teams routinely ask and verify.

Micro Skill

Before you ask

Identify the problem where you need help, try two resources first (notes and video). Write one sentence: "I'm stuck at ___ after trying ___."

SMART Ask

Specific: I am unsure how to calculate this patient's insulin dose.
Measurable: Could you review my calculations for two examples?
Action-ready: I've used the chart and obtained 12 units; I'm unsure about the correction factor.
Respect time: Is now a good time, or should I come back at 4 pm?
Thanks: Thank you, this helps me avoid mistakes.

Clinical escalation script: SBAR

Situation: Sir, Ward C, bed 12, has increasing breathlessness.
Background: Post-op day 1, saturation has dropped from 96% to 89%.
Assessment: Bilateral crepitations; likely fluid overload.
Request: May I initiate oxygen therapy and request an urgent review? Clear, concise, respectful, and safe.

With peers & seniors

Create a Help Circle: 3–5 friends, no-judgment questions.
Offer reciprocity: You explain acid–base today, I will teach ABG on Friday.
For faculty: Ask during office hours or after rounds, providing a brief context and a precise question. Act on advice within 24 hours.

I wanted to send a quick update: I applied your tip, and the ECG axis makes sense now. Thanks!

Case Snapshot: The Quiet Struggle

Aarav is sitting in the library, struggling with pharmacology. Riya notices and offers, do you want to discuss it together? I struggled last month. He uses the SMART ask: I have read Katzung and class notes, but I'm still confused about partial agonists. Could you explain it to me with an example? They sketch one dose–response curve.

Why it worked: Specific request, respect for time, application and shared learning.

Boundaries & Wellbeing

Emergency vs. elective: escalate immediately for patient safety; address non-urgent concerns in batches.
Privacy: never share patient identifiers on open groups.
When to seek professional help: persistent low mood, panic, sleep loss, or thoughts of self-harm → approach student counsellor/mentor; asking here is lifesaving. (2,3)

Learning Points

Courage develops through practice; every good doctor has a mentor—and asks for help. Asking is a professional behaviour that improves safety and speeds learning.
Come prepared, be specific, respect time, and close the loop with thanks and action.
Use SBAR for clinical issues and SMART for academic concerns.
Develop small peer networks where asking questions is a normal practice.

☕ Coffee Moment

After rounds, you whisper to a senior, "Could you spare five minutes to check my fluid plan?" She nods, scans your sheet, and corrects one step that is more appropriate for the index child. One humble ask, that is how 'safe doctors' are made.

References

1. Kilminster S, Cottrell D, Grant J, Jolly B. AMEE Guide No. 27: Effective educational and clinical supervision. Med Teach. 2007;29(1):2–19.
2. Sutkin G, Wagner E, Harris I, Schiffer R. What makes a good clinical teacher in medicine? A review of the literature. Acad Med. 2008;83(5):452–66.
3. Gordon M, Darbyshire D, Baker P. Non-technical skills training to enhance patient safety: a systematic review. Med Educ. 2012;46(11):1042–54.

Chapter 105: Doctor, Heal Thyself- Self Compassion

Introduction

Hospitals are loud, fast, and unforgiving. In those moments that feel like hours, the most valuable drug is composure. (1) Calm is not the absence of stress; it's the choice to act steadily despite it. In a calm environment, teams think clearly, and patients remain safe. (2,3) In your long, demanding journey, self-talk and self-compassion are essential tools. (4) This chapter shows how to turn an inner critic into a steady coach, so you can learn faster, recover after mistakes, and care for people without draining your energy.

Key Concepts

Stay calm

- **Prioritise:** Name the priority (airway, breathing, circulation); keep the rest for next.
- **Beat cognitive load:** Short cues and checklists beat long speeches when adrenaline is high. (1)
- **Closed-loop communication:** Name → task → confirmation. "Aarav, oxygen 10 L/min." Then Aarav confirms, "Oxygen on, 10 L/min."
- **Role clarity:** One leader, clear roles, minimal cross-talk.
- **Debrief:** Two minutes afterwards, turn chaos into learning and release tension. (2)

Self-talk

The running commentary in your head.
It can be harsh, 'I always mess up,' helpless, 'Nothing will change,' or helpful, 'I made an error, I can fix the step.'
Your performance and mood depend on the voice you practice most.

Identify Common distortions

- Always/never statements: You are always late; I can never understand this.
- Catastrophising like, "This one viva ruins my career."
- Mind-reading "Sir thinks I'm useless" and
- Comparison traps: I can never match Pankaj in history-taking skills.
- Naming the distortion weakens it. Understand, this is not the truth; this is a story in your mind; this is a distortion.

Self-compassion doesn't mean making excuses. It is an honest and kind self-assessment that includes accountability. You still own the mistake. (4)

Mindfulness

Notice and name the feeling without exaggeration.
I am feeling something wrong → Name the feeling, such as 'I am anxious' or 'I have pain.'
The moment you name the problem, it becomes smaller, and you gain a direction to solve it. (5)

Common humanity

Remember, others struggle too; you are not uniquely broken.

Self-kindness

Speak to yourself as you would talk to a good friend. (6)

Stay Steady

- **Simulation & Drills:** Rehearse ABC, defibrillator setup, and arrest algorithms to build muscle memory.
- **Checklists & cognitive aids:** Keep laminated CPR/ACLS/ALS cards and checklists on the crash cart.
- **Breath reset:** Box breathing 4–4–4–4 (4 sec inhale- 4 sec hold – 4 sec exhale – 4 sec hold) before giving orders.
- **Buddy system:** Pair up; a teammate quietly prompts the algorithm and times interventions.
- **Two-minute debrief:** "What went well? What will we change?" No blame, simply learning.
- **Self-care basics:** Get enough sleep, stay hydrated, and eat well. A depleted body tends to panic sooner.

The 60-second reset — S.T.O.P.

Stop (take a conscious one breath) → **T**ake stock 'My chest is tight; I'm anxious' → **O**bserve the thought 'I can never manage wards' → **P**roceed with a kinder, truer line: 'This is hard *today*. I can do the next step.'

Friendly phrases

Replace 'I'm useless.' with 'I'm new, and improving.'

Replace 'everyone is ahead of me' with 'we have different paces and are climbing the same mountain.'

Replace 'I am bad' with 'it was one bad day'. One data point does not define you.

The AND-Bridge: From But to And

Small words shape big conversations. 'But' often cancels what came before ("I agree, but..."). Replacing it with 'and' keeps both truths equally important and takes conversations toward solutions. This simple switch reduces defensiveness, supports teamwork, and generates a constructive mindset.

Whenever you face a 'but' situation, convert it to an 'and' situation and observe the difference. State the first truth, replace 'but' with 'and', and at the same time add the next step or action request. Keep tone calm. The word helps, but your voice gives real shape to the conversation.

Case Snapshot

A student tells the office, 'I want to register, but I don't have the money.' The clerk shrugs: Then come later.
Reframed with the AND-Bridge: I want to register, **and** I don't have money today. I'd like to apply for a fee waiver or split payment. Whom should I meet?
Result: The clerk directs the student to the welfare officer; registration is scheduled with a partial payment and a written plan.

Quick Conversions (before → after)

You're in pain, **but** the injection needs time.
→ You're in pain, **and** the injection needs about 20 minutes; I'll stay and monitor you.

I respect your view, **but** I see it differently.

→ I respect your view, **and** I see it differently—may I share why?

I want to help, **but** I need PPE.
→ I want to help, **and** I need PPE. Can we arrange a gown and gloves?

Cautions: 'And' is not a trick to dodge boundaries. Be honest: 'I want to help, and I'm not trained for central lines. Can the PICU fellow supervise?' Avoid stacking endless clauses; instead, be clear and concise.

Boundaries & Safety

- **Compassion and responsibility:** Say sorry, correct, document, and learn. Being kind to yourself does not mean avoiding issues.
- **Digital compassion:** Avoid doom-scrolling through your day; end with your 2-minute routine.
- **When to seek help:** If you experience persistent sadness, anxiety, insomnia, or hopeless thoughts; if you consider self-harm; or if stress disrupts your daily functioning—talk to your mentor, student counsellor, or a mental health

professional. Asking for help is a sign of strength.

Learning Points

- Calm leadership reduces errors, reassures teams, and strengthens the organization's overall performance.
- Short, specific commands with closed-loop confirmations are more effective than long instructions.
- Roles, checklists, and drills convert chaos into sequence.
- Debriefing turns pressure into progress and protects morale.
- You don't need to feel calm to sound and act calm; start with one breath.

Coffee Moment

Someone wrote on the hostel mirror: "Dear doctor-in-making, you are allowed to struggle and that makes you strong." You add a small note underneath: "I care, I learn, I grow." Tomorrow's voice became a little kinder, and tomorrow's doctor, a little stronger.

References

1. Flin R, O'Connor P, Crichton M. Safety at the sharp end: A guide to non-technical skills. Farnham: Ashgate; 2008.
2. Rudolph JW, Simon R, Dufresne RL, Raemer DB. There's no such thing as "nonjudgmental" debriefing: A theory and method for debriefing with good judgment. Simul Healthc. 2006;1(1):49–55.
3. Weinger MB, Slagle J. Human factors research in anesthesia patient safety: Lessons learned and gaps in knowledge. J Am Med Inform Assoc. 2002;9(Suppl 6):S58–63.
4. Neff KD. Self-compassion: An alternative conceptualization of a healthy attitude toward oneself. Self Identity. 2003;2(2):85–101.
5. Neff KD, Germer CK. A pilot study and randomized controlled trial of the mindful self-compassion program. J Clin Psychol. 2013;69(1):28–44.
6. Raab K. Mindfulness, self-compassion, and empathy among health care professionals: A review of the literature. J Health Care Chaplain. 2014;20(3):95–108.

Chapter 106: The Art and Science of Facing Exams

Introduction

Exams are an inevitable part of medical education. In MBBS, exams are like a crucible, testing not only knowledge but also endurance and resilience. Studies show that medical students consistently report higher levels of stress and anxiety compared to peers in other professional courses. (1) In India, surveys indicate that up to 50–70% of medical students experience significant exam-related stress. (2) While a certain degree of stress can sharpen performance, excessive stress impairs recall, reduces focus, and increases the risk of burnout.

The key, therefore, is not to eliminate stress but to manage it wisely with evidence-based strategies.

Understanding Exam Stress

- **Cognitive load:** A heavy syllabus and lack of prioritization lead to overload and "blanking out" despite preparation.
- **Psychological pressure:** Fear of failure, competition, expectations, and imposter syndrome amplify stress.
- **Contextual challenges:** Long study hours, poor sleep, irregular meals, and a lack of exercise can worsen stress resilience.
- **Physiological response:** Exams trigger the sympathetic nervous system, resulting in a faster heart rate, shallow breathing, and a cortisol surge. While this can sharpen alertness, it can also impair higher-order thinking if prolonged.

Recognizing this is the first step in scientifically addressing exam anxiety.

Evidence-Based Strategies to Face MBBS Exams

1. Structured Preparation: Time Management

Time blocking: As discussed earlier, 25–50 minutes of focused study followed by 5–10 minutes of rest improves concentration and reduces fatigue.

Spaced Repetition: Retrieval practice spaced over days to weeks is superior to cramming. (3)

Prioritization (Pareto Principle): 20% of topics often account for 80% of the exam marks. Focusing on high-yield subjects reduces cognitive overload.

Tip: Treat study sessions like clinical shifts: time-boxed, focused, and followed by recovery.

2. Cognitive-Behavioural Approaches

Cognitive behavioural therapy (CBT) related approaches are well-researched interventions for exam anxiety. (4) Key techniques include:

- **Cognitive reframing:** Replace "I will fail" with "I can attempt the questions I know, and partial credit matters."
- **Thought diaries:** Writing down fears and replacing them with rational counter-statements reduces catastrophic thinking.
- **Exposure:** Simulating exam conditions (timed mocks, viva practice) reduces anticipatory anxiety.

3. Mindfulness and Relaxation Techniques

- **Mindfulness meditation:** Brief daily sessions of mindful meditation improve focus and reduce anxiety and distress in medical students. (5)
- **Breath control (Box Breathing 4-4-4-4):** Slows heart rate, reduces sympathetic overdrive, and restores calm.
- **Progressive muscle relaxation:** Systematically tensing and releasing muscle groups decreases physical stress symptoms.

Even 5 minutes before an exam, mindful breathing can improve clarity.

4. Sleep, Exercise, and Nutrition

- **Sleep:** Research shows memory consolidation occurs during REM sleep. All-nighters impair recall and reasoning. (6)
- **Exercise:** Aerobic activity increases endorphins, reduces cortisol levels, and enhances cognitive performance. (7)
- **Nutrition:** Stable glucose from balanced meals prevents fatigue; dehydration reduces concentration by 10–15%.

Self-care is not indulgence: it is preparation.

5. Peer and Mentor Support

- **Study groups:** Small groups (3–4 students) improve accountability, clarify doubts, and provide emotional support.
- **Mentorship:** Faculty or senior guidance helps reduce uncertainty and build confidence. Studies show mentorship significantly improves medical students' stress handling and career satisfaction. (8)
- **Help-seeking:** Asking for support is a protective factor. Students who avoid seeking help are at higher risk of burnout.

6. Exam-Day Strategies

Pre-exam routine: Light meal, hydration, and 10 minutes of slow breathing.

Paper strategy:

First pass → Attempt easy questions to build confidence.

Second pass → Moderate ones.

Third pass → Tackle the difficult.

Viva calmness: Repeat the question aloud, pause, and answer stepwise. Saying "I'm not sure, but I would approach it this way…" shows reasoning.

Post-exam hygiene: Avoid ruminating or comparing answers obsessively, as it amplifies anxiety for subsequent exams.

Case Snapshot

Riya, an MBBS student, faces her final pathology paper. Her heart races as she opens the paper. She circles the 15 of 25 MCQs she knows well, then pauses to breathe before tackling the rest. In viva, she admits she doesn't know some rare syndromes, but outlines a logical approach. Later, she journals for 5 minutes and then joins friends for chai. She scores above average, not because stress has vanished, but because she has learned to use it, rather than be drowned by it.

Learning Points

- **Stress is natural but manageable**; calm is a practiced skill, not a gift.
- **Structured study methods** (spaced repetition, time block) outperform cramming.
- **CBT, mindfulness, and exercise** are scientific stress relievers.
- **Sleep and self-care** are as vital as study hours.
- **Peer and mentor support** builds resilience and confidence.

On exam day, strategy beats panic.

☕ Coffee Moment

The night before exams, you and your friends gather in the hostel mess. Laughter mixes with last-minute mnemonics. Someone admits, "I'm scared." You realize, everyone is. You take a breath, sip chai, and say, "We do our best; God does the rest." In that moment, stress softens into solidarity, and calm returns.

References

1. Dyrbye LN, Thomas MR, Shanafelt TD. Systematic review of depression, anxiety, and psychological distress among US and Canadian medical students.

Acad Med. 2006;81(4):354–73.

2. Gupta S, Choudhury S, Das M, et al. Factors causing stress among students of a medical college in Kolkata, India. Educ Health (Abingdon). 2015;28(1):92–5.
3. Cepeda NJ, Pashler H, Vul E, et al. Distributed practice in verbal recall tasks: A review and quantitative synthesis. Psychol Bull. 2006;132(3):354–80.
4. Richardson T, Stallard P, Velleman S. Cognitive behaviour therapy for child and adolescent anxiety disorders: A systematic review and meta-analysis. Behav Cogn Psychother. 2012;40(3):221–36.
5. Shapiro SL, Schwartz GE, Bonner G. Effects of mindfulness-based stress reduction on medical and premedical students. J Behav Med. 1998;21(6):581–99.
6. Curcio G, Ferrara M, De Gennaro L. Sleep loss, learning capacity and academic performance. Sleep Med Rev. 2006;10(5):323–37.
7. Hillman CH, Erickson KI, Kramer AF. Be smart, exercise your heart: Exercise effects on brain and cognition. Nat Rev Neurosci. 2008;9(1):58–65.
8. Frei E, Stamm M, Buddeberg-Fischer B. Mentoring programs for medical students — a review of the PubMed literature 2000–2008. BMC Med Educ. 2010;10:32.

Chapter 107: Bonds- From Ragging to Mentorship

Introduction

Medicine is founded on dignity, safety, and trust. Any behaviour that humiliates, coerces, or harms a junior—offline or online—conflicts with these values. Ragging may have once been considered an "icebreaker," but when power replaces consent, it becomes violence, not tradition. (1)

Yet, we must also remember that healthy traditions of greeting seniors with a "Good morning" or exchanging respectful hellos created bonds of collegiality and humility. These gestures, simple but powerful, reflect the social practice and professional discipline that once defined medical colleges, and they remain worth reclaiming. This chapter reinterprets ragging through the AETCOM lens and demonstrates how to cultivate a welcoming culture without causing harm.

Key Concepts

Respect & Consent

Friendly interaction is invited and optional. Ragging uses pressure, hierarchy, or fear; "consent" under threat is not consent.

Positive Traditions

Greeting seniors and teachers respectfully, seeking guidance with courtesy, and building rapport through mentorship enhance belonging and instil discipline. These should be encouraged as professional behaviours, not confused with coercion. (2)

Power Imbalance

New entrants rely on seniors for notes, rotations, and hostels, increasing vulnerability.

Harms of Ragging

Anxiety, sleep disturbance, depression, academic withdrawal, self-harm; bystanders may also experience moral injury. (3)

Legal duties of Institutions

National and UGC anti-ragging regulations enforce zero tolerance, establish anti-ragging committees and squads, conduct orientation programs, and specify clear penalties (suspension, expulsion, FIR as applicable). Affidavits you sign are binding commitments. (1)

Professional Identity

Doctors are guardians of dignity. "Do no harm" begins with how we treat the colleague sitting next to us.

If you are a Bystander, Intervene

Interrupt: "Let's stop, this isn't okay." Extract: walk the junior out; don't argue on the scene. Escalate: inform the warden and committee. Bystander duty is part of professionalism.

Case Snapshot

During hostel hours, a group of seniors demand that newcomers sing loudly in the corridor and share "embarrassing secrets." A third-year mentor arrives, defines the boundary. "This is coercive; we are stopping" and escorts the juniors to the common room. He also reminds them that building respectful traditions like greeting seniors or sharing a morning chai together are genuine ways to bond. He informs the warden and files a brief note with names, time, and screenshots of the WhatsApp thread. The committee conducts a swift inquiry; counselling is offered to juniors; the seniors face graded disciplinary action and are enrolled in a supervised mentorship program the following month.

Why this works: Early interruption prevented escalation, reporting ensured accountability, and the remedy restored culture by nurturing respectful interaction rather than normalizing harm.

Learning Points

- Ragging is not an icebreaker; it is misconduct when dignity is breached.
- Professionalism = Respect + Safety + Accountability; AETCOM principles apply outside the ward as much as inside.
- Institutions have legal duties and clear processes; use them early. Reporting is protection, not betrayal.
- Seniors set the tone: replace hierarchy with mentorship; design opt-in welcome rituals.
- Bystanders are not neutral; interruption and escalation are part of your duty of care.
- Respectful traditions—like greeting seniors and teachers—should be preserved as professional discipline and social glue.

Role of Mentoring

A doctor is not built solely by textbooks. Growth in medicine often occurs through conversations in corridors, guidance during stressful times, and role models who set the way. This is the essence of mentorship: a professional relationship in which a senior (mentor) guides, supports, and inspires a junior (mentee).

Why Mentoring Matters

Personal transition: Helps new MBBS students adjust to campus, hostel, and clinical environments.

Academic support: Guidance on how to study, manage workload, and prepare for exams.

Professional growth: Insights into career choices, research opportunities, and long-term pathways.

Emotional resilience: A safe space to share anxieties, deal with stress, and find balance.

Ethics & professionalism: Mentors model values of compassion, respect, and responsibility.

The Mentor–Mentee Program

Many medical colleges in India now run formal mentor–mentee programs:

- **Structure:** Each faculty mentor is assigned a small group of students (2–6 usually).
- **Frequency:** Regular meetings (monthly/quarterly) in a non-judgmental, confidential environment.
- **Focus:** Academic difficulties, emotional well-being, professional guidance.
- **Integration:** Links with counselling services, student support cells, and anti-ragging committees.
- **Outcome:** Builds a culture where students feel supported, not isolated.

Mentor's Role

Listen actively, without judgment.
Guide, not dictate — share experiences, open options.
Encourage self-reflection and independent decision-making.
Recognize early signs of burnout or stress and direct students to help.

Mentee's Role

Be open to guidance, share struggles honestly.
Respect mentor's time and feedback.
Take initiative in follow-up and applying advice.
Grow into a future mentor for juniors.

Coffee Moment

Think back to your first weeks of MBBS — a maze of classrooms, Latin terms, and unfamiliar faces. A senior walking beside you says, "I was here once too, and you'll be fine. Let me show you how." That is mentorship, turning fear into confidence and juniors into future mentors. Remember the senior who first made you feel you belonged—not through intimidation, but with a smile and a "Good morning, how's your first week going?" That is the tradition worth defending. Let your welcome be the memory a junior carries into a lifetime of learning.

References

1. University Grants Commission (UGC). Regulations on curbing the menace of ragging in higher educational institutions. New Delhi: UGC; 2009.
2. McLean M, Gibbs T. Twelve tips to promote a positive learning environment for medical students. Med Teach. 2010;32(5):372–6.
3. Frank E, Carrera JS, Stratton T, et al. Experiences of belittlement and harassment and their correlates among medical students in the United States. BMJ. 2006;333(7570):682.

Continuum

A *Continuum* is a flow without end,
A seamless line where
one stage swiftly becomes another.
Medicine is a continuum of
science, skills and service.
You will witness the lifelong journey
from student to doctor,
and from local to global. You will also shoulder
the responsibility
of carrying the flame of
knowledge and compassion forward.

Chapter 108: Global Perspectives on Healthcare Systems

Different nations develop their healthcare system in accordance with their values, policies, economic status, and the needs of their population. Understanding global healthcare systems can help shape how Indian healthcare system.

This chapter introduces you to healthcare systems in four global contexts: the United Kingdom (UK), the United States (USA), the Middle East (specifically, Dubai and the UAE), and Australia/New Zealand.

United Kingdom – Healthcare as a Right

The UK's National Health Service (NHS) is one of the world's most well-known examples of universal health coverage. Established in 1948, it is designed to provide healthcare that is free at the point of use and is funded through general taxation. (1)

Key Features

- Publicly funded by taxes, with no out-of-pocket expenditure for the service.
- Patients register with a GP, who is the first contact in the system and acts as a gatekeeper to specialist referral.
- Uniform digital records enhance continuity and coordination of care.
- Prioritizes equity, providing the same level of care regardless of income or social status.

If you arrive at an NHS hospital with chest pain, you will receive the same care, regardless of your financial situation.

Challenges and Limitations

- Long wait times, particularly for non-emergency surgeries (e.g., knee replacements, cataract surgery).
- GP appointment backlogs - some patients wait days or weeks for a consultation.
- Staff shortages, particularly in nursing, emergency medicine, and critical care, among others.
- An ageing population and a chronic disease burden put immense pressure on capacity.
- Bureaucratic overload and administrative inefficiencies in hospital management.
- Limited investment in infrastructure and medical equipment compared to the rising demand.

Doctors Struggle

Although both the public and healthcare workers highly value the NHS, many doctors are increasingly expressing dissatisfaction with it.

- **Burnout and moral distress**: Excessive workloads, particularly following the COVID-19 pandemic, entail an emotional toll stemming from the need to make challenging decisions with limited resources.
- **Pay erosion and strikes**: Junior doctors and consultants have protested against real-term pay cuts over the past decade. The cost of living in cities like London often does not match NHS salaries.
- **Systems rigidity and a poor work-life balance:** Limited autonomy in the workplace and under-resourced teams.
- **Emigration and career shifts**: Many young doctors leave for Australia, New Zealand, or private sector roles, citing better pay, improved working conditions, and greater professional respect.

A 2023 BMA survey found that over 40% of junior doctors were planning to leave the NHS in the next five years. (2) The NHS symbolizes universal healthcare with dignity: can it balance access and equity for the people who make it work - its doctors, nurses, and staff?

United States: Healthcare as a Business

The USA's system is the most expensive in the world, but it does not have universal health coverage.

Key Features

- Private providers and insurance companies dominate it.
- Medicare provides health insurance for citizens aged 65 and older, and individuals with specific disabilities.
- Medicaid is a cooperative federal and state initiative to assist citizens with limited resources.
- High technological advancement and research output.

Realities

- **Uninsured population**: Over 30 million Americans remain uninsured, despite the Affordable Care Act (ACA) of 2010. The ACA significantly reduced the number of uninsured Americans. However, an estimated 27-30 million Americans still lack health insurance (2023). It includes people in states that did not expand Medicaid, immigrants without documentation, individuals who can't afford marketplace plans, even with subsidies and people who fall into the "coverage gap" (too rich for Medicaid, too poor for subsidies).

- **Bankruptcy due to medical bills is common:** A 2019 study published in the *American Journal of Public Health* estimated that nearly 66.5% of all bankruptcies in the U.S. involved medical issues, either due to bills or time lost from work due to illness. (3) The Consumer Financial Protection Bureau reported that over $88 billion in medical debt was listed in 2022, and even insured individuals often face high additional charges.

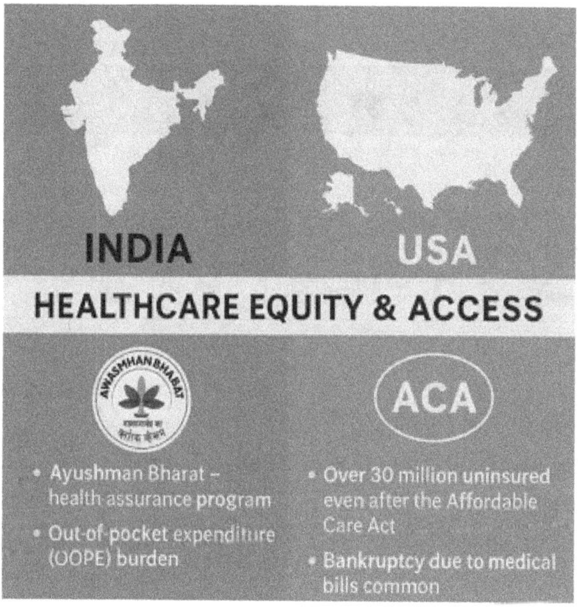

Figure 108.1: Healthcare Equity and Access in India and USA

Lesson

A highly advanced healthcare system may not guarantee universal access as healthcare equity includes not only financial resources but also policies and priorities.

United Arab Emirates: Healthcare as Prestige and Priority

Dubai has a high-quality healthcare infrastructure emerging for medical tourism. (4)

Key Features

- Dual system: Public (for Emirati citizens) and private (for expats and visitors).
- World-class private hospitals, many of which are internationally accredited.
- Mandatory health insurance for residents.
- Huge government investment in health infrastructure.

Lesson

Growth must be inclusive to reach the last man in the queue.

Australia & New Zealand: Blended Models

These countries have universal health coverage that is well accessible to indigenous communities. (5)

Table 108.1: Universal health coverage in Australia and New Zealand

Aspect	Australia – Medicare	New Zealand – Health NZ
Funding	General taxation + levy	General taxation
Private sector	Allowed but regulated	Less dominant
Indigenous health	Focus on Aboriginal & Torres Strait Islander health equity	Strong Māori-focused services
Mental health	Community-based care	Integrated with primary care

- Indigenous communities in these countries have historically faced poorer health outcomes and limited access to care.
- Aboriginal and Torres Strait Islander people in Australia.
- Māori people in New Zealand.
- Governments operate specialised programs and clinics that respect their cultures and traditional healing practices. Healthcare services are accessible to all, reducing disparities in life expectancy, maternal health, and chronic illnesses.

Lesson

A sound healthcare system doesn't merely treat everyone the same; it makes an extra effort where the need is greater.

Where Does India Stand ?

India is unique. You have gone through the infrastructure and function of healthcare system in India.

- Low public health spending.
- Huge private sector.
- Rapid digital innovation.
- Enormous human resource potential.

Yet, our goals are aligned with the best systems

- Equity, like the UK.
- Technology, like the US.

- Infrastructure ambition, like Dubai.
- Community care, like Australia and NZ.

We need

- More investment.
- More governance.
- And doctors who care beyond the hospital walls.

Table 108.2: Comparative overview of major healthcare systems

Aspect	United Kingdom	United States	India
Underlying philosophy	Healthcare as a right	Healthcare is market-driven se	Healthcare as a mixed responsibility
Coverage model	Universal Health Coverage (UHC)	No universal coverage	Public coverage + private sector
Funding source	General taxation	Government and private insurance programs	Out-of-pocket payments, Ayushman Bharat, Private insurance
Out-of-pocket expenditure	Minimal	High (even for insured patients)	High (among the highest globally)
Primary care role	GP as gatekeeper	Direct specialist access common	Variable; weak gatekeeping
Equity in access	High equity by design	Significant inequities	Urban–rural and socioeconomic gaps
Technology & innovation	Moderate, centrally regulated	World-leading innovation & research	Rapid digital innovation, uneven penetration
Financial risk protection	Strong	Weak	Improving but still limited
Doctor experience	High workload, burnout, pay dissatisfaction	High income, administrative and litigation stress	Overburdened public sector, fragmented private sector
Major challenge	Waiting times, workforce stress	Cost, inequity, medical debt	Underfunding, access gaps, regulation
Key lesson	Equity can coexist with quality	Technology alone doesn't ensure access	Scale and equity must grow together

☕ Coffee Moment

You're attending a global conference as a student delegate.
A young doctor from New Zealand says,
"We track each newborn's health from day one. How about you?"
You pause! Then you smile. We are developing digital health cards for all citizens under the Ayushman Bharat Scheme, which will also include newborn babies. A significant amount of work has been accomplished, but much remains to be done. This will be one of the biggest health databases in the world.
Because the story of Indian healthcare is being written now.
You will help write it!!

References

1. Anderson M, Pitchforth E, Edwards N, Alderwick H, McGuire A, Mossialos E. United Kingdom: Health System Review. Health Syst Transit. 2022 May;24(1):1-194.
2. Armitage R. Junior doctors leaving the NHS: what would it mean for general practice? Br J Gen Pract. 2023 Feb 23;73(728):126-127.
3. Himmelstein DU, Lawless RM, Thorne D, Foohey P, Woolhandler S. Medical Bankruptcy: Still Common Despite the Affordable Care Act. Am J Public Health. 2019 Mar;109(3):431-433.
4. Alshamsi AI. A review of the United Arab Emirates healthcare systems on medical tourism and accreditation. Front Health Serv. 2024 Feb 21;4:1329252.
5. Khatri RB, Assefa Y. Drivers of the Australian Health System towards Health Care for All: A Scoping Review and Qualitative Synthesis. Biomed Res Int. 2023 Oct 20;2023:6648138.

How to Use the Competency Mapping Table

The competency mapping table is a bridge between the NMC Foundation Course outcomes and the chapters in this book. It helps to connect each mandated competency with the corresponding chapters and learning resources designed to develop the specific skill, knowledge, or attitude.

The table lists the competency, domain (Knowledge, Skill, Attitude or Communication) and level of learning. The final column suggests the section or chapter where that topic is addressed, along with appropriate learning methods or resources, such as interactive lectures, small-group discussions, simulations, reflections, or field visits, aligned with competency-based medical education.

While the table is structured around the prescribed competencies, this book goes far beyond the minimum requirements.

Use this table as your guide:

For students, it helps locate chapters linked to specific competencies or to prepare for assessments.

For faculty, it provides a straightforward guide for planning sessions, reflections, and evaluations during the Foundation Course.

Together, this mapping and the accompanying chapters will help you transition from acquiring competencies to truly embodying them.

Domains of Learning

Domain	Common action verbs
K: Knowledge (Cognitive domain)	Describe, discuss, define, enumerate, classify, choose, differentiate, elicit, etc.
S: Skill (Psychomotor domain)	Demonstrate, identify, present, perform, document, record, interpret etc.
A: Attitude and Behaviour (Affective domain)	Inform, demonstrate understanding of, act etc.
C: Communication (Affective domain)	Counsel, display, lead, practice, advocate etc.

Levels of Competency

Competency Level	Meaning	Example
K: Knows	A knowledge attribute - Understanding concepts, facts, and principles.	Describing health systems or disease mechanisms.
KH: Knows How	Higher level of knowledge. Applying and integrating knowledge in context .	Applying theory of communication to patient care.
S: Shows	A skill attribute: ability to identify or demonstrate the steps.	Showing steps of respiratory system examination in skill lab.
SH: Shows How	A skill attribute: ability to interpret or demonstrate a complex procedure requiring thought, knowledge and behaviour.	Perform hand hygiene following all steps when entering in PICU.
P: Perform (under supervision or independently)	Performed under supervision for a pre-specified number of times leads to certification or capacity to perform independently. Mastery: when performed independently for multiple times.	Demonstrating different domains of CPR training leading to provider level certification. Mastery: Perform CPR in ER with team.

Competency Mapping

Code	Competency	Domain - Level	Chapter map and additional Resource
FC 1	Orientation		
FC 1.1	Demonstrate understanding of the role of doctors in the society and their impact.	A- KH	Inception – 2 Genesis -2, 3 Interactive lecture, role play, reflection writing.
FC 1.2	Demonstrate understanding of the Roles of an Indian Medical Graduate and relate it to the societal impact.	A- KH	Inception-2 Genesis - 2, 3 Small group discussion, panel discussion, self-reflection.
FC 1.3	Discuss and appreciate the expectations of the students from the Nation, society, Institution, peers, colleagues and patients and vice versa.	A- KH	Inception – 2 Group discussion, facilitated reflection, peer interaction.
FC 1.4	Demonstrate understanding of the rules and regulations of the institution.	A- SH	Inception – 7 Campus tour, orientation briefing, Q&A with administration.
FC 1.5	Orient themselves to the college campus, facilities, faculty, administrative structure, support systems and processes of the institution.	A- KH	Inception – 5 Guided institutional walk, introduction session, orientation video.
FC 1.6	Discuss the various career pathways and opportunities for personal growth.	A- KH	Inception – 2 Interactive lecture, guest talk by alumni/senior faculty, career counseling session.
FC 1.7	Demonstrate understanding of the overview of MBBS curriculum, its structure and outcomes and its relation to the career pathways.	K- KH	Inception – 3 Interactive lecture, flowchart discussion, group quiz.
FC 1.8	Demonstrate understanding the role of physician at various levels	K- KH	Inception, Genesis Lecture, field visit to CHC/PHC, case-based

	of Health care delivery.		discussion.
FC 1.9	Discuss the principles of family practice.	K- KH	Synthesis-7 Interactive lecture, role play, family health case scenario.
FC 1.10	Demonstrate awareness of the History of Medicine and alternate systems of Medicine.	K- K	Genesis - 7- Synthesis Lecture, documentary review, group presentation on traditional systems.
FC 2	Skills		
FC 2.1	Perform Basic Life support in Skills lab.	Skill- SH	Revive Skills lab demonstration, simulation practice, checklists/OSCE.
FC 2.2	Perform First Aid in a simulated environment.	Skill- SH	Resonance Simulation, peer demonstration, first aid workshop.
FC 2.3	Follow bio-safety and universal precautions.	Skill- SH	Illumination – 6 Demonstration, poster-based discussion, skills lab practice.
FC 2.4	Demonstrate handling and safe disposal of Biohazardous materials in a simulated environment.	Skill- SH	Illumination – 5 Skills lab demonstration, hands-on practice.
FC 2.5	Demonstrate proper hand washing and use of personal protective equipment.	Skill- SH	Illumination – 6 Demonstration, skills lab training, return demonstration.
FC 2.6	Demonstrate appropriate response to needle stick injuries.	Skill- SH	Illumination – 5 Skills lab simulation, video-based learning, debrief.
FC 2.7	Demonstrate Biomedical Waste segregation (BMW), observe and explain the process of management of BMW in accordance with National Regulations.	Skill- SH	Illumination – 5 Field visit to waste management unit, demonstration, discussion.
FC 2.8	Discuss the Immunization requirements of Health care professionals.	K- KH	Inception – 4 Lecture, case discussion, schedule exercise (WHO/National).
FC	Demonstrate awareness of	Skill- SH	Covenant – 2

2.9	significance of documentation in patient care and the proper method of documentation.		Case-based discussion, documentation workshop, role play.
FC 3	Community Orientation		
FC 3.1	Demonstrate understanding of the National Health Goals and Policies.	K- KH	Matrix – 1 Lecture, group discussion, policy review activity.
FC 3.2	Discuss the national health scenario, demographic, socio-cultural and epidemiological issues.	K- KH	Matrix Interactive lecture, infographic discussion, field-based observation.
FC 3.3	Demonstrate understanding of the health care systems in India with reference to primary, secondary and tertiary level care.	K- KH	Matrix – 2 Lecture, field visit to PHC/CHC, debriefing.
FC 3.4	Discuss the basic principles of community health and its impact on health and disease.	Skill- SH	Matrix Group discussion, field activity, community case study.
FC 3.5	Demonstrate understanding of structure and functioning of the community health center.	K- KH	Matrix, Inception – 6 Field visit, debrief, interaction with CHC staff.
FC 3.6	Demonstrate ability to obtain patient experiences through patient and family interactions and relate these experiences to impact of environment and diseases.	Skill- SH	Resonance 2 Patient/family interview, reflection writing, facilitated discussion.
FC 4	Professional Development		
FC 4.1	Demonstrate the concept of Professionalism and ethics among health care professionals and discuss the consequences of unprofessional and unethical behaviour.	Skill-KH	Genesis and Inception – 7 Interactive lecture, case discussion, role play.
FC 4.2	Demonstrate understanding that compassion, altruism,	K- KH	Covenant – 4 Reflective discussion,

	integrity, duty, responsibility and trust are the core values that defines the nature of the physician's work.		storytelling, interactive lecture.
FC 4.3	Discuss the value, honesty and respect during interaction with peers, seniors, faculty, other health care workers and patients.	Skill-KH	Resonance – 5, 14 Role play, group discussion, reflection log.
FC 4.4	Discuss the significance of working in a health care team.	Skill-KH	Revive – 4 Team-based exercise, simulation, debriefing.
FC 4.5	Discuss disability competencies.	K-KH	Genesis – 5 Lecture, video trigger, empathy-building activity.
FC 4.6	Demonstrate understanding and respect of cultural diversities and interact with those with different cultural values.	K/A-KH	Inception – 7 Role play, cultural immersion activity, group reflection.
FC 4.7	Discuss the significance and methods of stress management and risk-taking behaviour.	K- KH	Resonance – 8, 12, 13 Small group session, stress management workshop, mindfulness exercise.
FC 4.8	Understand the role of Yoga and meditation in personal health.	Skill- S	Synthesis – 3, 5 Yoga and meditation demonstration, supervised practice.
FC 4.9	Discuss the significance and appropriate ways of Time management.	K-KH	Resonance – 10 Workshop on time management, reflection diary.
FC 4.10	Demonstrate importance of interpersonal relationship while working in a health care team.	Skill-KH	Resonance – 9,11,14 Group exercise, communication workshop, reflection session.
FC 4.11	Understand the role of mentoring.	Skill-KH	Resonance – 14 Mentor–mentee meeting, small group reflection.
FC 4.12	Demonstrates understanding of the	Skill-KH	Inception – 4 Group activity, collaborative

	process of group learning and group dynamics.		task, reflection.
FC 4.13	Comprehend the learning pedagogy and its role in learning skills.	Skill-KH	Inception – 4 Interactive lecture on learning styles, SDL planning session.
FC 4.14	Demonstrates understanding of different methods of self-directed learning.	Skill-KH	Inception – 4 Self-directed learning module, mentor feedback.
FC 4.15	Understand collaborative learning.	Skill-KH	Inception – 4 Peer learning session, collaborative assignment.
FC 5	Communication		
FC 5.1	Demonstrate ability to communicate with patient and families, be aware of barriers to communication and appropriate ways to respond.	C- SH	Genesis – 2, Illumination – 2, 3, 12 Role play, standardized patient interaction, video feedback.
FC 5.2	Demonstrate use of local language in patient and peer interactions.	C- SH	Practice Role play in vernacular, peer-practice sessions.
FC 5.3	Demonstrate ability to communicate and learn in English.	C- SH	Practice Communication drills, English writing workshop.
FC 5.4	Demonstrate basic computer skills.	Skill- SH	Practice Computer skills workshop, hands-on digital literacy session.
FC 5.5	Demonstrate ability for accessing online resources.	Skill- SH	Illumination – 4 Guided PubMed/ Cochrane search exercise, hands-on tutorial on UpToDate/Embase.

Beyond Competence

Competencies bring structure to learning. They tell us *what* to learn, *how* to demonstrate it, and *when* we are ready to move forward. But medicine, in its deepest essence, cannot be fully contained within tables or codes.

What truly defines a doctor is not only the ability to perform, but the willingness to care; not only to know, but to listen; not only to treat, but to heal.

Competency mapping marks the completion of the Foundation Course and the beginning of the lifelong process of learning, unlearning, and relearning. Furthermore, you grow not only in competence, but also in conscience, as you evolve from student to intern and from clinician to healer.

Keep your First Book of Medicine as your companion. Each time you return, you will find new meanings waiting for you because the book, like medicine itself, changes every time you do.

Competence is the beginning of mastery; compassion is its final form.

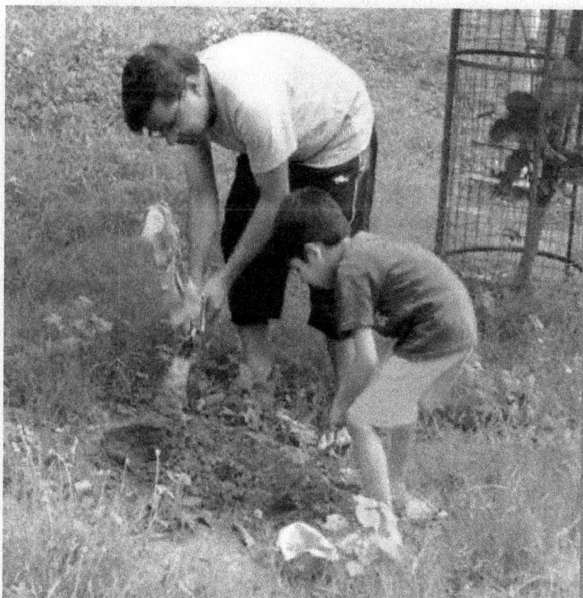

www.ingramcontent.com/pod-product-compliance
Lightning Source LLC
LaVergne TN
LVHW052018200926
848481LV00005B/1525

* 9 7 9 8 9 0 3 9 2 1 3 5 5 *